Gabrijela Kocjan

Fine Needle Aspiration Cytology

Gabrijela Kocjan

Fine Needle Aspiration Cytology

Diagnostic Principles and Dilemmas

With 527 Figures

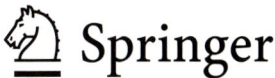

Dr. Gabrijela Kocjan
University College London
Medical School
Dept. of Histopathology
Rockefeller Building
WC1E 6JJ London

United Kongdom

Library of Congress Control Number: 2005937513

ISBN-10 3-540-25639-3 Springer Berlin Heidelberg New York
ISBN-13 978-3-540-25639-7 Springer Berlin Heidelberg New York

This work is subject to copyright. All rights are reserved, whether the whole or part of the material is concerned, specifically the rights of translation, reprinting, reuse of illustrations, recitation, broadcasting, reproduction on microfilm or in any other way, and storage in data banks. Duplication of this publication or parts thereof is permitted only under the provisions of the German Copyright Law of September 9, 1965, in its current version, and permission for use must always be obtained from Springer. Violations are liable for prosecution under the German Copyright Law.

Springer is a part of Springer Science+Business Media
springeronline.com
© Springer-Verlag Berlin Heidelberg 2006
Printed in Germany

The use of general descriptive names, registered names, trademarks, etc. in this publication does not imply, even in the absence of a specific statement, that such names are exempt from the relevant protective laws and regulations and therefore free for general use.

Product liability: the publishers cannot guarantee the accuracy of any information about dosage and application contained in this book. In every individual case the user must check such information by consulting the relevant literature.

Editor: Gabriele Schröder
Desk Editor: Ellen Blasig
Typesetting and Production: LE-TEX Jelonek, Schmidt & Vöckler GbR, Leipzig
Cover design: estudio calamar, Frido Steinen-Broo, Calamar, Spain

Printed on acid-free paper   24/3100/YL - 5 4 3 2 1 0

To my parents, Hilda and Franc
For encouraging my independence

To Tony and Arabella,
For being proud of me

Preface

The urge to write this book arose after years of storing glass slides from difficult cases into plastic folders where they have been breaking and fading. When discussing these cases at the weekly teaching for trainee pathologists, some of the observations that arose, made it obvious that experience cannot compensate for methodical approach, careful observation, clinical information and honest conclusion. Hence in writing this book, I had two major aims: firstly, to reiterate the importance of the approach to cytodiagnosis and, secondly, to expose diagnostic dilemmas in some of the most difficult areas of Fine Needle Aspiration Cytology (FNAC).

FNAC had become a well established diagnostic component in pathology. Within any pathology laboratory, FNAC has its dedicated proponents but also those who are practicing it occasionally, perhaps only to cover the absence of a colleague, or, alongside histopathology, as part of the subspecialty reporting. The differences in expertise often mean that the standard of reporting varies, the latter group being reluctant to ask some of the basic as well as more difficult questions for fear of appearing ignorant. Cytology training is variable in different institutions, depending on the local circumstances. Trainees without any prior experience in cytology may be exposed to difficult FNAC cases early in their career.

In order to help the approach to FNAC samples for those with and without any prior experience, the first part of this book lists principles of cytological diagnosis. The importance of a methodical approach to interpreting cytological material cannot be overstated. However, cytological interpretation is not merely a mathematical algorithm where numerical values are added up. In majority of cytology cases, the whole is more than the sum of parts: the interpretation of morphological features is complex. It needs careful observation of morphology but also, crucially, it needs to be taken in the clinical context. Without the clinical information, morphology alone may be misleading.

Chapters on diagnostic dilemmas in FNAC practice discuss potentially difficult morphological features. As well as to educate, the aim of these chapters is to expose difficult areas of diagnosis where FNAC has its limitations. To that end and in line with the developing area of medical litigation affecting all areas of practice, there is a chapter on medico-legal issues associated with FNAC. This is a growing field that has been addressed in a number of legal references but has thus far not been addressed extensively from a cytologicl standpoint.

In preparing this manuscript, I would like to thank, first of all, my patients for allowing me to use their clinical histories and photomicrographs. I would also like to thank my colleagues in the Department of Histopathology, University College London, in particular Dr. Mary Falzon for their help in sharing some of the diagnostic dilemmas presented in this manuscript. The ability to share problems with clinicians and fellow pathologists is the essential requirement for ensuring a good night's sleep and one's professional reputation. I would also like to thank my clinical colleagues by their supportive approach to cytology in sending their patients for FNAC. The experience I have accumulated on these sound clinical grounds had been shared with generations of postgraduate trainee pathologists. I thank them for being a source of inspiration through curiosity and enthusiasm. Many went on to become dedicated cytopathologists and made me immensely proud of them. I would also like to give special thanks to Eva Kauerova for her help in the past five years.

I hope that you, the reader, will use this book in your daily practice, if only to find that there are no straight answers to difficult questions.

G Kocjan
September 2005
London

Contents

Preface.................................VII

Contents...............................IX

Introduction and Historical Perspective.... 1

References.................................. 3

FNAC Technique and Slide Preparation 7

2.1 Informed Consent......................... 7

2.2 Location of the FNAC Procedure........... 8
2.2.1 The FNAC Clinic........................ 9
2.2.2 Inpatient FNAC........................ 12
2.2.3 Image-Guided and Other FNAC Procedure Locations...................... 12

2.3 The Importance of the Aspirator......... 14

2.4 Aspiration Techniques................... 15
2.4.1 Suction FNAC.......................... 15
2.4.2 The Capillary Method.................. 16

2.5 Slide Preparation....................... 17
2.5.1 Conventional Preparations............. 17
2.5.2 Liquid-Based Preparations............. 18
2.5.3 Cell Block............................ 18

2.6 Fixation Techniques..................... 19
2.6.1 Air Drying............................ 19
2.6.2. Alcohol Fixation..................... 20
2.6.3 Transport Medium...................... 20

2.7 Staining Methods........................ 20
2.7.1 Papanicolaou Staining................. 20
2.7.2 Romanowsky Staining................... 22
2.7.3 Other Stains.......................... 23

2.8 Ancillary Techniques.................... 23
2.8.1 Cytochemistry......................... 23
2.8.2 Immunocytochemistry................... 24
2.8.3 Molecular Markers in Cytology......... 26

2.9 Safety.................................. 27

References................................. 28

Diagnostic interpretation of FNAC material.............................. 35

3.1 Slide Background........................ 35
3.1.1 Cystic Background..................... 39
3.1.2 Inflammatory Background............... 40
3.1.3 Necrotic Background................... 42
3.1.4 Myxoid and Mucinous Background........ 42
3.1.5 Lymphoid Background................... 43
3.1.6 Other Background Features............. 43

3.2 Cell Arrangement........................ 44
3.2.1 Clusters.............................. 46
3.2.2 Sheets................................ 46
3.2.3 Single Cells.......................... 47
3.2.4 Papillary Arrangement................. 47
3.2.5 Other Features........................ 48

3.3 Cellular Features: the Nucleus.......... 49
3.3.1 Nuclear Size.......................... 50
3.3.2 Nuclear Shape......................... 51
3.3.3 Position of the Nucleus............... 52
3.3.4 Chromatin Pattern..................... 53
3.3.5 Number of Nuclei...................... 54
3.3.6 Nucleoli.............................. 54
3.3.7 Mitoses............................... 55

3.4	Cellular Features: Cytoplasm	55
3.4.1	Relative Amount	55
3.4.2	Quality and Contents	55
3.4.3	Shape and Definition	56

| 3.5 | Criteria of Malignancy | 57 |

| 3.6 | Cytology Report | 57 |

References 58

Diagnostic Dilemmas in FNAC Practice: Cystic Lesions 59

4.1	Cysts in the Neck	59
4.1.1	Thyroglossal Duct Carcinoma	60
4.1.2	Branchial Cleft Cysts	61
4.1.3	Salivary Gland Lesions	62
4.1.4	Lymphoepithelial Cysts	63
4.1.5	Cystadenolymphoma	64
4.1.6	Acinic Cell Carcinoma	66
4.1.7	Pleomorphic Adenoma	67
4.1.8	Dermoid Cyst	68
4.1.9	Thyroid Cysts	68
4.1.10	The Lymph Nodes	70
4.1.11	Parathyroid Cysts	71
4.1.12	Cysts of the Jaw	72
4.1.13	Teratoid Cyst	72

4.2	Cysts in the Abdomen	73
4.2.1	Cystic Lesions of the Pancreas	73
4.2.2	Cystic Lesions of the Liver	77
4.2.3	Adrenal and Renal Cystic Lesions	78
4.2.4	Cystic Lesions of the Peritoneum	79

| 4.3 | Thoracic Cysts | 79 |

| 4.4 | Breast Cysts | 80 |

| 4.5 | Other Cysts and Artefacts | 82 |

References 85

Diagnostic Dilemmas in FNAC Practice: Lymphoid Infiltrates 91

5.1.	Granulomatous Infiltrates	91
5.1.1	Tuberculous Lymphadenitis	91
5.1.2	Sarcoidosis	92
5.1.3	Kikuchi-Fujimoto Disease	92
5.1.4	Cat-Scratch Disease	94
5.1.5	Leishmania Lymphadenitis	94
5.1.6	Kimura's disease	95
5.1.7	Sinus Histiocytosis with Massive Lymphadenopathy	96
5.1.8	Foreign-Body Granulomatous Inflammatory Response	96
5.1.9	Malignant Lymphomas	97

5.2	Lymphoid Infiltrates in Extranodal Sites	99
5.2.1	Lymphoid Infiltrates in the Thyroid	99
5.2.2	Lymphoid Processes in the Salivary Gland	103
5.2.3	Lymphoid Infiltrates of the Orbit	105
5.2.4	Lymphoid Lesions in the Breast	107

5.3	Neoplasms Containing Lymphocytes	107
5.3.1	Dilemmas in the Cytological Diagnosis of Lymphomas	108
5.3.2	Solid Neoplasms Containing Lymphocytes	109

References 110

Diagnostic Dilemmas in FNAC Practice: Metastatic Tumours 117

6.1	Metastatic Carcinomas	118
6.1.1	Establishing the Diagnosis of Malignancy	118
6.1.2	Determining the Nature of the Tumour	120
6.1.3	Finding the Primary Tumour	124
6.1.4	The Role of Imaging in the FNAC of Metastases	129

| 6.2 | Metastases of Non-Epithelial Tumours | 129 |

References 130

Diagnostic Dilemmas in FNAC Cytology: Small Round Cell Tumours 133

7.1	Small Round Cell Tumours of Childhood	133
7.1.1	Ewing's Sarcoma/Primitive Neuroectodermal Tumour	134
7.1.2	Neuroblastoma	136
7.1.3	Ganglioneuroblastomas	136

7.1.4	Rhabdomyosarcoma	137
7.1.5	Acute Lymphoblastic Leukaemia and LBL	139
7.1.6	Small Round Cell Tumours of Kidney	141
7.1.7	Hepatoblastoma	141
7.1.8	Pleuropulmonary Blastoma	142
7.1.9	Small-Cell Synovial Sarcoma	142
7.2	**Small Round Cell Tumours in Adults**	**142**
7.2.1	Desmoplastic Small Round Cell Tumour	143
7.2.2	Small-Cell Carcinoma of the Lung	144
7.2.3	Burkitt's Lymphoma	144
7.2.4	Lymphoglandular Bodies	145
7.2.5	Merkel Cell Carcinoma	146
7.2.6	Olfactory Neuroblastoma	147
References		**148**

Diagnostic Dilemmas in FNAC Cytology: Soft-Tissue Lesions ... 151

8.1	Introduction	151
8.2	**Spindle-Cell Lesions**	**153**
8.2.1	Spindle-Cell Lesions of the Lung	156
8.2.2	Spindle-Cell Lesions of the Salivary Gland	156
8.2.3	Spindle-Cell Lesions of the Breast	157
8.2.4	Myofibrosarcoma	157
8.3	**Myxoid and Chondroid Lesions**	**157**
8.3.1	Low-Grade Fibromyxoid Sarcoma	159
8.3.2	Leiomyosarcoma	160
8.3.3	Ossifying Fibromyxoid Tumour	161
8.3.4	Myxoid Mucinous Neoplasms	161
8.3.5	Intramuscular Myxoma	162
8.3.6	Chondrosarcoma	162
8.3.7	Chondroblastoma	162
8.4	**Pseudosarcomatous Lesions**	**162**
8.4.1	Nodular Fasciitis	165
8.4.2	Nodular Myositis	165
8.4.3	Proliferative Fasciitis and Myositis	165
8.4.4	Fibromatoses	166
8.4.5	Fibrous histiocytoma	167
8.4.6	Pseudoangiomatous Stromal Hyperplasia	167
8.4.7	Pleomorphic Lipoma	168
8.4.8	Atypical Lipoma	168
8.4.9	Spindle-Cell Lipoma	169
8.4.10	Ancient Schwannoma	169
8.4.11	Angioleiomyoma	169
8.4.12	Calcifying Aponeurotic Fibroma	169
8.4.13	Lipomatous Haemangiopericytoma	169
8.5	**Tumours of Low or Borderline Malignancy**	**169**
8.5.1	Dermatofibrosarcoma Protuberans	170
8.5.2	Haemangiopericytoma	170
8.5.3	Acral Myxoinflammatory Fibroblastic Sarcoma	171
8.6	**Soft-Tissue Deposits of Non-Sarcomatous Lesions**	**171**
8.6.1	Malignant Lymphoma and Leukaemia	171
8.6.2	Calcinosis Cutis	171
8.7	**Sarcomas Mimicking Other Lesions**	**171**
8.7.1	Epithelioid Sarcoma	171
8.7.2	Metastatic Soft-Tissue Sarcomas	172
8.7.3	Well-Differentiated Liposarcoma	172
8.8	**Rare and Difficult Sarcomas**	**172**
8.8.1	Alveolar Soft-Part Sarcoma	172
8.8.2	Angiosarcoma	172
8.8.3	Kaposi's Sarcoma	174
8.8.4	Clear-Cell Sarcoma of Soft Parts	175
8.8.5	Haemangioendothelioma	175
8.8.6	Giant-Cell Fibroblastoma	175
8.8.7	Rhabdomyosarcoma	175
8.8.8	Synovial Sarcoma	176
References		**177**

Diagnostic Dilemmas in FNAC Cytology: Difficult Breast Lesions ... 181

9.1	Fibroadenoma	182
9.2	Papillary Lesions	188
9.3	Apocrine Changes	193
9.4	Mucinous Lesions	195
9.5	Lobular Carcinoma	196
9.6	In Situ or Invasive Carcinoma?	198
9.7	Rare Lesions	202

9.7.1	Radial Scar/Complex Sclerosing Lesion	202	10.11	Transrectal Digitally Guided FNAC......... 219
9.7.2	Collagenous Spherulosis	203		
9.7.2	Ductal Adenoma	203	10.12	FNAC in Gynaecology 219
9.7.3	Gynaecomastia	203		
9.7.5	Spindle-Cell and Mesenchymal Lesions of the Breast	204	10.13	Diagnostic Accuracy and Cost-Effectiveness of FNAC 219
9.7.6	Pseudoangiomatous Stromal Hyperplasia	205		
9.7.7	Metaplastic Tumours	205		References.................................... 220
9.7.8	Secretory Carcinoma	205		
9.7.9	Tumoral Calcinosis	205		

Principles of Safe FNAC Practice: FNAC versus Core Biopsy 225

9.7.10	Clear-Cell Hidradenoma	206
9.7.11	Tubular Adenoma	206
9.7.12	Adenomyoepithelioma	206
9.7.13	Squamous Cells	206
9.7.14	Inflammatory Myofibroblastic Tumour	207

11.1	Breast Lesions	225
11.2	Lung Lesions	227
11.3	Hepatic Lesions	227
11.4	Abdominal Lesions	227
11.5	Prostate Cancer	228
11.6	Thyroid Lesions	228
11.7	Gynaecological Lesions	228
11.8	Soft-Tissue Lesions	228
11.9	Skeletal Lesions	228
11.10	Summary	229

9.8	FNAC or core biopsy?	207
9.9	Radiation Changes	207

References.................................... 207

References.................................... 229

Principles of Safe Practice: the Role of FNAC in Clinical Management 213

Principles of Safe FNAC Practice: Medicolegal Issues..................... 231

10.1	FNAC Breast Lesions	214
10.2	FNAC Thyroid	215
10.3	FNAC Head and Neck Conditions	216
10.4	FNAC Lymph Nodes	216
10.5	FNAC Adrenal and Kidney	217
10.6	FNAC Gastrointestinal Tract	217
10.7	FNAC Soft Tissue	218
10.8	FNAC Bone	218
10.9	FNAC in Children	218
10.10	FNAC for HIV-Related Lesions	219

References.................................... 235

Subject Index........................ 237

Chapter 1

Introduction and Historical Perspective

First reports of fine-needle aspiration cytology (FNAC) as a technique for obtaining diagnostic material date back to the 19th century when, at St Bartholomew's Hospital, London, aspiration was undertaken on a large mass in the liver by the surgeons Stanley and Earle [1]. Sir James Paget advocated the use of aspiration as an investigative technique in his lectures [2]. Menetrier was probably the first to use aspiration to investigate lung cancer [3]. Some years later, at the beginning of the 20th century, Griegg and Gray published the results of a lymph node aspirate for tripanosomiasis [4]. In 1921, Guthrie described using a 21-guage needle and a technique similar to that used today, but the first large-scale study was carried out at the Memorial Hospital, New York, by the pioneering team of Martin, Ellis and Stewart [5,6]. Stewart published the results of 2,500 tumours biopsied by an aspiration method using an 18-gauge needle [7]. Stewart emphasised the importance of the technique of aspiration, sample preparation and close cooperation between clinician and pathologist to assure the degree of diagnostic accuracy achievable with needle aspiration. Despite the pioneering work of American pathologists, the technique initially did not have a following amongst all American pathologists, most of who viewed it with scepticism. The historical background of FNAC has been researched by Webb [8] and Grunze and Spriggs [9].

True fine needles for aspiration (22- to 27-gauge vs. 18-gauge) were first introduced in Europe in the 1950s by Lopez-Cardozo in The Netherlands [10] (Fig. 1.1) and Soderström in Sweden [11]. It was, however, publications by Zajicek, from the Karolinska Hospital in Stockholm, that brought aspiration cytology to international attention [12, 13] (Fig. 1.2). Linsk described the work of the aspiration cytology pioneers Zajicek, Esposti and Lowhagen [14]. At that time, the European clinicians, mainly from the ranks of haematologists (Fig. 1.3) developed the Romanowsky and May-Grünwald Giemsa stains for use on air-dried smears to allow for rapid interpretation (Fig. 1.4). Despite their success, it was not until the 1980s that FNAC became widely used. The reasons included lack of confidence in the sensitivity and specificity of the procedure, fear of tumour implantation in the needle track, apprehension of lawsuits and the reluctance of surgeons to relinquish the use of the formal histological biopsy technique [15].

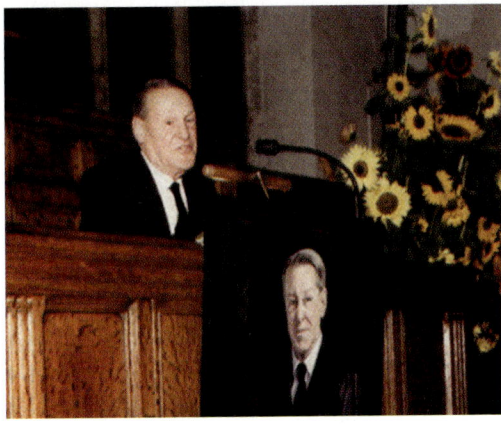

Fig. 1.1
True fine needles used for aspiration (22- to 27-gauge vs. 18-gauge) were first introduced in Europe by Paul Lopez-Cardozo in The Netherlands

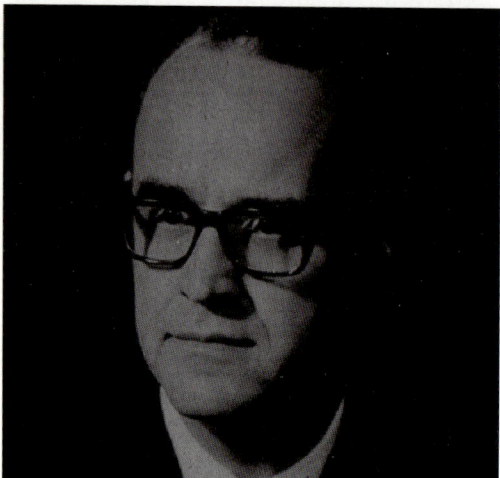

Fig. 1.2
The publications by Zajicek, from the Karolinska Hospital in Stockholm, have brought aspiration cytology to international attention

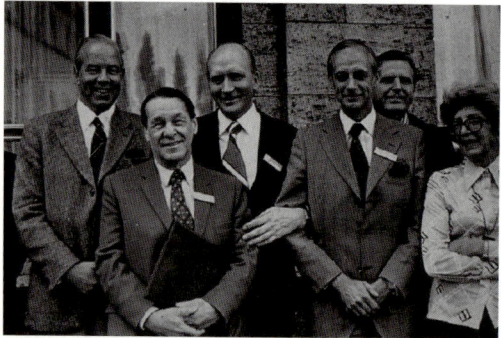

Fig. 1.3
Despite their success, it was not until the 1980s that fine-needle aspiration cytology (FNAC) became widely used, particularly in Europe. The pioneers of European cytology: Dr J. Jenny, Dr N. Husain, Dr E. Wachtel

FNAC is best understood as a method where a fine needle is used to remove a sample of cells from a suspicious mass for diagnostic purposes. The material obtained is made into a cytological sample suitable for microscopic examination. This is an aspiration cytology rather than a tissue biopsy technique. The architectural arrangement of the cells in the smear may also provide information about the histology of the tissue from which the sample was removed.

Cytopathologists have the skill to translate cytological features into the tissue patterns needed for diagnosis. William Frable, a renowned American cytologist, said „good surgical pathologists who have expressed a negative reaction to FNAC simply do not realise how closely allied recognition patterns are between aspiration biopsy cell spread and its tissue section counterpart" [16]. However, FNAC biopsy is not a substitute for conventional surgical histopathology. Instead, it should be regarded as being complementary to it, part of the diagnostic processes in combination with clinical, radiological and other laboratory data.

FNAC biopsy is regarded as a minimally invasive, cost-effective technique with diagnostic accuracy in the range of 90–99%. The scepticism of some histopathologists about the technique has largely abated along with fears that it may replace tissue diagnosis. Moreover, the task of convincing clinicians of the value of the technique has been extremely successful, since their expectations of a high level of accuracy have been met. While the use of the FNAC biopsy technique has widened, there are pressures for specialisation in this area, and a good balance between expertise and the availability of the test has to be achieved.

The advantages of FNAC are that it is safe, gives a rapid report, is sensitive and specific for the diagnosis of malignancy, requires little equipment, cause minimal discomfort to the patient, is an outpatient procedure, reduces bed occupancy, allows preoperative diagnosis, avoids the use of frozen sections, reduces the incidence of exploratory procedures, allows a definitive diagnosis on inoperable patients, does not result in fibrosis (which may interfere with future investigations), does not require wound healing and is readily repeatable and cost effective [15].

The disadvantages of FNAC are that the aspiration technique requires practice and skill, a certain percentage of the aspirates are unsatisfactory, interpretation requires experience and diagnostic material is limited [15].

The diagnostic accuracy of FNAC depends on several factors, including the site and type of lesion, the experience of the aspirator, the quality of the specimen preparation and the diagnostic skills of the cytopathologist [17–53]. Various studies have reported a greater accuracy in diagnosis when the same person performs the aspiration procedure, prepares the smears and provides the interpretation. Regardless of the general uniformity of the procedure (a clinically suspicious mass, fine needle, palpation, aspiration, smearing, staining and adequate reading of the stained specimen) there are important site-specific considerations that should not be overlooked. The important gross distinction is between superficial and deep-seated lesions.

Superficial masses (breasts, lymph nodes, head and neck, thyroid and salivary gland) are palpable and usually do not pose a risk of a sampling error. In the case of a suspicious mass in the thyroid, for example, the most cost-effective diagnostic test for its evaluation is FNAC. It is the test of choice for the triage of patients requiring surgery, thus avoiding approximately 80% of all thyroid surgery. FNAC of deep-seated lesions is usually performed using radiographic image guidance. There is a general agreement that the diagnostic yield of the FNAC of deep-seated lesions increases when a radiologist and a cytopathologist work together.

FNAC of palpable lesions is performed by pathologists with special expertise in both the aspiration technique and specimen preparation. This increases the diagnostic yield, because pathologists are able to make an on-site assessment of specimen cellularity. It also enhances the clinicopathological correlation, since the pathologist interpreting the specimen has also seen and examined the patient. The pathologists may obtain additional tissue at the time of the initial biopsy for special diagnostic studies that may help to further refine the diagnosis. Patients are typically seen in the FNAC clinic on the same day that they are seen in other clinics. The pathologist performs the aspiration and contacts the referring physician with a preliminary diagnosis, typically within 1 hour of patient's arrival at the clinic. Performed on an outpatient basis or at patient's bedside, FNAC has the best safety record of any method of obtaining material for a morphological diagnosis.

References

1. Cited by Deeley TJ. Needle Biopsy. London: Butterworths, 1974
2. Paget J. Lectures on Tumours. London. Longman, 1983
3. Menetrier P. Cancer primitif du poumon. Bull Soc Anat Paris 1886; 11:643
4. Griegg EDW, Gray ACH. Note on the lymphatic gland in sleeping sickness. Lancet 1904; 1:1570
5. Guthrie CG. Gland puncture as a diagnostic measure. Bull Johns Hopkins Hosp 1921; 32:266–9
6. Martin HE, Ellis EB. Biopsy by needle puncture and aspiration. Ann Surg 1930; 92:169–81
7. M Stewart FW. Diagnosis of tumours by aspiration. Am J Pathol 1933; 9:801-13
8. Webb AJ. Through a glass darkly: the development of needle aspiration biopsy. Bristol Med Chir J 1974; 89:59–68
9. Grunze H, Spriggs AJI. History of Clinical Cytology: A Selection of Documents. Darmstadt: Ernst Giebeler, 1980
10. Lopez-Cardozo P. Clinical Cytology. Leiden; Stafleu, 1954.
11. Soderstrom N. Puncture of goitres for aspiration biopsy. Acta Med Scand 1952; 144:235–44.
12. Zajicek J. Aspiration biopsy cytology: cytology of supradiaphragmatic organs. S Karger, New York, 1974
13. Zajicek J. Aspiration biopsy cytology: cytology of infradiaphragmatic organs. S Karger, New York, 1979
14. Linsk JA. Aspiration cytology in Sweden: the Karolinska group. Diagn Cytopathol 1985; 1:332–5
15. Young J. Fine Needle Aspiration Cytopathology. Blackwell, 1993
16. Frable WJ. The history of fine needle aspiration biopsy: the American experience. In: Schmidt W, Miller T, eds. Cytopathology Annual; ASCP Press, Chicago, 1994; 91–9.
17. Bakshi NA, Mansoor I, Jones BA. Analysis of inconclusive fine-needle aspiration of thyroid follicular lesions. Endocr Pathol 2003; 14(2):167–75
18. Brown LA, Coghill SB, Powis SA. Audit of diagnostic accuracy of FNA cytology specimens taken by the histopathologist in a symptomatic breast clinic. Cytopathology 1991 ;2(1):1–6
19. Joseph L, Edwards JM, Nicholson CM, Pitt MA, Howat AJ. An audit of the accuracy of fine needle aspiration using a liquid-based cytology system in the setting of a rapid access breast clinic. Cytopathology 2002; 13(6):343–9
20. Crystal BS, Wang HH, Ducatman BS. Comparison of different preparation techniques for fine needle aspiration specimens. A semiquantitative and statistical analysis. Acta Cytol 1993; 37(1):24–8

21. Stanley MW. Cost benefit and outcomes analysis for fine-needle aspiration. Why do we know so little? Clin Lab Med 1999; 19(4):773–81, vi
22. Brown LA, Coghill SB. Cost effectiveness of a fine needle aspiration clinic. Cytopathology 1992; 3(5):275–80
23. Nasuti JF, Gupta PK, Baloch ZW. Diagnostic value and cost-effectiveness of on-site evaluation of fine-needle aspiration specimens: review of 5,688 cases. Diagn Cytopathol 2002; 27(1):1–4
24. Robinson IA, Cozens NJ. Does a joint ultrasound guided cytology clinic optimize the cytological evaluation of head and neck masses? Clin Radiol 1999; 54(5):312–6
25. Kocjan G. Evaluation of the cost effectiveness of establishing a fine needle aspiration cytology clinic in a hospital out-patient department. Cytopathology 1991; 2(1):13–8
26. Padel AF, Coghill SB, Powis SJ. Evidence that the sensitivity is increased and the inadequacy rate decreased when pathologists take aspirates for cytodiagnosis. Cytopathology 1993; 4(3):161–5
27. Renshaw AA. Evidence-based criteria for adequacy in thyroid fine-needle aspiration. Am J Clin Pathol 2002; 118(4):518–21
28. Lazda EJ, Kocjan G, Sams VR, Wotherspoon AC, Taylor I. Fine needle aspiration (FNA) cytology of the breast: the influence of unsatisfactory samples on patient management. Cytopathology 1996; 7(4):262–7
29. Pennes DR, Naylor B, Rebner M. Fine needle aspiration biopsy of the breast. Influence of the number of passes and the sample size on the diagnostic yield. Acta Cytol 1990; 34(5):673–6
30. Brown LA, Coghill SB. Fine needle aspiration cytology of the breast: factors affecting sensitivity. Cytopathology 1991; 2(2):67–74
31. Lee KR, Foster RS, Papillo JL. Fine needle aspiration of the breast. Importance of the aspirator. Acta Cytol 1987; 31(3):281–4
32. Phadke DM, Lucas DR, Madan S. Fine-needle aspiration biopsy of vertebral and intervertebral disc lesions: specimen adequacy, diagnostic utility, and pitfalls. Arch Pathol Lab Med 2001; 125(11):1463–8
33. Fessia L, Botta G, Arisio R, Verga M, Aimone V. Fine-needle aspiration of breast lesions: role and accuracy in a review of 7,495 cases. Diagn Cytopathol 1987; 3(2):121–5
34. Lieu D. Fine-needle aspiration: technique and smear preparation. Am Fam Physician 1997; 55(3):839–46, 853–4
35. Lee HC, Ooi PJ, Poh WT, Wong CY. Impact of inadequate fine-needle aspiration cytology on outcome of patients with palpable breast lesions. Aust N Z J Surg 2000; 70(9):656–9
36. Hamill J, Campbell ID, Mayall F, Bartlett AS, Darlington A. Improved breast cytology results with near patient FNA diagnosis. Acta Cytol 2002; 46(1):19–24
37. Dray M, Mayall F, Darlington A. Improved fine needle aspiration (FNA) cytology results with a near patient diagnosis service for breast lesions. Cytopathology 2000; 11(1):32–7
38. Mayall F, Denford A, Chang B, Darlington A. Improved FNA cytology results with a near patient diagnosis service for non-breast lesions. J Clin Pathol 1998; 51(7):541–4
39. Rubenchik I, Sneige N, Edeiken B, Samuels B, Fornage B. In search of specimen adequacy in fine-needle aspirates of nonpalpable breast lesions. Am J Clin Pathol 1997; 108(1):13–8
40. Singh N RD, Berney M, Calaminici MT, Sheaff T, Wells A. Inadequate rates are lower when FNAC samples are taken by cytopathologists. Cytopathology 2003; 14(6):327–31
41. Young NA, Mody DR, Davey DD. Misinterpretation of normal cellular elements in fine-needle aspiration biopsy specimens: observations from the College of American Pathologists Interlaboratory Comparison Program in Non-Gynecologic Cytopathology. Arch Pathol Lab Med 2002; 126(6):670–5
42. MacDonald L, Yazdi HM. Nondiagnostic fine needle aspiration biopsy of the thyroid gland: a diagnostic dilemma. Acta Cytol 1996; 40(3):423–8
43. McHenry CR, Walfish PG, Rosen IB. Non-diagnostic fine needle aspiration biopsy: a dilemma in management of nodular thyroid disease. Am Surg 1993; 59(7):415–9
44. Vural G, Hagmar B, Lilleng R. A one-year audit of fine needle aspiration cytology of breast lesions. Factors affecting adequacy and a review of delayed carcinoma diagnoses. Acta Cytol 1995; 39(6):1233–6
45. Saxe A, Phillips E, Orfanou P, Husain M. Role of sample adequacy in fine needle aspiration biopsy of palpable breast lesions. Am J Surg 2001; 182(4):369–71
46. Snead DR, Vryenhoef P, Pinder SE, Evans A, Wilson AR, Blamey RW, et al. Routine audit of breast fine needle aspiration (FNA) cytology specimens and aspirator inadequate rates. Cytopathology 1997; 8(4):236–47
47. Boerner S, Sneige N. Specimen adequacy and false-negative diagnosis rate in fine-needle aspirates of palpable breast masses. Cancer 1998; 84(6):344–8
48. Boerner S, Fornage BD, Singletary E, Sneige N. Ultrasound-guided fine-needle aspiration (FNA) of nonpalpable breast lesions: a review of 1885 FNA cases using the National Cancer Institute-supported recommendations on the uniform approach to breast FNA. Cancer 1999; 87(1):19–24
49. Stephenson TJ, Cross SS, Underwood JC, Reed MW, Shorthouse AJ. Why pathologists should not take fine needle aspirates. Cytopathology 1995; 6(5):358–60
50. Polacarz SV. Why pathologists should take needle aspirates. Cytopathology 1995; 6(5):358

51. Coghill SB, Brown LA. Why pathologists should take needle aspiration specimens. Cytopathology 1995; 6(1):1–4
52. Hoda RS. Why pathologists should take needle aspiration specimens. Cytopathology 1995; 6(6):419–20
53. Howat AJ. Why pathologists should take needle aspiration specimens. Cytopathology 1995; 6(6):419

Chapter 2

FNAC Technique and Slide Preparation

Contents

2.1 Informed Consent 7

2.2 Location of the FNAC Procedure 8
2.2.1 The FNAC Clinic 9
2.2.2 Inpatient FNAC 12
2.2.3 Image-Guided and Other FNAC Procedure Locations 12

2.3 The Importance of the Aspirator 14

2.4 Aspiration Techniques 15
2.4.1 Suction FNAC 15
2.4.2 The Capillary Method 16

2.5 Slide Preparation 17
2.5.1 Conventional Preparations 17
2.5.2 Liquid-Based Preparations 18
2.5.3 Cell Block 18

2.6 Fixation Techniques 19
2.6.1 Air Drying 19
2.6.2. Alcohol Fixation 20
2.6.3 Transport Medium 20

2.7 Staining Methods 20
2.7.1 Papanicolaou Staining 20
2.7.2 Romanowsky Staining 22
2.7.3 Other Stains 23

2.8 Ancillary Techniques 23
2.8.1 Cytochemistry 23
2.8.2 Immunocytochemistry 24
2.8.3 Molecular Markers in Cytology 26

2.9 Safety 27

References 28

2.1 Informed Consent

The ethical and legal requirement to obtain informed consent prior to performing a medical procedure is becoming a mandatory process, thus replacing the paternalistic relationship between doctor and patient that has prevailed for centuries [1]. The patient, after being explained the procedure, its format, purpose, risks, benefits and the alternative approach, makes a voluntary and informed decision to proceed. The modern concept of informed consent is a process of mutual communication rather than a signature on a standardised form [2, 3].

The idea of modern informed consent dates back to 1914 when a judicial ruling stated: "Every human being of adult years and sound mind has a right to determine what shall be done with his body" [2]. Further legal developments included emphasis on the information given to the patient in order for a decision to be truly informed rather than just consented to. The patient should be allowed the opportunity to ask questions and the doctor should be satisfied that the patient understands what they are signing [4]. Although there are different legal interpretations as to who has a duty to inform, it is generally accepted that the duty to inform lies with the person who performs the procedure.

A consent form usually has two parts, the first part explaining the procedure and the second underlining the risks (Fig. 2.1). Both need to be read and understood by the patient prior to the procedure [5]. It has been shown that twice as many patients read the information leaflet explaining the commencement of procedure when information is disseminated in advance rather than on the day of the procedure [6]. It is suggested that the consent forms should be written in simple terms, using larger print and in duplicate copy. Patients should be given copies of the consent forms they sign so that they can re-read them at home. For true patient autonomy to exist in informed consent, patients should be given the form in a language they understand or else be provided with a competent interpreter [7]. Patient recall of the list of complications has been used as a measure of comprehension of the informed consent procedure [8].

CONSENT FORM FOR FNA CYTOLOGY DIAGNOSTIC PROCEDURE

I,_____
(PRINT NAME AND SURNAME)

Authorise DR_____

To perform Fine Needle Aspiration Cytology Diagnostic Procedure.

Fine Needle Aspiration Cytology (FNAC) is a simple diagnostic test, performed by a doctor, with a thin needle in order to obtain cells for microscopic analysis. It involves minimal pain for which a local anaesthetic may be used in some instances. It may be need to be repeated id multiple sites are sampled or more material is needed. The results are usually available within one week and are sent by post to the referring doctor. You will not need a period of rest after the procedure.

The alternative to FNAC is a tissue biopsy. This is a surgical procedure involving obtaining a piece of tissue and may require a stay in hospital. This may need to be performed later, if FNAC is unable to provide the full answer. FNAC involves minimal risk of bleeding which occurs only very rarely. The level of pain after the procedure is usually such as not to require medication.
In some instances, a photograph may be taken of the lesion for teaching and discussion purposes.

I have read and understand this consent form, and my question have been answered.

Date:_____
(Patient/Responsible Party):

PLEASE SIGN HERE _____
Date:_____
(Witness):

DOCTOR!S DECLARATION: I have explained this procedure, risk and alternatives to the patient and believe he/she has been adequately informed and has consented.
(Doctor!s signature):

Date:_____

Fig. 2.1
Sample patient consent form

Aspects of informed consent that are important to the patient and the doctor include (1) the nature of the procedure, (2) the purpose, (3) risks and complications, (4) benefits and (5) alternatives [9]. Doctors are also interested in the consequences of the procedure as regards management [10]. There are also ethical issues related to each of these aspects of informed consent. Similarly, the patient's privacy and confidentiality are not to be underestimated [11].

In FNAC practice, patients generally lack knowledge of the procedure. Once explained, they frequently query the level of pain, invariably expecting a much more painful procedure than the one subsequently experienced. Concern is often voiced as to whether the needle may have an adverse effect on any pathology, for example whether it will disseminate a malignant disease. Sometimes there is a perception that FNAC may be a curative procedure, particularly if the lesion is cystic. Very few patients understand the reason for the procedure, its place in the diagnostic workup or the impact of the result on further management. They frequently confuse the tissue biopsy with the fine-needle biopsy, as FNAC is sometimes known.

Pathologists, when obtaining FNAC consent and performing the procedure, are experiencing a near-patient episode, aspects of which they have not been trained for. They may lack communication skills, which are important in gaining the patient's confidence. Pathologists occupy a unique place in the management process; they make a diagnosis but do not discuss the results with the patient. This is usually the task of the referring physician. This approach must be explained to the patient in advance of the procedure.

Providing information is an important part of the doctor-patient relationship [12]. To that end, informed consent is an integral part of that communication. Importantly, it is offering professional protection. Ensuring that all elements of informed consent are met will result in fewer negligence claims, greater patient satisfaction and improved professional image [7]. The process of informed consent has led to the empowerment of the patient. The current information revolution is expected to bring further changes in the doctor-patient relationship [1].

2.2 Location of the FNAC Procedure

One of the advantages of FNAC is that it can be performed at various locations. Most frequently it is performed in the hospital outpatients department, but it can also be performed in hospital wards, in a dedicated room within a pathology laboratory or in imaging or endoscopy suites.

FNAC need not be confined to the hospital environment and may be performed almost anywhere, provided the basic conditions of safety are satisfied. Using FNAC in rural North West Australia, Zardawi advocates a multidisciplinary setting with the direct involvement of pathologists, radiologists and clinicians and finds it an extremely accurate, well-tolerated, relatively non-invasive and low-risk test that obviates the need for surgical intervention in most benign conditions and disseminated malignancies [13].

2.2.1 The FNAC Clinic

The name FNAC clinic usually refers to the outpatient FNAC service offered to patients with lumps that need investigation. Patients are initially seen by a specialist and are subsequently referred to the FNAC clinic. Patients are usually booked in advance, with a letter of referral or a request form being available at the time of the appointment. The minimum staff and equipment required for the FNAC clinic room is an assistant (usually a cytotechnologist), an examination couch with access from both sides, a writing desk, a work surface, a microscope, a sink, an examination tray for instruments and good lighting and air conditioning (Fig. 2.2). A cytotechnologist, who puts the patient in the optimal position for the procedure, usually assists the aspirator. In most cases patients lie on their back, but they may have additional requirements, for example in the case of thyroid FNAC they will have to extend their neck over the support cushion (Fig. 2.3). Patients having difficulty lying flat may remain seated with support or may have the couch elevated to a comfortable position. Every effort should be made to put the patient at ease, since success of the procedure depends on their cooperation. In some cases, an additional chaperone/nurse may be needed to assist patients with special needs, for example those who are wheelchair bound, poorly mobile, blind or children. Patients who wish their partners or companions to be present during the procedure are allowed to do so, making sure that they are seated comfortably and not in the way of the procedure being carried out. In cases where there is limited space, this recommendation may be modified in that the accompanying person(s) will help to settle the patient and then leave the room, to return immediately after the procedure is over. In some instances it is advised that there should be access to a recovery room in the vicinity of the FNAC room where the patient may be observed for a short period after the procedure, particularly in cases of bleeding.

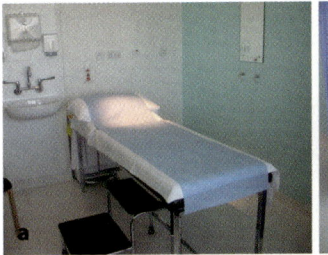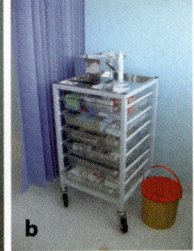

Fig. 2.2
a A layout of the clinic room with easy access to the examination table from all sides. **b** The instrument trolley should contain all that is necessary for the FNAC procedure

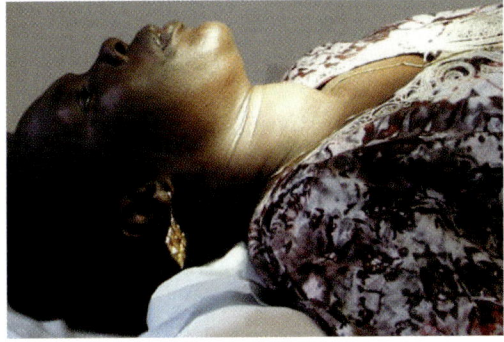

Fig. 2.3
FNAC for the thyroid is best performed with the patient's neck extended over a support

An FNAC clinic is the ideal place for the aspirator to obtain a first-hand clinical history. The patient is usually asked about their symptoms and any relevant medical history that may not have been recorded in the referring letter. The anatomical position of the lesion is carefully assessed and, subject to the patient's consent, may be photographed in order to gain a more precise insight into the pathology (Fig. 2.4). In the course of examination, particularly after the preliminary microscopy, it may be useful to ask additional questions in reaching a final diagnosis (e.g. is there a history of an excised mole?).

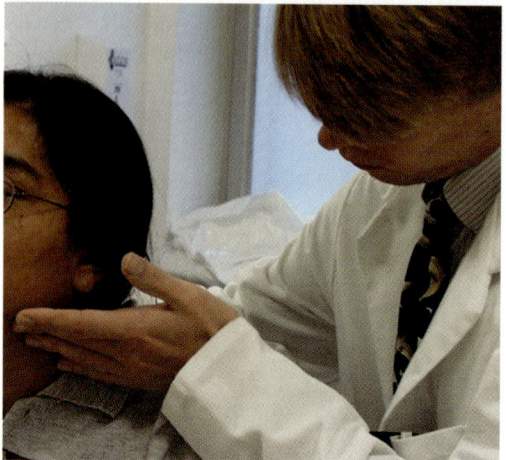

Fig. 2.4
FNAC clinic. The aspirator can palpate the lesion and assess its consistency, mobility and realtionship to other anatomical structures

With regard to equipment, the examination trolley/FNAC box should ideally contain the following: needles of various calibres, not larger than 21 gauge (Fig. 2.5), syringes (20, 10 and 5 ml), a syringe holder (e.g. Cameco; Fig. 2.6a), glass slides (coated and non-coated) – preferably with a frosted end, alcohol swabs, anaesthetic (e.g. 2% lignocaine without adrenalin), universal containers (empty and containing transport medium), gauze swabs, Elastoplast, a pencil, rubber gloves, a protective mask and an apron. The contents should be clearly listed in the laboratory manual and checked before each clinic. Slides are stained using one of the rapid stains (Fig. 2.6b). The aspirator should have a writing surface and a microscope available to record the macroscopic findings and check the adequacy of the aspirated material whilst the patient is still present in the clinic (on-site evaluation; Fig. 2.7). Nasuti et al. report the average rate of non-diagnostic FNAC without on-site evaluation to be 20%. The non-diagnostic rate for FNAC with on-site evaluation is 0.98% [14].

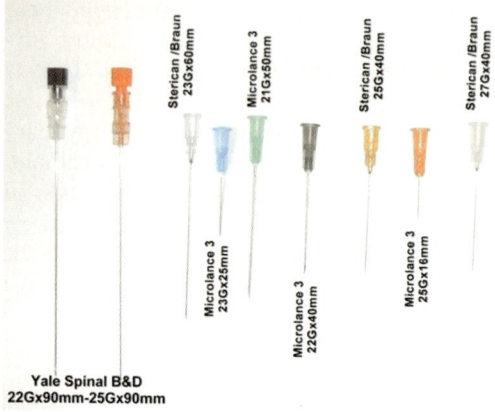

Fig. 2.5
Various types of needles available for performing the aspiration. Most frequently used are those of 22 gauge (G) and less

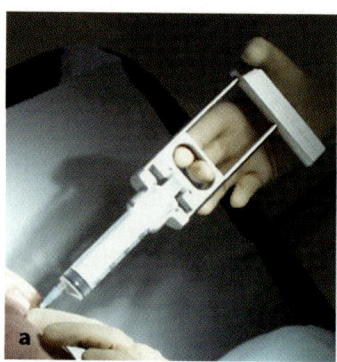

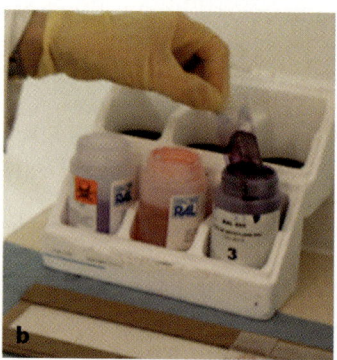

Fig. 2.6
a Fine needle aspiration with the aid of a Cameco syringe holder is used mainly for cystic lesions. **b** Rapid stains should be available in the clinic for assessment of material adequacy

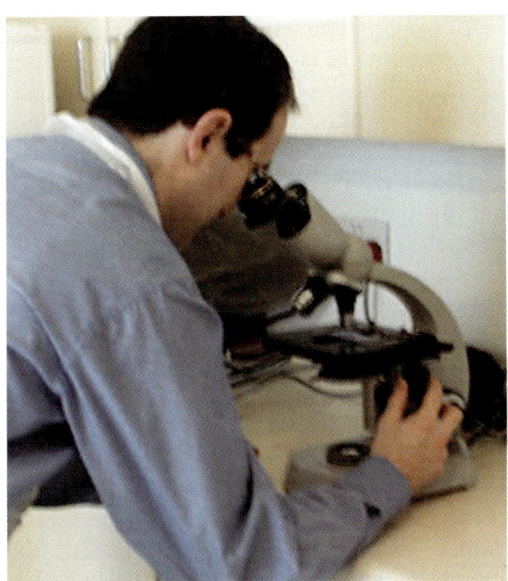

Fig. 2.7
FNA material can be checked for cellularity immediately after rapid staining, preferably whilst the patient is still present

The other advantage of on-site evaluation is that results in terms of material adequacy may be given to the patient immediately, whilst the discussion of the final pathology result and management is usually left to the referring clinician. In cases where the FNAC clinic is a one-stop clinic, the results are usually immediately available to the referring clinician and given to the patient in the same session. This practice is particularly common in cases of breast FNAC, where patients obtain the results the same day. However, the views amongst surgeons as to the appropriateness of giving the bad news in the first clinical session are not unanimous. One-stop clinics are cost effective and beneficial, particularly for patients with benign disease who do not need further follow up. These clinics are currently most frequently used for breast lumps, although there are also centres where head and neck lesions are managed in this way.

The reliability and efficiency of the FNAC service depends on the quality of the specimens [15–17]. A combined approach of ultrasound-guided fine-needle aspiration of head and neck masses, with an immediate assessment of the material by a pathologist was found to be 24% more accurate than specimens obtained by clinicians, with an 84% reduction in inadequate specimens [18]. FNAC at a surgical symptomatic breast clinic where the pathologist takes, stains and immediately reports the aspiration cytology smears achieved high levels of complete sensitivity (95.7%) and specificity (100%) for aspiration cytodiagnosis. Significant reductions of unnecessary biopsy procedures and outpatient revisits have allowed major resource savings to be made. Brown et al. recommend that in view of the high degree of accuracy obtained by this approach to the investigation of palpable breast lesions, combined clinics, with their benefits for the patient, both physical and psychological, should be encouraged [19]. FNAC performed by a dedicated specialist and immediate reporting should be an integral part of a breast diagnostic service [20]. Rapid stains are usually good for the assessment of cellularity, but are not always optimal for detailed morphology. They may have specific artefacts that one should be familiar with prior to reporting. This applies particularly to lymphoid cells in all their forms.

The duration and frequency of FNAC clinics is variable and depends on demand. The aspirator can usually see between eight and ten patients in one session. Patients are seen at approximately 25-min intervals, with the assistance of a dedicated cytotechnologist.

The introduction of pathologist-led FNAC clinics has been found to be cost effective. The average reported rate of non-diagnostic FNAC without on-site evaluation is 20%. In our experience, the establishment of an FNAC clinic (and the concomitant reduction in inadequate specimen rates) results in a threefold reduction in the cost of diagnosing breast lesions within 12 months [21]. If one assumes that patients will undergo a repeat FNAC for each non-diagnostic specimen, the estimated additional cost in direct institutional charges is US $2,022,626 over 5-year period, or US $404,525 per year, without on-site evaluation. There are similar reports from others who set out the economic benefits of FNAC clinics [14, 22–28]. (see chapter 10.13)

2.2.2 Inpatient FNAC

Inpatients have their FNAC samples taken in hospital wards. Ward staff usually have very little experience of what is needed, so it is useful to advise them in advance as to what the procedure entails and what equipment is needed, making sure that the patient is present on the ward at the time the FNAC is planned for. In some cases, a nurse may be asked to assist with the FNAC procedure. In our experience, an FNAC instruments box is brought from the laboratory so that only minimum equipment is needed from the ward (e.g. an examination trolley and a sharps container). The optimal way of performing FNAC on inpatients would be in a treatment room attached to the ward. Alternatively, optimal conditions have to be created by the patient's bedside in order for the procedure to succeed; the procedure is explained to the patient and then clear access to the lesion is achieved by positioning the patient and the equipment around them, at the same time making every effort to maintain their privacy and dignity. The FNAC tools need to be easily accessible, close to the bedside and ensuring good lighting of the working areas. All of the relevant staff should wear protective clothing (aprons, gloves and masks), where appropriate. Glass slides should be transported in specimen boxes and liquid material in sealed containers. The FNAC procedure and ward visit should be recorded on the patient's request form as well as in the hospital records along with the signature of the aspirator and the date of the procedure.

2.2.3 Image-Guided and Other FNAC Procedure Locations

2.2.3.1 Ultrasound-Guided FNAC

Ultrasound-guided FNAC is practiced in some centres. This is the preferred method in some centres and is particularly useful in the staging of head and neck lesions, non-palpable breast lesions and thyroid lesions, in the case of the latter by helping to avoid surgery in 37% of cases [29–31]. FNAC is performed either by a radiologist with or without the presence of a cytopathologist, or by a cytopathologist who has acquired ultrasonographic skills. The room is usually dark and there may be twice as many staff involved as when performing a non-image-guided FNAC. Unless this is performed by a well-trained team, an overlap of activity may occur. Image-guided FNAC is particularly advantageous in cases of small, non-palpable or multiple lesions. In the case of the thyroid, some centres advocate the use of image-guided FNAC. Karstrup et al. report ultrasound-guided FNAC of the thyroid to be superior to both ultrasound-guided core biopsy (CB) and the combination of ultrasound-guided FNAC and CB. They recommend the use of CB in a few selected patients only [32]. It has been shown that ultrasound-guided breast FNAC contributed to a change of clinical staging from N0 to N1 in 75% and from N1 to N0 in 30% of cases, and multicentricity/multifocality was identified sonographically and proved by FNAC in 21% of patients [33]. In addition, ultrasonographically guided percutaneous FNAC is a particularly useful, safe and reliable method of establishing the cytological diagnosis of intrathoracic tumours [34].

2.2.3.2 Endoscopy-Guided Ultrasound FNAC

The use of endoscopy-guided ultrasound (EUS) FNAC (EUS-FNAC) of the pancreas, mediastinum, duodenum, bile ducts, hypopharynx, rectum, lung and other sites accessible through the endoscope is increasing [35–43]. After localising the lesion by endosonography, a 22-gauge aspiration needle (Olympus, Pentax, Wilson-Cook) device is placed into the mass under real-time control (Fig. 2.8). A metallic central stylet crosses the entire length of the needle catheter assembly. The catheter is passed through the aspiration channel of the endoscope and the needle with the stylet is advanced through the gastrointestinal wall. The stylet is then removed and continuous suction is applied using a 20-ml syringe. After this, the needle is moved back and forth within the lesion for 1–2 min. When the aspiration is complete, suction is released and the catheter system is removed through the aspiration channel. The entire contents of the needle are collected with the stylet, which is reintroduced into the needle. Multiple aspirates from different sites ensure the adequacy of the material. A minimum of two and a maximum of four passes per patient are advised. After slide preparation, the syringe and the needle are rinsed with a fixative and are used for a Shandon Cytospin preparation (Thermo Electron Corporation) or liquid-based cytology (LBC). Any visible tissue fragments should be gently removed with forceps or the tip of a needle and transferred to formalin or alcohol-formalin-acetic acid (AFA) fixative for cell block preparation, if needed [44]. The diagnostic accuracy of the method appears to be directly related to the availability of a cytopathologist in the endoscopy suite during the procedure to assess the cellularity of the aspirate [45]. The costs involved, however, may prevent some centres from using cytopathologists during the procedure [46]. EUS-FNAC is technically challenging and requires long training in centres with a high volume of EUS procedures. The accuracy of EUS-FNAC is dependent on the experience of both the endoscopist and the pathologist [47].

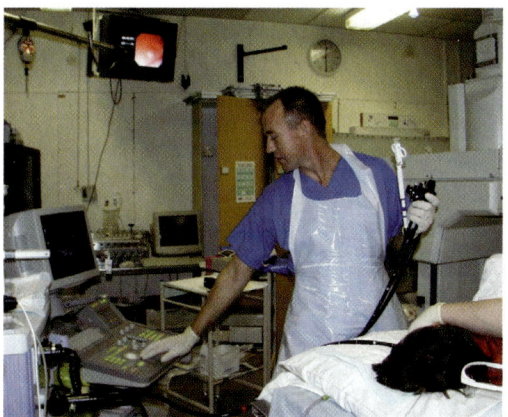

Fig. 2.8
Endoscopy-guided FNAC (EUS-FNAC) is a highly skilled procedure, the accuracy of which is directly related to the experience of the aspirator

2.2.3.3 Computed Tomography (CT)-Guided FNAC

CT-guided FNAC is associated with high diagnostic accuracy and a low rate of complications, particularly in the diagnosis of pulmonary lesions [48]. It has been shown that an accurate diagnosis from FNAC of intrathoracic cancer is more likely when a cytopathologist is present than when not present during the procedure [49–51]. Kucuk et al. found that there is no significant difference between single-pass needle and multiple-pass coaxial needle systems with respect to the diagnostic accuracy and the complication rate [50]. When a radiologist who is trained in head and neck imaging identifies a possible early recurrence of a tumour by CT, the prompt use of CT-guided FNAC is an effective way to diagnose these tumours so that appropriate treatments can be initiated [52].

2.2.3.4 Other FNAC Procedure Locations

FNAC can be performed almost anywhere, provided the aforementioned conditions are met. As a first-line investigation, FNAC should have a place in primary care practices and hospital diagnostic units. (see chapter 10.11) This would introduce a means of triage for patients with lumps and bumps that would otherwise need specialist referral.

It is not advisable to perform FNAC within pathology laboratories since these are not usually equipped for seeing patients. Patients require, for example, an adequately equipped waiting room, public facilities, lifts, telephones, access to general information provided by a receptionist who is trained to handle enquiries and refreshments. Pathology laboratories, by the nature of their work and with staff not trained in dealing with the general public, are usually not suitable for outpatient clinical activity, although it may appear convenient for the cytopathology team. There may be exceptions to this where the system works well within the pathology department.

2.3 The Importance of the Aspirator

Although FNAC is a simple technique, it is not banal. The importance of the aspirator in locating the lesion, correctly inserting the needle and collecting cells for analysis is a sequence of events that requires operator skills that are sometimes underestimated. Many a junior doctor has been given the task of performing FNAC without prior training or experience. This is reflected in the difference in the proportion of adequate material received from hospitals as compared with that taken in FNAC clinics by a trained hand. The experience needed to perform FNAC is gained through many repeated attempts; somewhere in the region of 250 passes are needed before good results can be expected. Why is the performance so variable for such a simple method? The effects of various factors on the sensitivity of the technique have been explored. Small tumour size, certain types of tumour and lesions that are difficult to palpate are causes of reduced sensitivity.

There are several steps in the procedure, all of which are equally important. In performing FNAC without image guidance on palpable lumps, confidence and experience is needed to palpate small lesions. No results will be obtained from a vaguely palpable area where the aspirator is not convinced of a lesion. Those patients are best left alone and their management discussed with the referring clinician. If palpable, the lump needs to be fixed in order to stay in position during the passage of the needle in several different directions. This is usually achieved by the fingers of a non-dominant hand, holding the lump between the index and the third finger. Sometimes, if a lump (usually a lymph node) is small and slippery, a firm base like a rib or muscle must be found in order to stabilise it, making sure at the same time to approach it tangentially in order to avoid reaching the ribs/vessels/trachea or similar supporting structures. The aspirator needs to have a good knowledge of the local anatomy to avoid complications, namely bleeding, but also to understand the presence of possible contaminants in the aspirate (e.g. respiratory epithelium in FNAC of the thyroid, if the trachea is aspirated by mistake).

Who should perform FNAC? This debate has been going on for a long time, and the consensus is that the cytopathologist is the best person to perform this procedure. The immediate availability of the patient's history and macroscopic appearance including size, anatomical site, consistency and the contents (solid, cystic, firm, soft, calcified, mucoid or purulent) makes interpretation of the results easier (Fig. 2.9). In addition, on-site checking of adequacy is a preferred way of handling the procedure. However, the presence of a cytopathologist on-site cannot be guaranteed in all situations. In these cases, practices have developed whereby material is aspirated by the clinician or a radiologist. In the United Kingdom, in some instances nurses may be trained to take appropriate samples. Whoever is to perform the FNAC should have had training in the technique. This may be achieved in the first instance by using teaching aids available for this purpose or by shadowing a senior colleague in the clinic and performing one of the several FNAC passes that are made at the time, subject to the patient's consent. Trainee aspirators can achieve good results early in their experience. Brown and Coghill found that after 1 year each trainee aspirator had improved to the level of an experienced aspirator [19]. Snaed et al. found that there was a significant improvement in the performance of individual junior aspirators when their 1st year was compared with their last year on the unit [53].

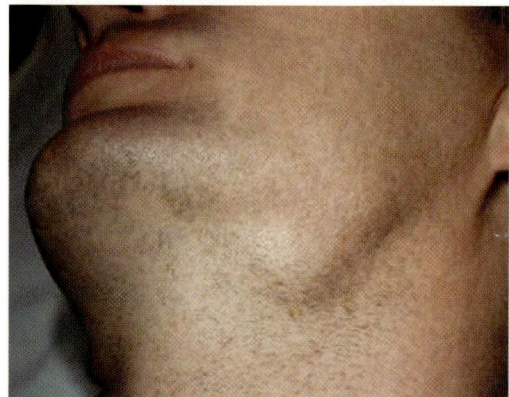

Fig. 2.9
Patient with a submandibular lump referred for FNAC with a suspicion of a lymphoma. The lesion is an inflamed salivary gland

How many FNAC passes per lesion should be performed? The sensitivity of FNAC biopsy of the breast as a function of the number of aspirations performed on any given lesion has been investigated. A mathematical extrapolation of the data indicated that three or four aspirations of any given lesion provide the optimal yield within the limits of practicality. This performance of multiple FNAC procedures is particularly important when the pathologist either does not perform the FNAC or is unable to assist in the immediate interpretation of the specimen to assess its adequacy [54].

As FNAC has become a critical component of the investigation of palpable masses, false-negative diagnoses have become a major concern, prompting a re-evaluation of the definition of specimen adequacy. After excluding inadequate preparations, FNAC interpretations of definite cancer or as benign are highly accurate [55]. Although cytopathologists agree that several parameters relate to the adequacy of an FNAC specimen, there is no unanimity on the role of epithelial cell quantification in the determination of an adequate FNAC [22]. Aspirates of the breast are classified as adequate if a total of five or six epithelial cell clusters (each comprising at least five to ten well-preserved cells) are present on all slides, or as inadequate if fewer than five or six such clusters are present [22, 56]. Although a definition of adequacy based on cellularity is useful in reducing false negative results, cellularity alone cannot be relied upon in the management of non-palpable lesions [57]. The aspirator's performance should be monitored and audited. By identifying poor aspirators who may benefit from targeted training and advice, the quality of FNAC specimens, and ultimately patient care, would improve [53]. The rate of inadequate samples is variable in various sites, but should generally be kept below 10% and ideally not be above 5%. Dray et al. made an audit of the comparison of a rapid diagnosis FNAC service with consultant pathologist aspirators to a conventional FNAC service with clinician aspirators of varied experience [24]. There were statistically significant differences in specificity (biopsy cases only), with 73% for pathologists and 49% for clinicians, specificity (full) of 74% and 56%, respectively, an inadequate sampling rate of 23% and 37%, respectively, and complete sensitivity with 76% and 67%, respectively. The use of pathologist aspirators allowed the specimens to be reported in a few minutes. Specimens taken by clinicians took at least 30 min to report. When compared with clinician aspirators, pathologist aspirators obtained better quality results that were reported more quickly [24, 58–62]. Complete sensitivity rose by 15% and the number of missed malignancies fell by half when breast FNAC specimens were taken by the pathologist in a joint surgical clinic, compared with those taken by a surgeon alone [63].

LBC may bring improvements to the adequacy of the material in terms of the quality of the material preservation. The onus for specimen preparation artefacts will no longer be only on the aspirator, but also on the laboratory. However, LBC will not make up for inefficient material collection, often masked by large amounts of blood. LBC will involve a fewer number of slides, which, unless they are representative, will enable easier decisions about material adequacy. Improvements in the sample quality are expected following the removal of blood from LBC preparations. Diagnosis of FNAC material using the LBC method is feasible, accurate and reliable, even in the rapid-diagnosis clinic [55].

2.4 Aspiration Techniques

2.4.1 Suction FNAC

In this method, the needle is passed into the lesion and negative pressure is applied, usually by virtue of a syringe attached to the needle, and often with the help of a syringe holder (Cameco). In image-guided FNAC, most of the apparatus is designed to obtain material with the aid of negative-pressure suction. This method is particularly useful when draining a liquid from the lesion (e.g. cyst fluid, ascites or pleural fluid; Fig. 2.10). However, it is important that the negative pressure is released prior to exiting the lesion. If this is forgotten, after exiting the lesion the material from the needle may be accidentally aspirated into the syringe and it becomes more difficult to expel it in the traditional manner. In this case, making a cell solution would salvage the material. If, however, negative pressure is appropriately released before exiting the lesion, the cellular material is contained within the needle and its hub. The needle is then detached from the syringe and the material expelled onto a glass slide (or into a solution if an LBC sample is being made). tor and the nature of the lesion. If fresh blood is drawn immediately after entering the lesion, the attempt is abandoned and pressure applied to the needle penetration site to stop bruising. It may be possible to repeat the FNC in a different site of the same lesion. Otherwise, it is advisable to abandon further attempts to obtain specimens for fear of haemorrhage. FNC sampling was found to be diagnostic in a greater number of cases than FNAC sampling, although no clear superiority over FNAC has been found [64].

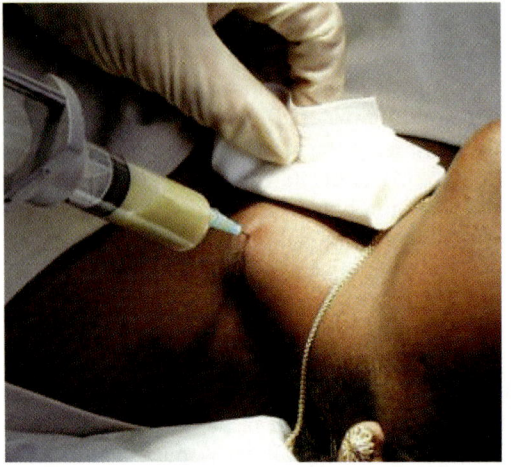

Fig. 2.10
FNAC technique with suction applied is useful for draining abscesses or cysts. This patient has TB lymphadenopathy from which the pus is being drained. The aspirated material is sent for TB culture

2.4.2 The Capillary Method

In the past decade, FNAC has been performed increasingly without the aid of suction, with a needle alone, the so-called fine needle capillary (FNC) technique or non-aspiration aspiration (Fig. 2.11). The needle is passed into the lesion and multiple fast jabbing movements in and out of the lesion as well as in different directions are performed. Once the material is seen in the hub of the needle, there is usually sufficient material. Several passes may be performed safely, although the average number of passes may vary according to the experience of the aspira-

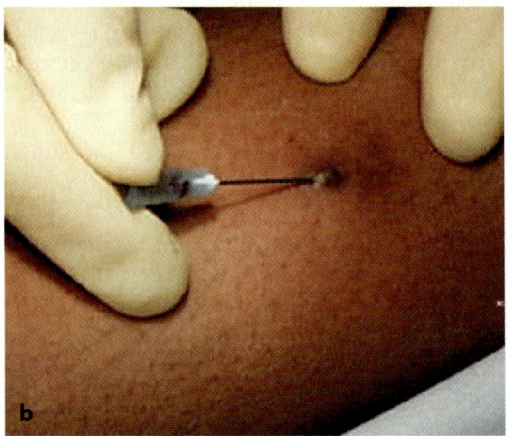

Fig. 2.11
a Capillary technique using needle only, without aspiration, is currently the preferred method for FNAC.
b FNAC skin. Non-aspiration technique in a case of cutaneous Kaposi's sarcoma

The complication rate of FNAC is low and is mainly minor haemorrhage. Complications are avoided by the scrupulous use of thin needles (less than 21 gauge, preferably 23 and 25 gauge) and haemostasis after the procedure. Tumour seeding, feared by some patients and clinicians, is not a complication of FNAC performed in the manner described here.

2.5 Slide Preparation

2.5.1 Conventional Preparations

Material obtained with a fine needle is expelled onto appropriately labelled glass slides. This is usually performed by using a 20-ml syringe filled with air, attaching the needle to it and pushing the contents out of the needle. Sometimes, if the hub of the needle is full, it is possible to tap the hub against the glass and obtain the material directly from there. In this case, caution is needed to avoid needle-stick injury. The needle is discarded immediately into a special sharps container before spreading the material onto the slides.

The expelled material is ideally spread over several slides in small amounts rather than deposited in one large pool on a single slide. This way it is easier to obtain a thin-layer preparation that will be uniformly fixed or dried and will stain evenly throughout. Large amounts of blood are to be avoided because it clots, fibrin trapping the cells and creating large cracks on the slide (Fig. 2.12).

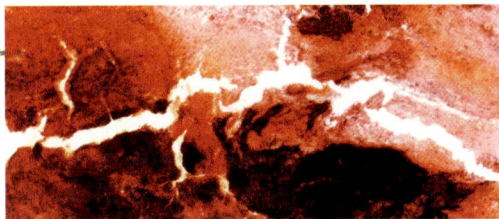

Fig. 2.12
Large amounts of blood should be avoided because it clots, fibrin trapping the cells and creating large cracks on the slide

Spreading of the material is usually performed with the help of another glass slide by sliding it over the FNAC material gently to avoid crush artefacts. This technique needs practice since accurate morphology depends on good cell preservation. Hence, the main cause of failure of smear preparations is inadequate smears made by inexperienced aspirators.

Glass slides preferably have a frosted end onto which the patient's details and the details of the procedure are written (e.g. side –left or right, pass number, any other significant information that may be helpful in interpretation). Slide labelling is usually performed by an assistant but has to be checked by the aspirator because wrongly labelled slides may become a liability and the aspirator is ultimately responsible for its correctness. It is particularly important when multiple sites are sampled or in a busy clinic where many patients are seen in rapid succession. The advice in this case is that for every patient, a new set of slides is laid out, the previous ones having been safely stored away from the immediate working area. If an unlabelled slide or container is discovered later, it should be discarded, even if this means repeating the procedure. For immunocytochemistry, it is advisable to use pre-coated slides to help cell adhesion. The decision as to which slides are to be stained and which are to be kept for special stains rests with the cytopathologist. The name of the aspirator should be recorded on the request form. If the slides are received from elsewhere, the decision may depend on the number of slides received, the method of fixation and cell preservation, and has also to be made by the interpreting cytopathologist.

Cystic fluid contents need to be handled as liquid-based preparations. No conventional smears are used because of low cellularity (see 2.5.2). If the fluid content is thick or gelatinous, some drops of fluid may be smeared onto glass slides and immediately air-dried and stained with rapid stains.

Heavily bloodstained fluids can be processed with the help of some of the red blood cell lysing fixatives (e.g. Devine's lysing solution or Cyto-Rich Red; TriPath Care Technologies, Burlington, North Carolina, USA) that increase the diagnostic utility of FNAC by lysing the red blood cells whilst preserving the cellular morphology and retaining the suitability for use in immunocytochemistry.

Macroscopic findings are recorded at the time of the aspiration, in particular the site, consistency, mobility and size of the lump as well as the description of the aspirated contents (e.g. mucinous, tenacious, clear, fatty). The number of slides and the name of the aspirator are also recorded. Patients are usually curious as to the macroscopic finding and the information that it may convey. It is advisable to reassure them that the quantity of material is sufficient for analysis, but it may be misleading to discuss the macroscopic appearances [65].

2.5.2 Liquid-Based Preparations

Liquid based cytology (LBC) was introduced initially for cervical smears, but some laboratories are increasingly processing other specimens, including FNAC, using this technology. After aspiration, the syringe and needle are thoroughly rinsed with either saline or a fixative and for Shandon Cytospin preparations (Thermo Electron Corporation) or liquid-based preparations (LBC). Some laboratories prepare all FNAC specimens as Cytospin preparations. Howat et al. have shown that the Cytospin method of FNAC in palpable breast disease has a favourable sensitivity and specificity, and is therefore an alternative to conventional FNAC using direct smears [66]. In order to enable a wider range of aspirators to obtain adequate FNAC samples, the specimen may be collected in a liquid preservative solution. The aspiration is performed in the usual way. The aspirate is then ejected directly into a container filled with 20 ml of CytoLyt or CytoRich transport solution; the syringe is also flushed thoroughly with either solution. CytoLyt is an alcohol-based solution. If a fresh, non-alcohol-fixed specimen is indicated clinically, the specimen is put into a balanced electrolyte solution. In the laboratory, material is processed further following the manufacturer's instructions [67, 68].

The initial reports of LBC FNAC preparations are encouraging. When conventional preparations are compared with ThinPrep (Cytic Corporation) processing, there is no significant difference in diagnostic accuracy [69]. One of the advantages of monolayer preparations is that the diagnostic material is spread evenly amongst the slides and that ancillary techniques can be performed (Fig. 2.13) [70, 71].

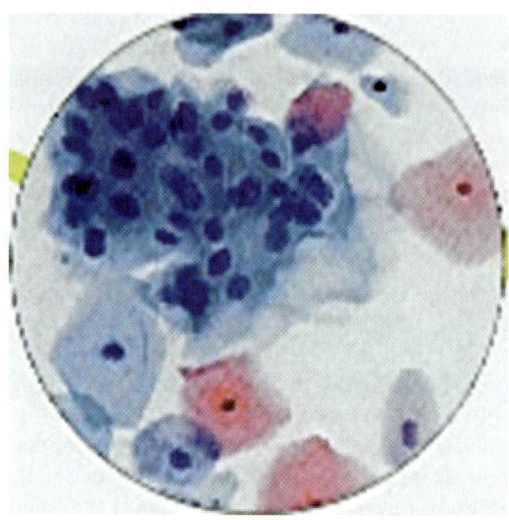

Fig. 2.13
A monolayer cell preparation of cervical cells shows crisp cellular detail with no overlapping or background contamination (ThinPrep ×400)

Cystic fluid contents need to be handled like fluids. Conventional smears are not used because of the low cellularity. Fluid concentration is obtained by either the Cytospin or LBC methods [72]. If the fluid content is thick or gelatinous, some drops of fluid may be smeared onto glass slides and immediately air dried and stained with rapid stains (Fig. 2.10).

2.5.3 Cell Block

If the FNAC material is very bloody and paucicellular, a cell-block technique may be helpful [73]. The cell block is prepared with small tissue fragments or cell deposits after centrifugation. The side surfaces of a Coplin jar where the contents of the needle have been expelled are examined carefully; any thick tissue fragments observed are scraped from the surface and resuspended in AFA solution for postfixation. The sample is transferred to a centrifuge tube and centrifuged at 1,500 rpm (400×g) for 5 min. The supernatant is discarded and two drops of reagent 2 (coloured fluid) and of reagent 1 (clear fluid) (Shandon Cytoblock, Thermo Electron Corporation) are added to produce a firm cell button, which is processed as for microbiopsy samples and embedded in a paraffin mould. The gel is solidified by using alcohol as the fixative. This system is designed to enable the preparation of paraffin-embedded cell suspensions, cell aggregates and small tissue fragments. Processing a cell block on residual ThinPrep Pap Test material, using a thrombin-based technique, was useful in augmenting the diagnosis [74].

2.6 Fixation Techniques

2.6.1 Air Drying

Immediate fixation of the FNAC specimen is crucial. The fixative depends on the choice of stain to be used, and the stain used depends on the preference within the laboratory; some prefer alcohol fixation followed by the Papanicolaou (Pap) stain, and some air-dried smears followed by Romanowsky staining (Diff Quick, May Grünwald Giemsa).

In conventional cell preparations, if slides are to be fixed by air drying, they need to be thinly spread and be dry to the naked eye within 5 min. If the specimen is very thick and does not visibly dry within that period, or if it is put into a sealed container before it is completely dry, air-drying artefacts will occur. Under the microscope, this is reflected by enlarged nuclei, fuzzy cell boundaries and the chromatin pattern assuming grotesque shapes, all of which may be misleading (Fig. 2.14). Air-drying artefact may be the cause of false positive or false negative diagnosis. It is sometimes difficult to establish strict criteria as to what degree of cell distortion constitutes an inadequate sample due to the air-drying artefact. It is advisable in these cases to try to compare material on other slides from the same case, although these may not have been prepared in the same way. In case of doubt, before a diagnostic decision is made on sub-optimal material, a repeat FNAC may be advised.

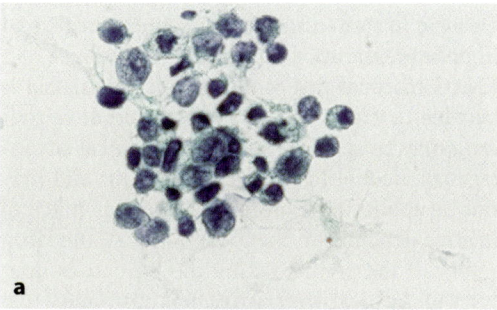

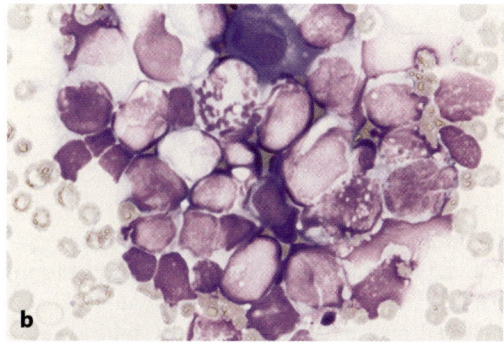

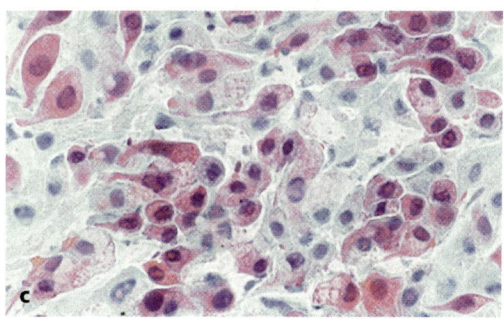

Fig. 2.14
a Alcohol-fixed cells from a small cell carcinoma (SCC) of the lung. Cells are small and show a crisp chromatin pattern. **b** The same cells prepared using the air-drying technique and stained with MGG stain. Cells are much larger and may show air drying artefact. **c** Bile duct epithelium showing the effects of delayed alcohol fixation. The cytoplasmic staining is uneven and the cell shapes are distorted.

2.6.2. Alcohol Fixation

Some laboratories prefer wet-fixed FNAC preparations. Alcohol or wet fixation may be achieved either by using a spray fixative or dipping the slides in 95% ethyl alcohol, to be followed by Pap stain. In either case, immediate fixation is crucial. Delay in fixation results in cellular distortion and in poor preservation of nuclear detail (Fig. 2.15). FNAC material that is not fixed immediately is best left to dry in the air so that alternative staining may be applied. The morphological advantages of alcohol fixation are subjective and may not be applicable to all materials. The choice of fixative depends on the local policy of the laboratory. If the person taking the aspirate is unaware of the local preferences, it is customary that some slides are alcohol fixed and some are air dried, thus enabling the advantages of each stain to be maximised.

2.6.3 Transport Medium

In order to avoid the technical issues associated with poor material preparation and fixation, particularly by inexperienced aspirators, FNAC material may be expelled directly into a transport medium (Cytolyt) and sent to a laboratory for further preparation to be handled as a fluid. Sediment may be fixed in CytoRich Red (TriPath Imaging, Burlington, North Carolina, USA) prior to centrufugation [75].

2.7 Staining Methods

2.7.1 Papanicolaou Staining

The Pap stain uses a standard nuclear stain, haematoxylin, and two cytoplasmic counterstains, OG-6 and EA [76, 77]. The outcome of this method is crisp nuclear detail and transparency of the cytoplasm, which allows the examiner to clearly visualise the cellular morphology (Fig. 2.15) [78, 79]. Either a progressive or regressive technique may be used for nuclear staining. Several automatic programmable stainers are available. Each laboratory must develop a written staining protocol for manual, automated, or for both methods, which results in the optimal staining of the specimen [80].

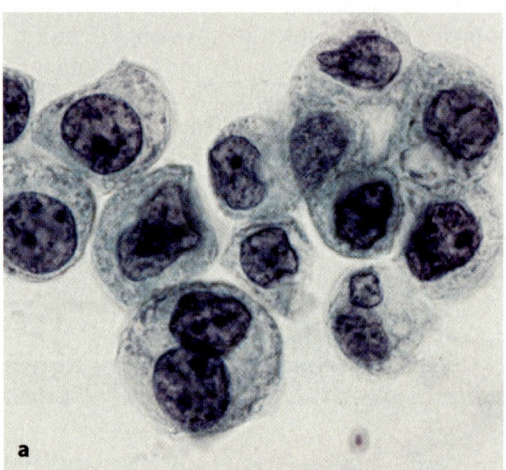

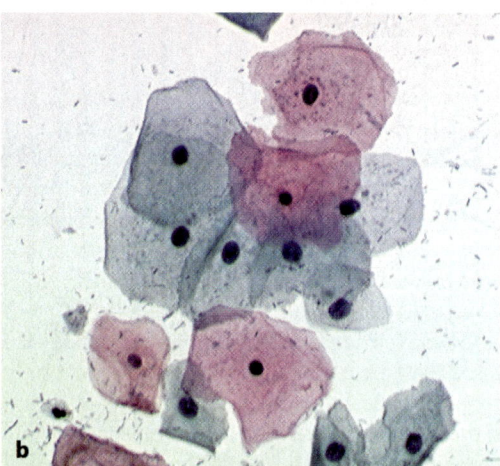

Fig. 2.15
a Cells from alveolar carcinoma are often difficult to differentiate from alveolar macrophages. The Papanicolaou (Pap) stain allows the study of nuclear and cytopalsmic detail to cofirm the diagnosis. b Pap staining of cervical epithelium shows delicate nuclear and cytoplasmic detail (Pap ×600)

In FNAC practice, the use of Pap vs. Romanowsky stains is subjective and depends on regional or local preferences. Most cytological books and atlases contain images of both stains. The analysis of false positive and false negative salivary gland FNAC samples shows the importance of using both a Romanowsky-type stain (Fig. 2.16) such as Diff-Quik (Mercedes Medical, Sarasota, Florida, USA) and the Pap stain when examining FNAC material from the salivary gland, because stromal components may be more readily identified on the Romanowsky stain (Fig. 2.17) [52].

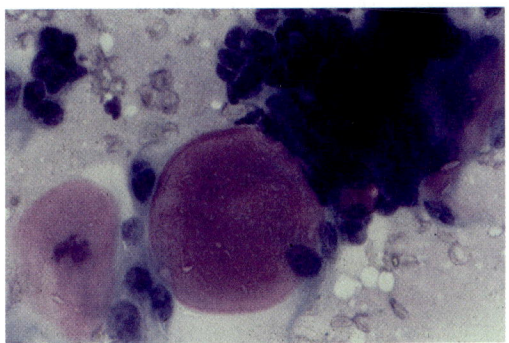

Fig. 2.16
FNAC breast. MGG staining of metachromatic globules seen in collagenous spherulosis (MGG x600)

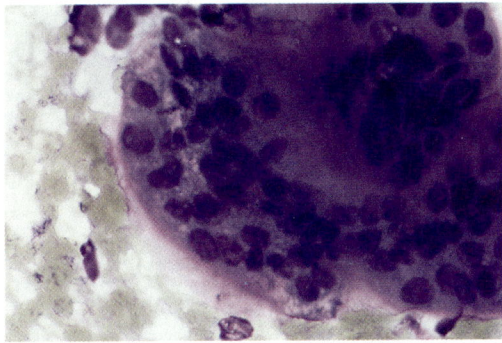

Fig. 2.17
FNAC of an epimyoepithelial carcinoma of the parotid gland shows a double cell layer and metachromatic stroma associated with cells (MGG x600)

Different options exist for preparing FNAC specimens. In order to compare direct smears and cytocentrifugation specimens, Crystal et al. prospectively obtained FNAC from 38 operative cases, making alcohol-fixed and air-dried direct smears and collecting additional passes in 50% ethanol, Saccomano's solution and Hanks' Balanced Salt Solution [81]. They evaluated cellularity, nuclear and cytoplasmic preservation, the percentage of single cells, background and the degree of three-dimensionality for each medium. Cellularity was significantly decreased for ethanol, Hanks' and Saccomano preparations as compared to alcohol-fixed direct smears. Nuclear preservation was best for alcohol-fixed direct smears. Background was best seen in direct alcohol and air-dried smears. There were no significant differences in cytoplasmic preservation and percent single cells. Direct smears made by cytotechnologists or pathologists are better than Cytospin specimens. However, despite their inherent disadvantages, rinse techniques may be advantageous when specimens are collected solely by clinicians [81].

A Pap stain, as fast as Diff-Quik yet with cytomorphology as exquisite as that processed by ThinPrep for the optimal evaluation of FNAC, was described by Yang [82, 83]. Satisfactory results were obtained after three modifications were made: (1) rehydration of air-dried smears with normal saline, (2) use of a 4% formaldehyde/65% ethanol fixative, (3) and use of Richard-Allan haematoxylin 2 and Cyto-stain. The first modification restored the transparency of the cells and haemolysed red blood cells, the second modification reduced the time needed for proper fixation and staining from minutes to seconds, and the third modification simplified the procedure. This 90-s protocol yields a transparent, polychromatic stain with crisp nuclear and cytoplasmic features. The cytomorphology processed by this protocol is superior to those processed by the standard Pap procedure [83]. A quick cytological diagnosis using the Ultrafast Papanicolaou stain (Richard Allan Scientific, Kalamazoo, Michigan, USA) has become useful, as are its modifications when the nucleus is stained with Gill-5 haematoxylin (modified Ultrafast stain) rather than with Richard-Allan haematoxylin 2 in Ultrafast stain [75, 84–86]. This preparation, which was originally designed for the immediate assessment of rapid FNAC preparations, can also be adapted for permanent slides [82]. It involves the addition of three simple steps prior to the conventional Pap procedure: the first step is to make the cells appear larger, thus increasing the resolution for analysis of cellular details; the second step is to haemolyse the background blood, thus unmasking tumour cells; the third step is to bring out the vibrant colours in the cells and the nucleoli, which stain red [82]. Other rapid Pap staining methods have been developed, such as the Shandon Rapid-Chrome Papanicolaou Staining Kit (Thermo Electron Corporation).

2.7.2 Romanowsky Staining

Romanowsky stains, mixtures of eosin and methylene blue, are a family of polychrome stains that achieve their effect by the production of azure dyes as a result of demethylation of thiazines and the acidic component, eosin [80]. Unlike the Pap stain they are metachromatic. Most Romanowsky stains used in cytology are aqueous stains as opposed to the methyl-alcohol-based stains of haematology. Many commercial stains are available, and most consist of a methanol-based fixative and two dyes, which result in the differentiation of cytoplasmic and nuclear components. Most Romanowsky stains are rapid and are useful in enhancing pleomorphism and distinguishing extracellular from intracytoplasmic material (Fig. 2.18).

Romanowsky stains are usually used for air-dried FNAC material [79]. Diff Quik is usually used for rapid staining and the assessment of material adequacy, whilst May Grünwald Giemsa MGG is used for traditional laboratory staining in making a final diagnosis. The advantages of the Romanowsky staining are in a good definition of the cell outline and cytoplasmic contents. Nuclear detail may also be seen, although it is more difficult to appreciate than in Pap staining (Figs. 2.19 and 2.20). The preference for either Romanowsky or Pap stains is subjective and largely depends on local practices and an individual's training. Both methods are widely accepted as valid, and trainee pathologists are expected to be proficient in interpreting FNAC material stained with either or both of the stains. Training should include learning about air-drying artefacts, which may cause distortion of nuclear and cytoplasmic detail and cause pitfalls in interpretation.

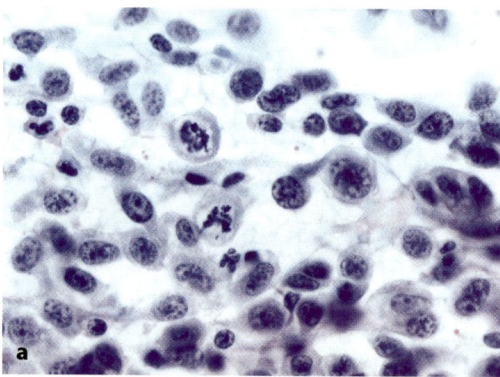

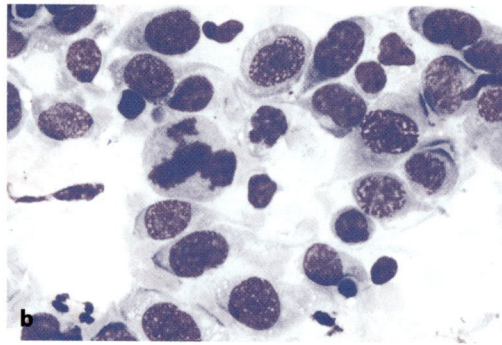

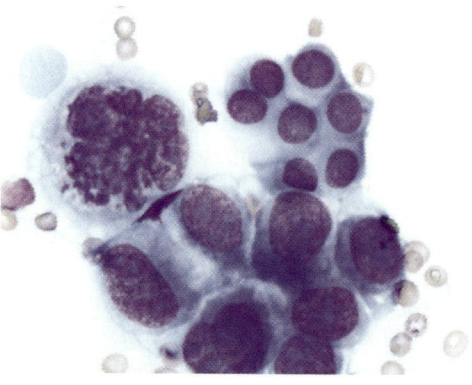

Fig. 2.18
Fluid containing metastatic adenocarcinoma cells stained with MGG stain shows nuclear and cytopalsmic detail well

Fig. 2.19
a Non-Hodgkin's lymphoma (NHL). Pap stain shows clear nuclear detail. **b** MGG stain shows better cytoplasmic detail

2.8 Ancillary Techniques

2.8.1 Cytochemistry

FNAC samples may on occasion need further special stains to be performed. These are the same as applied in histopathology and should be available in the routine laboratory. The most frequently used stains are periodic acid-Schiff (PAS) for detection of glycogen, PAS distase (PAS-d) and alcian blue for the detection of mucins, methenamine silver (Grocott) for the detection of fungi, Ziehl Nielsen stain for acid-fast bacilli and Perls for detection of haemosiderin (Figs. 2.21–2.24).

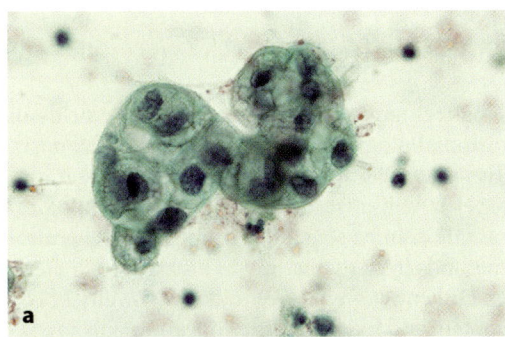
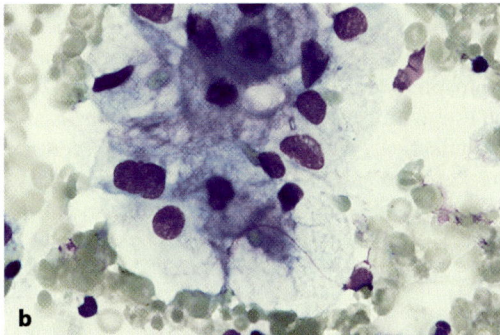

Fig. 2.20
a Pap stain of the fluid containing cells from a metastatic clear cell carcinoma of the kidney. Nuclear and cytoplasmic detail are clearly seen. **b** MGG stain of similar cells as shown in the Pap stain. Nuclear deatils is more difficult to appreciate

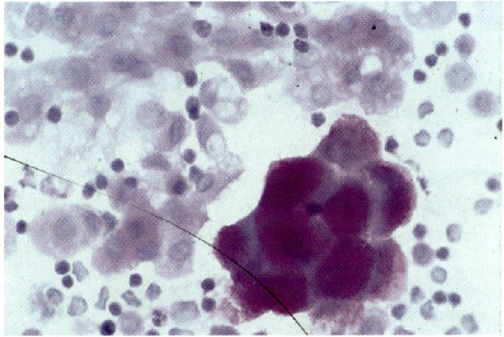

Fig. 2.21
Malignant cells from an adenocarcinoma stain postively with periodic acid-Schiff (PAS) diastase (PAS-d) staining, confirming the epithelial nature of the cells in the ascitic fluid (PAS-d x400)

2.7.3 Other Stains

Apart from the routine stains, it is possible to stain FNAC material differently. Toluidine Blue is sometimes used for the assessment of material adequacy but is not recommended as a definitive stain. Haematoxylin and Eosin, a largely histological stain, is sometimes applied to alcohol-fixed material. It is used particularly in centres that practice mainly histology so that it is easily available and familiar to the reporting pathologist. Difficulty may arise if such smears need further assessment or consultation with specialist cytopathologists because it is not considered as a cytological stain and the preparation may be rejected on the grounds of lack of familiarity with such staining in difficult cases.

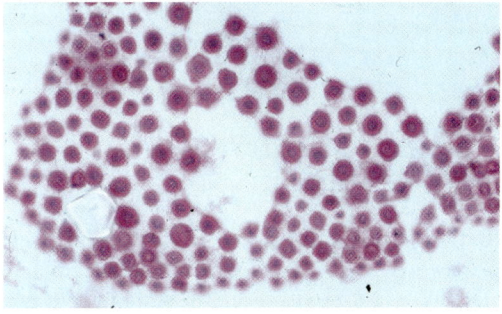

Fig. 2.22
PAS stain highlights cryptococcus in the cerebrospinal fluid of an immunocompromised patient (PAS x400)

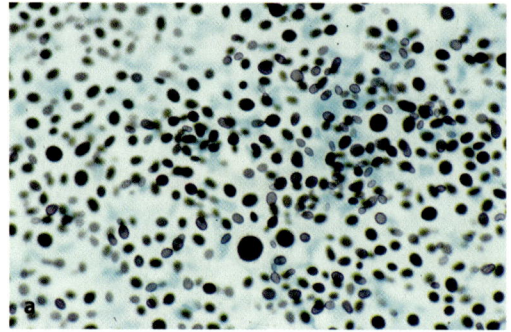

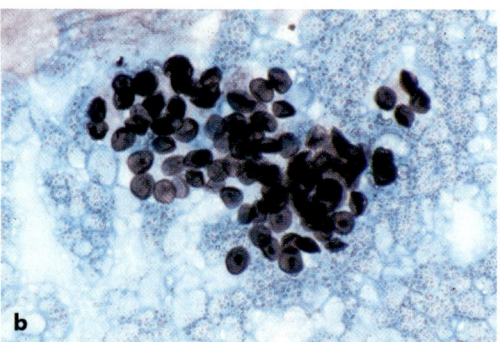

Fig. 2.23
Methenamine silver staining (Grocott) of a lymph node with cryptococcus infection in an HIV-positive patient

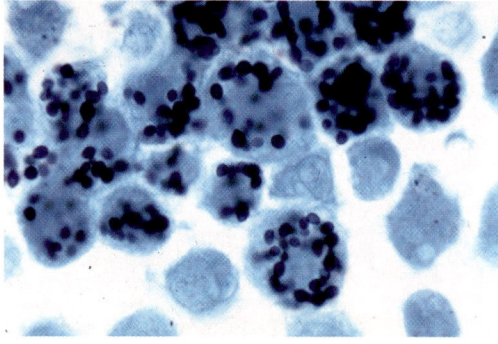

Fig. 2.24
Gomori staining to highlight the histoplasma in macrophages

Routine stains have in the last 2 decades been replaced in many cases with immunocytochemistry (see 2.8.2). However, the simplicity of use and low cost of some of the traditional cytochemical stains should encourage their continued use.

2.8.2 Immunocytochemistry

This technique has revolutionised the fields of histopathology and cytopathology diagnosis. The principle of antibodies staining target epitopes is very attractive and effective. Cytological samples can be stained by immunocytochemical methods in the same way as histological material. Difficulty often arises in the variability of cell content and fixation of the conventionally prepared cytological slides. The use of coated slides is helpful because it prevents washing off of the cell content during processing. Similarly, the use of Cytospin preparations is recommended because these are made with suspensions of cells and are effectively washouts of cells, thus preventing background staining. The choice of immunocytochemical signal may vary. Both alkaline phosphatase and peroxidase may be used successfully (Fig. 2.25).

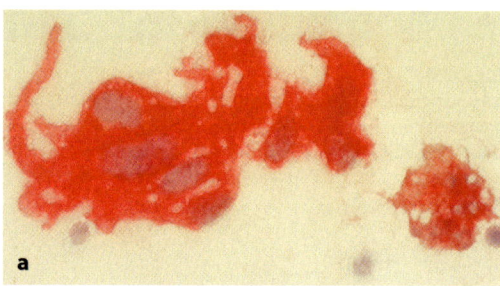

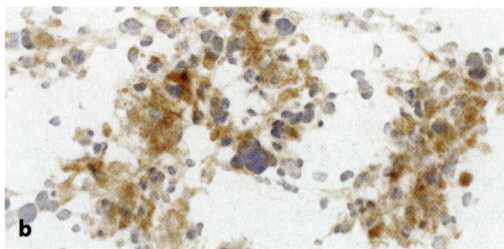

Fig. 2.25
a CD34 staining of cells from an angiosarcoma of the scalp confirming the vascular origin of the tumour. (immuno-alkaline phosphatase)
b FNAC neck. Chromogranin confirms the lesion to be a carotid body tumour (immuno peroxidase)

The more commonly used antibodies in FNAC preparations are various epithelial and stromal markers, lymphoproliferative markers, cell proliferation markers, specific viral markers and specific tumour markers (e.g. anti-prostate-specific antigen or anti-thyroglobulin; Figs. 2.26–2.28). MUC1 can be used as an ancillary marker for diagnosing pancreatic ductal carcinoma in cytological preparations [87]. Immunocytochemical study for anaplastic lymphoma kinase (ALK) protein, which provides useful prognostic information, can also be demonstrated satisfactorily using cytology samples (Figs. 2.29 and 2.30) [88].

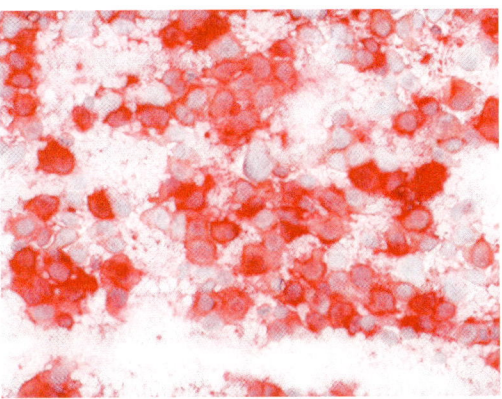

Fig. 2.28
Melanocyte-specific antigen (HMB 45) staining confirms the malignant cells to be from a melanoma

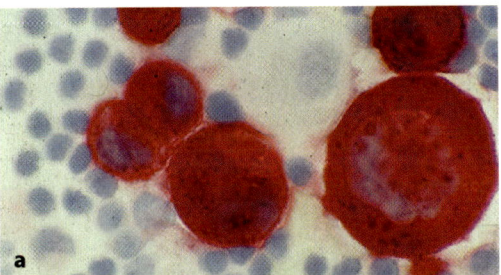

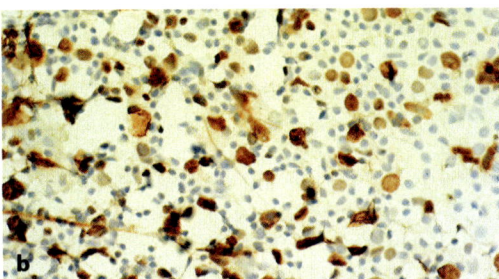

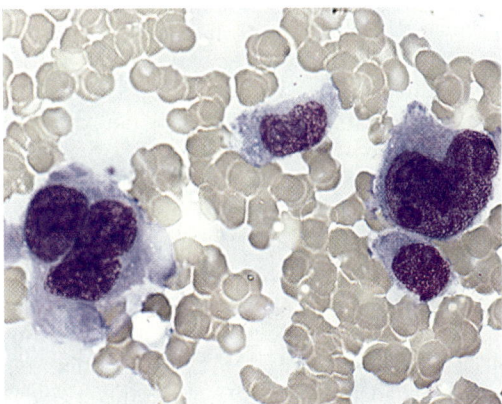

Fig. 2.29
FNAC of anaplastic, large-cell NHL (ALCL)

Fig. 2.26
a AUA1 staining of epithelial cells in the fluid. b MIB 1 proliferation marker in a lymph node aspirate

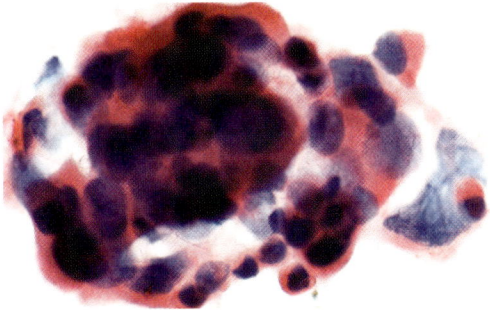

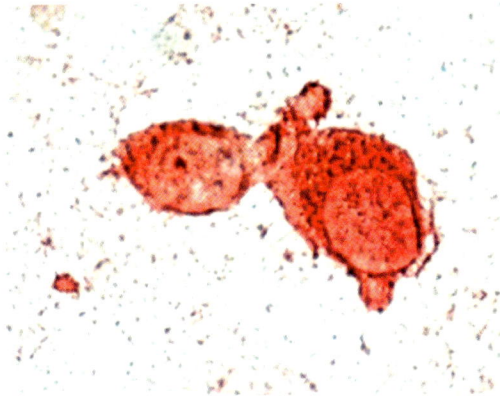

Fig. 2.27
Prostate-specific antigen staining of lung FNAC material confirms that the tumour is not a primary lesion but a metastasis from the prostate

Fig. 2.30
Anaplastic lymphoma kinase (ALK-1) staining of the ALCL shown in Fig. 2.28

2.8.3 Molecular Markers in Cytology

FNAC samples are suitable for several of the ancillary studies that are currently available, such as flow cytometry, polymerase chain reaction (PCR) fluorescence in situ hybridisation (FISH) and gene microarray analysis [89–95]. DNA cytometry has the potential to support the differential diagnosis of breast lesions, and sampling of free cells increases sensitivity. Cells from benign breast lesions (fibrocystic disease, fibroadenoma) include DNA-cytometrically abnormal cell clones and show a tendency toward polyploidy, characteristics that should be included in the diagnostic criteria [96].

FNAC samples often have variable and poor cellularity, but Howes et al. have developed a method involving the use of PCR and subsequent direct sequencing that enables analysis of the p53 gene from a relatively few malignant or suspicious cells in a background of normal cells [97]. DNA and protein analyses show that samples stored for periods of several months, either at room temperature, 4°C or −20°C, can be processed reliably. For RNA-based diagnosis, samples were still intact after 5 months of storage in PreservCyt (Cytyc, Boxborough, MA, USA) at 4°C. In addition, using FNAC material that was stored for 16 months at 4°C, Tisserand et al. detected p53 mutations with either a functional assay for separating alleles in yeast (an RNA-based functional assay) or direct cDNA sequencing. FNAC samples stored in PreservCyt at 4°C are very good material for molecular diagnosis techniques. In addition, it is feasible to adopt a strategy of storing excess FNAC material to create cellular banks that will be invaluable for future gene studies [98, 99].

Expression profiling of tumours from cancer patients has uncovered several genes that are critically important in the progression of a normal cell to an oncogenic phenotype. Leading the way in these discoveries is the use of a technology that is currently in transition from basic science applications to use in the clinic. Microarrays can determine the global gene regulation of an individual cancer, which may be useful in formulating an individualised therapy for the patient. Currently, cells used in breast cancer microarray studies often come from either homogenous cultures or heterogeneous biopsy samples. Both cell sources are at a disadvantage in determining the most accurate gene profile of cancer, which often consists of multiple subspecies of cancerous cells within a background of normal cells. Therefore, the acquisition of small, but highly specific biopsy samples for analysis may be required for an accurate expression analysis of the disease. Amplification methods, such as PCR and amplified antisense RNA amplification, have been used to amplify the mRNA signal from very small samples, which can then be used for microarray analysis. Glanzer and Eberwine describe the acquisition, amplification and analysis of very small samples (<10,000 cells) for expression analysis and demonstrate that the ultimate resolution of cancer expression analysis, one cell, is both feasible and practical [100]. When comparing the relative merits of FNAC vs. core biopsy samples for use in the genomic studies, Symmans et al. showed that both yield a similar quality and quantity of total RNA and are suitable for cDNA microarray analyses in approximately 70–75% of single-pass samples [101]. Transcriptional profiles from FNAC and core biopsy samples of the same tumour are generally similar. The authors concluded that each technique has relative advantages: FNAC provides transcriptional profiles that are a purer representation of the tumour cell population, whereas transcriptional profiles from core biopsy samples include more representation from non-lymphoid stromal elements. Selection of the preferred needle biopsy sampling technique for genomic studies of breast carcinomas should depend on whether variable stromal gene expression is desirable in the samples [101]. A comprehensive transcriptional profile made on FNAC material can reliably measure conventional single-gene prognostic markers such as oestrogen receptor (ER) and HER-2/neu. A complex pattern of genes (not including ER) can also be used to predict clinical ER status. FNAC-based diagnostic microarray tests may be developed that could not only capture conventional prognostic information, but may also contain additional clinical information that cannot currently be measured with other methods

[102]. cDNA microarray techniques may also be useful and applicable for the pre-operative FNAC diagnosis of salivary gland tumors [103]. There are numerous studies showing the potential of gene microarray analysis on FNAC of the breast [100–102, 104–126].

Ancillary techniques are particularly helpful in the diagnosis of lymphoproliferative diseases [127]. FNAC of lymph nodes is an adequate method for chromosomal analysis. The specific cytogenetic abnormality associated with cytological diagnosis provides an opportunity to make a definitive diagnosis [128]. With proper handling and management of specimens, FNAC can routinely provide samples that are adequate for molecular genetic studies, in addition to cytomorphology and flow cytometry, making it possible to consistently render accurate and definitive diagnoses in a subset of B-cell non-Hodgkin lymphomas (NHL). By incorporating the FISH and PCR methods, FNAC may assume an expanded role for the primary diagnosis of B-cell NHL [129, 130]. Salto Tellez et al. report the application of microsatellite analysis in cytological samples for detection of the origin of metastatic tumours [131].

Cytological specimens have been used successfully for genomic and proteomic studies. Such investigational studies are under way and offer great potential for revolutionising the prediction of patient outcomes and disease response to therapy, as well as assessment of the risk of developing breast cancer [132]. FISH remains the most objective and powerful technique for HER-2/neu assessment on breast cancer FNAC material [133]. Lymph node micrometastases can be detected by gene promoter hypermethylation in samples obtained by EUS-FNAC [134].

Real-time PCR assay using FNAC and tissue biopsy specimens can be used for the rapid diagnosis of mycobacterial lymphadenitis in children [135], and DNA amplification can be used for the diagnosis of cat-scratch disease in small-quantity clinical specimens [136].

2.9 Safety

The FNAC method is simple, painless and cost effective. In order for it to be safe both for the patient and for the aspirator, several rules need to be observed. The patient's safety is ensured by obtaining appropriate clinical history and conducting a thorough clinical examination prior to taking a sample. History of anticoagulation is a contraindication for FNAC. Lesions near or abutting onto large vessels need to be aspirated only by experts and only with a 25-gauge needle. Vessels should be approached tangentially to avoid penetration and haemorrhage. After every procedure, the cytology assistant is asked to apply pressure to the aspiration site for 1 min to avoid bruising and prevent haemorrhage. Very vascular organs like the thyroid should be aspirated with the needle pointing only in one direction, not in the fan-shaped manner usually practiced. Fewer passes may be advised in some instances where blood is drawn at the first pass. In case of liver cysts where hydatid disease is suspected, FNAC is usually not recommended in case of anaphylaxis (Fig. 2.31). The patient may be given specific instructions, for example not to swallow, breathe or talk during the FNAC procedure. In our experience, the pain associated with FNAC is more often triggered by its anticipation than the actual pain due to needle penetration. Sympathetic handling of the situation and provision of a clear explanation of the procedure in advance may relieve this type of pain. In the case of a needle-phobic patient or a child, an anaesthetic can be applied by means of a needle-free system that is commercially available (Fig. 2.32). Alternatively, anaesthetic cream can be applied following the manufacturer's instructions, usually 1 h prior to the FNAC procedure.

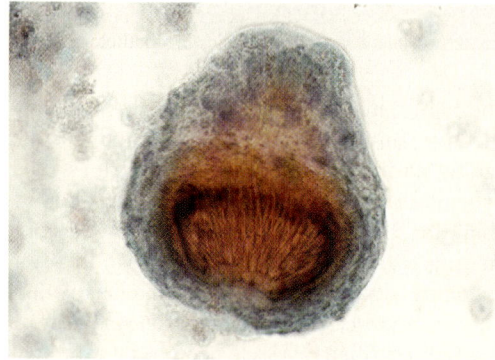

Fig. 2.31
Pap stain showing the clear structure of Echinoccocus granulosus parasite

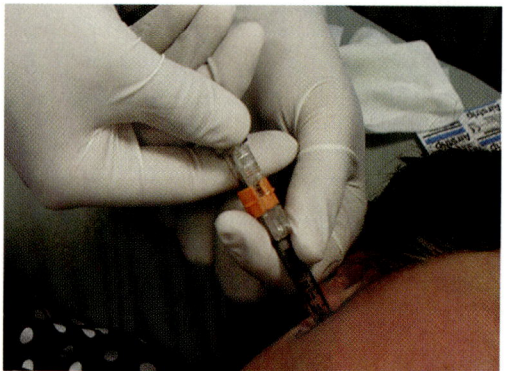

Fig. 2.32
FNAC clinic. A needle-free system is used to adminster anaesthetic in some cases

The aspirator's safety is achieved by following standard Health and Safety guidelines that apply to hospital and laboratory staff. Gloves and a mask should be worn when handling FNAC material. Since FNAC slide preparation is carried out on site, usually without the benefit of a safety cabinet, care is needed not to create aerosol spray when expelling the material. Similarly, the use of electric fans in the FNAC room is not advised. The examination tray should be cleaned with a commercially available surface cleaner after every patient. Only those instruments needed for individual FNAC procedures should be laid out in advance. The gloves used for patient examination and specimen preparation should be taken off when writing a report and using a microscope.

Needle-stick injuries of the aspirator are rare and need to be avoided. Re-sheathing of the used needle is one of the most common causes of needle stick injury and is therefore strictly forbidden. Needle needs to be disposed of safely immediately after the material is expelled from it and prior to specimen preparation in case the needle gets entangled amongst the glass slides causing a possible injury. If needle-stick injury occurs, this needs to be reported following the local Occupational Health policies. The United Kingdom Chief Medical Officer's Expert Advisory Group on AIDS now recommend use of combination antiretroviral therapy as prophylaxis following occupational exposure to HIV [137]. Post-exposure prophylaxis (PEP) should be started as soon as possible after the event, ideally within the first 1 or 2 h. For this to be achieved, many hospitals have PEP starter packs available, which are kept in easily accessible sites. Healthcare workers receiving PEP should have follow up counselling, post-exposure HIV testing and a medical evaluation [137]. They should also be monitored for any of the potential adverse effects of PEP. This follow up should be carried out by the local occupational health physician in liaison with a physician experienced in the use of antiretroviral therapy (usually a genitourinary physician).

References

1. Balicer RD, Fadlon J. The information age and its effect on the doctor-patient relationship. Harefuah 2004;143(10):749–52, 764
2. Feld AD. Informed consent: not just for procedures anymore. Am J Gastroenterol 2004;99(6):977–80
3. Kuczewski MG, Marshall P. The decision dynamics of clinical research: the context and process of informed consent. Med Care 2002;40(9 Suppl):V45–54
4. Cericola SA. Understanding informed consent. Plast Surg Nurs 1998;18(4):249–51
5. Gasparini G, Boniello R, Longobardi G, Pelo S. Orthognathic surgery: an informed consent model. J Craniofac Surg 2004;15(5):858–62
6. Pereira SP, Hussaini SH, Wilkinson ML. Informed consent for upper gastrointestinal endoscopy. Gut 1995;37(1):151–3

7. Pape T. Legal and ethical considerations of informed consent. AORN J 1997;65(6):1122–7
8. White CS, Mason AC, Feehan M, Templeton PA. Informed consent for percutaneous lung biopsy: comparison of two consent protocols based on patient recall after the procedure. AJR Am J Roentgenol 1995;165(5):1139–42
9. Plaut EA. The ethics of informed consent: an overview. Psychiatr J Univ Ott 1989;14(3):435–8
10. Newton-Howes PA, Bedford ND, Dobbs BR, Frizelle FA. Informed consent: what do patients want to know? N Z Med J 1998;111(1073):340–2
11. Mullenix PS, Carter PL, Martin MJ, Steele SR, Scott CL, Walts MJ, et al. Predictive value of intraoperative touch preparation analysis of sentinel lymph nodes for axillary metastasis in breast cancer. Am J Surg 2003;185(5):420–4
12. Perez-Moreno JA, Perez-Carceles MD, Osuna E, Luna A. Preoperative information and informed consent in surgically treated patients. Rev Esp Anestesiol Reanim 1998;45(4):130–5
13. Zardawi IM. Fine needle aspiration cytology in a rural setting. Acta Cytol 1998;42(4):899–906
14. Nasuti JF, Gupta PK, Baloch ZW. Diagnostic value and cost-effectiveness of on-site evaluation of fine-needle aspiration specimens: review of 5,688 cases. Diagn Cytopathol 2002;27(1):1–4
15. Lazda EJ, Kocjan G, Sams VR, Wotherspoon AC, Taylor I. Fine needle aspiration (FNA) cytology of the breast: the influence of unsatisfactory samples on patient management. Cytopathology 1996;7(4):262–7
16. Lee HC, Ooi PJ, Poh WT, Wong CY. Impact of inadequate fine-needle aspiration cytology on outcome of patients with palpable breast lesions. Aust N Z J Surg 2000;70(9):656–9
17. MacDonald L, Yazdi HM. Nondiagnostic fine needle aspiration biopsy of the thyroid gland: a diagnostic dilemma. Acta Cytol 1996;40(3):423–8
18. Robinson IA, Cozens NJ. Does a joint ultrasound guided cytology clinic optimize the cytological evaluation of head and neck masses? Clin Radiol 1999;54(5):312–6
19. Brown LA, Coghill SB. Fine needle aspiration cytology of the breast: factors affecting sensitivity. Cytopathology 1991;2(2):67–74
20. Hamill J, Campbell ID, Mayall F, Bartlett AS, Darlington A. Improved breast cytology results with near patient FNA diagnosis. Acta Cytol 2002;46(1):19–24
21. Kocjan G. Evaluation of the cost effectiveness of establishing a fine needle aspiration cytology clinic in a hospital out-patient department. Cytopathology 1991;2(1):13–8
22. Boerner S, Sneige N. Specimen adequacy and false-negative diagnosis rate in fine-needle aspirates of palpable breast masses. Cancer 1998;84(6):344–8
23. Brown LA, Coghill SB. Cost effectiveness of a fine needle aspiration clinic. Cytopathology 1992;3(5):275–80
24. Dray M, Mayall F, Darlington A. Improved fine needle aspiration (FNA) cytology results with a near patient diagnosis service for breast lesions. Cytopathology 2000;11(1):32–7
25. Lieu D. Fine-needle aspiration: technique and smear preparation. Am Fam Physician 1997;55(3):839–46, 853–4
26. Mayall F, Denford A, Chang B, Darlington A. Improved FNA cytology results with a near patient diagnosis service for non-breast lesions. J Clin Pathol 1998;51(7):541–4
27. Stanley MW. Cost benefit and outcomes analysis for fine-needle aspiration. Why do we know so little? Clin Lab Med 1999;19(4):773–81
28. Young NA, Mody DR, Davey DD. Misinterpretation of normal cellular elements in fine-needle aspiration biopsy specimens: observations from the College of American Pathologists Interlaboratory Comparison Program in Non-Gynecologic Cytopathology. Arch Pathol Lab Med 2002;126(6):670–5
29. Knappe M, Louw M, Gregor RT. Ultrasonography-guided fine-needle aspiration for the assessment of cervical metastases. Arch Otolaryngol Head Neck Surg 2000;126(9):1091–6
30. Sack MJ, Weber RS, Weinstein GS, Chalian AA, Nisenbaum HL, Yousem DM. Image-guided fine-needle aspiration of the head and neck: five years' experience. Arch Otolaryngol Head Neck Surg 1998;124(10):1155–61
31. Liao J, Davey DD, Warren G, Davis J, Moore AR, Samayoa LM. Ultrasound-guided fine-needle aspiration biopsy remains a valid approach in the evaluation of nonpalpable breast lesions. Diagn Cytopathol 2004;30(5):325–31
32. Karstrup S, Balslev E, Juul N, Eskildsen PC, Baumbach L. US-guided fine needle aspiration versus coarse needle biopsy of thyroid nodules. Eur J Ultrasound 2001;13(1):1–5
33. Selinko VL, Middleton LP, Dempsey PJ. Role of sonography in diagnosing and staging invasive lobular carcinoma. J Clin Ultrasound 2004;32(7):323–32
34. Knudsen DU, Nielsen SM, Hariri J, Christensen J, Kristensen S. Ultrasonographically guided fine-needle aspiration biopsy of intrathoracic tumors. Acta Radiol 1996;37(3 Pt 1):327–31
35. Byrne MF, Gerke H, Mitchell RM, Stiffler HL, McGrath K, Branch MS, et al. Yield of endoscopic ultrasound-guided fine-needle aspiration of bile duct lesions. Endoscopy 2004;36(8):715–9
36. Varadarajulu S, Hoffman BJ, Hawes RH, Eloubeidi MA. EUS-guided FNA of lung masses adjacent to or abutting the esophagus after unrevealing CT-guided biopsy or bronchoscopy. Gastrointest Endosc 2004;60(2):293–7

37. Erickson RA. EUS-guided FNA. Gastrointest Endosc 2004;60(2):267–79
38. Afify AM, al-Khafaji BM, Kim B, Scheiman JM. Endoscopic ultrasound-guided fine needle aspiration of the pancreas. Diagnostic utility and accuracy. Acta Cytol 2003;47(3):341–8
39. Agarwal B, Abu-Hamda E, Molke KL, Correa AM, Ho L. Endoscopic ultrasound-guided fine needle aspiration and multidetector spiral CT in the diagnosis of pancreatic cancer. Am J Gastroenterol 2004;99(5):844–50
40. Chen VK, Eloubeidi MA. Endoscopic ultrasound-guided fine needle aspiration is superior to lymph node echofeatures: a prospective evaluation of mediastinal and peri-intestinal lymphadenopathy. Am J Gastroenterol 2004;99(4):628–33
41. Frossard JL, Amouyal P, Amouyal G, Palazzo L, Amaris J, Soldan M, et al. Performance of endosonography-guided fine needle aspiration and biopsy in the diagnosis of pancreatic cystic lesions. Am J Gastroenterol 2003;98(7):1516–24
42. Jhala NC, Jhala D, Eltoum I, Vickers SM, Wilcox CM, Chhieng DC, et al. Endoscopic ultrasound-guided fine-needle aspiration biopsy: a powerful tool to obtain samples from small lesions. Cancer 2004;102(4):239–46
43. Weynand B, Deprez P. Endoscopic ultrasound guided fine needle aspiration in biliary and pancreatic diseases: pitfalls and performances. Acta Gastroenterol Belg 2004;67(3):294–300
44. Fabre M. Comment reussir une ponction a l'aiguille fine sous echoendoscopie digestive? Acta Endoscopica 2005;35:65–75
45. Ylagan LR, Edmundowicz S, Kasal K, Walsh D, Lu DW. Endoscopic ultrasound guided fine-needle aspiration cytology of pancreatic carcinoma: a 3-year experience and review of the literature. Cancer 2002;96(6):362–9
46. Layfield LJ, Bentz JS, Gopez EV. Immediate on-site interpretation of fine-needle aspiration smears: a cost and compensation analysis. Cancer 2001;93(5):319–22
47. Harewood GC, Wiersema LM, Halling AC, Keeney GL, Salamao DR, Wiersema MJ. Influence of EUS training and pathology interpretation on accuracy of EUS-guided fine needle aspiration of pancreatic masses. Gastrointest Endosc 2002;55(6):669–73
48. Arslan S, Yilmaz A, Bayramgurler B, Uzman O, Nver E, Akkaya E. CT- guided transthoracic fine needle aspiration of pulmonary lesions: accuracy and complications in 294 patients. Med Sci Monit 2002;8(7):CR493–7
49. Austin JH, Cohen MB. Value of having a cytopathologist present during percutaneous fine-needle aspiration biopsy of lung: report of 55 cancer patients and metaanalysis of the literature. AJR Am J Roentgenol 1993;160(1):175–7
50. Kucuk CU, Yilmaz A, Akkaya E. Computed tomography-guided transthoracic fine-needle aspiration in diagnosis of lung cancer: a comparison of single-pass needle and multiple-pass coaxial needle systems and the value of immediate cytological assessment. Respirology 2004;9(3):392–6
51. Padhani AR, Scott WW, Jr., Cheema M, Kearney D, Erozan YS. The value of immediate cytologic evaluation for needle aspiration lung biopsy. Invest Radiol 1997;32(8):453–8
52. Hughes JH, Volk EE, Wilbur DC. Pitfalls in salivary gland fine-needle aspiration cytology: lessons from the College of American Pathologists Interlaboratory Comparison Program in Nongynecologic Cytology. Arch Pathol Lab Med 2005;129(1):26–31
53. Snead DR, Vryenhoef P, Pinder SE, Evans A, Wilson AR, Blamey RW, et al. Routine audit of breast fine needle aspiration (FNA) cytology specimens and aspirator inadequate rates. Cytopathology 1997;8(4):236–47
54. Pennes DR, Naylor B, Rebner M. Fine needle aspiration biopsy of the breast. Influence of the number of passes and the sample size on the diagnostic yield. Acta Cytol 1990;34(5):673–6
55. Joseph L, Edwards JM, Nicholson CM, Pitt MA, Howat AJ. An audit of the accuracy of fine needle aspiration using a liquid-based cytology system in the setting of a rapid access breast clinic. Cytopathology 2002;13(6):343–9
56. NHS. Breast Screening Programme : Guidelines for Cytology procedures and reporting in breast cancer screening. NHS Publication 1992;22:18
57. Rubenchik I, Sneige N, Edeiken B, Samuels B, Fornage B. In search of specimen adequacy in fine-needle aspirates of nonpalpable breast lesions. Am J Clin Pathol 1997;108(1):13–8
58. Coghill SB, Brown LA. Why pathologists should take needle aspiration specimens. Cytopathology 1995;6(1):1–4
59. Hoda RS. Why pathologists should take needle aspiration specimens. Cytopathology 1995;6(6):419–20
60. Fessia L, Botta G, Arisio R, Verga M, Aimone V. Fine-needle aspiration of breast lesions: role and accuracy in a review of 7,495 cases. Diagn Cytopathol 1987;3(2):121–5
61. Howat AJ. Why pathologists should take needle aspiration specimens. Cytopathology 1995;6(6):419
62. Singh N RD, Berney M, Calaminici MT, Sheaff T, Wells A. Inadequate rates are lower when FNAC samples are taken by cytopathologists. Cytopathology 2003 Dec;14(6):327–31
63. Padel AF, Coghill SB, Powis SJ. Evidence that the sensitivity is increased and the inadequacy rate decreased when pathologists take aspirates for cytodiagnosis. Cytopathology 1993;4(3):161–5
64. Kamal MM, Arjune DG, Kulkarni HR. Comparative study of fine needle aspiration and fine needle capillary sampling of thyroid lesions. Acta Cytol 2002;46(1):30–4

65. CM K. Cytopreparatory techniques. In: Bibbo M (ed) Comprehensive Cytopathology 1991;Philadelphia: WB Saunders
66. Howat AJ, Armstrong GR, Briggs WA, Nicholson CM, Stewart DJ. Fine needle aspiration of palpable breast lumps: a 1-year audit using the Cytospin method. Cytopathology 1992;3(1):17–22
67. Cytic. Thin Prep Non Gyn FNA. http://www.thinprep.com/lab/lab_thinprep_nongyn_fna.shtml;ThinPrep Processor Operator's Manual. P/N 85489-002 Rev. G
68. TriPath Imaging I. http://www.tripathimaging.com/usproducts/surepath.htm CytoRich preservative
69. Bedard YC, Pollett AF. Breast fine-needle aspiration. A comparison of ThinPrep and conventional smears. Am J Clin Pathol 1999;111(4):523–7
70. TriPath Imaging I. Prep Stain System Operator's Manual. (Burlington, NC)
71. Cytic. System Operator's Manual. Cytic Corporation, Boxborough, MA, USA 1995
72. Cattoretti G. Preparation of cytospin from single cell suspension. Lab Protocols 2002:http://icg.cpmc.columbia.edu/cattoretti/Protocol/immunohistochemistry/CytospinPreparation.html
73. Zito FA, Gadaleta CD, Salvatore C, Filotico R, Labriola A, Marzullo A, et al. A modified cell block technique for fine needle aspiration cytology. Acta Cytol 1995;39(1):93–9
74. Rowe LR, Marshall CJ, Bentz JS. Cell block preparation as an adjunctive diagnostic technique in ThinPrep monolayer preparations: a case report. Diagn Cytopathol 2001;24(2):142–4
75. Yang GC, Papellas J, Wu HC, Waisman J. Application of Ultrafast Papanicolaou stain to body fluid cytology. Acta Cytol 2001;45(2):180–5
76. Papanicolaou G. A new procedure for staining vaginal smears. Science 1942;5:432
77. Street C. Papanicolaou Techniques in Exfoliative Cytology. In: Cawdry EV (ed) Laboratory Technique in Biology and Medicine, 3rd edn, Williams and Wilkins 1952:253
78. NHS. External Quality Assessment Scheme for the Evaluation of Papanicolaou Staining in Cervical Cytology. NHS CSP Handbook 2004;vesrion 1
79. Boon M. Routine cytologic staining procedures. In: Weid GL, Bibbo M, Keebler CM, Koss LG, Patten SM, Rosenthal DL (eds) Tutorials of Cytology, International Academy of Cytology, Chicago 1992
80. ASC CPC. Non Gynaecological Cytology Practice Guidelines. 2004;para III c
81. Crystal BS, Wang HH, Ducatman BS. Comparison of different preparation techniques for fine needle aspiration specimens. A semiquantitative and statistical analysis. Acta Cytol 1993;37(1):24–8
82. Yang GC. Ultrafast Papanicolaou stain is not limited to rapid assessments: application to permanent fine-needle aspiration smears. Diagn Cytopathol 1995;13(2):160–2
83. Yang GC, Alvarez, II. Ultrafast Papanicolaou stain. An alternative preparation for fine needle aspiration cytology. Acta Cytol 1995;39(1):55–60
84. Bandlish U, Kapoor K, Shukla S. Efficacy of a modified ultrafast Papanicolaou (UFP) stain for breast aspirates. J Indian Med Assoc 2004;102(6):309, 312, 326
85. Maruta J, Hashimoto H, Yamashita H, Noguchi S. Quick aspiration cytology for thyroid nodules by modified Ultrafast Papanicolaou staining. Diagn Cytopathol 2003;28(1):45–8
86. Zu Y, Gangi MD, Yang GC. Ultrafast Papanicolaou stain and cell-transfer technique enhance cytologic diagnosis of Hodgkin lymphoma. Diagn Cytopathol 2002;27(5):308–11
87. Chhieng DC, Benson E, Eltoum I, Eloubeidi MA, Jhala N, Jhala D, et al. MUC1 and MUC2 expression in pancreatic ductal carcinoma obtained by fine-needle aspiration. Cancer 2003;99(6):365–71
88. Ng WK, Ip P, Choy C, Collins RJ. Cytologic and immunocytochemical findings of anaplastic large cell lymphoma: analysis of ten fine-needle aspiration specimens over a 9-year period. Cancer 2003;99(1):33–43
89. Dong HY, Harris NL, Preffer FI, Pitman MB. Fine-needle aspiration biopsy in the diagnosis and classification of primary and recurrent lymphoma: a retrospective analysis of the utility of cytomorphology and flow cytometry. Mod Pathol 2001;14(5):472–81
90. Fiegl M, Haun M, Massoner A, Krugmann J, Muller-Holzner E, Hack R, et al. Combination of cytology, fluorescence in situ hybridization for aneuploidy, and reverse-transcriptase polymerase chain reaction for human mammaglobin/mammaglobin B expression improves diagnosis of malignant effusions. J Clin Oncol 2004;22(3):474–83
91. Gong JZ, Williams DC, Jr., Liu K, Jones C. Fine-needle aspiration in non-Hodgkin lymphoma: evaluation of cell size by cytomorphology and flow cytometry. Am J Clin Pathol 2002;117(6):880–8
92. Henrique RM, Sousa ME, Godinho MI, Costa I, Barbosa IL, Lopes CA. Immunophenotyping by flow cytometry of fine needle aspirates in the diagnosis of lymphoproliferative disorders: A retrospective study. J Clin Lab Anal 1999;13(5):224–8
93. Katz RL, Wojcik EM, el-Naggar AK, Ordonez NG, Johnston DA. Proliferation markers in non-Hodgkin's lymphoma. A comparative study between cytophotometric quantitation of Ki-67 and flow cytometric proliferation index on fine needle aspirates. Anal Quant Cytol Histol 1993;15(3):179–86
94. Lavarino C, Corletto V, Mezzelani A, Della Torre G, Bartoli C, Riva C, et al. Detection of TP53 mutation, loss of heterozygosity and DNA content in fine-needle aspirates of breast carcinoma. Br J Cancer 1998;77(1):125–30
95. Salto-Tellez M, Koay ES. Molecular diagnostic cytopathology: definitions, scope and clinical utility. Cytopathology 2004;15(5):252–5

96. Elzagheid A, Kuopio T, Collan Y. Implementation of DNA cytometric measurements in fine-needle aspiration biopsy diagnostics of breast disease. Cancer 2004;102(6):380–8
97. Howes GP, Stephenson J, Humphreys S. Sensitive and reliable PCR and sequencing used to detect p53 point mutations in fine needle aspirates of the breast. J Clin Pathol 1996;49(7):570–3
98. Tisserand P, Fouquet C, Marck V, Mallard C, Fabre M, Vielh P, et al. ThinPrep-processed fine-needle samples of breast are effective material for RNA- and DNA-based molecular diagnosis: application to p53 mutation analysis. Cancer 2003;99(4):223–32
99. Jeffers MD MJ, Farquharson MA, Stewart CJ, Mutch AF. Analysis of clonality in cytologic material using the polymerase chain reaction (PCR). Cytopathology 1997;8(2):114–21
100. Glanzer JG, Eberwine JH. Expression profiling of small cellular samples in cancer: less is more. Br J Cancer 2004;90(6):1111–4
101. Symmans WF, Ayers M, Clark EA, Stec J, Hess KR, Sneige N, et al. Total RNA yield and microarray gene expression profiles from fine-needle aspiration biopsy and core-needle biopsy samples of breast carcinoma. Cancer 2003;97(12):2960–71
102. Pusztai L, Ayers M, Stec J, Clark E, Hess K, Stivers D, et al. Gene expression profiles obtained from fine-needle aspirations of breast cancer reliably identify routine prognostic markers and reveal large-scale molecular differences between estrogen-negative and estrogen-positive tumors. Clin Cancer Res 2003;9(7):2406–15
103. Kainuma K, Katsuno S, Hashimoto S, Suzuki N, Oguchi T, Asamura K, et al. Identification of differentially expressed genes in salivary gland tumors with cDNA microarray. Auris Nasus Larynx 2004;31(3):261–8
104. Assersohn L, Gangi L, Zhao Y, Dowsett M, Simon R, Powles TJ, et al. The feasibility of using fine needle aspiration from primary breast cancers for cDNA microarray analyses. Clin Cancer Res 2002;8(3):794–801
105. Ayers M, Symmans WF, Stec J, Damokosh AI, Clark E, Hess K, et al. Gene expression profiles predict complete pathologic response to neoadjuvant paclitaxel and fluorouracil, doxorubicin, and cyclophosphamide chemotherapy in breast cancer. J Clin Oncol 2004;22(12):2284–93
106. Blancato J, Singh B, Liu A, Liao DJ, Dickson RB. Correlation of amplification and overexpression of the c-myc oncogene in high-grade breast cancer: FISH, in situ hybridisation and immunohistochemical analyses. Br J Cancer 2004;90(8):1612–9
107. Cleator S, Ashworth A. Molecular profiling of breast cancer: clinical implications. Br J Cancer 2004;90(6):1120–4
108. Dunmire V, Wu C, Symmans WF, Zhang W. Increased yield of total RNA from fine-needle aspirates for use in expression microarray analysis. Biotechniques 2002;33(4):890–2, 894, 896
109. Garber K. Genomic medicine. Gene expression tests foretell breast cancer's future. Science 2004;303(5665):1754–5
110. Glinsky GV, Higashiyama T, Glinskii AB. Classification of human breast cancer using gene expression profiling as a component of the survival predictor algorithm. Clin Cancer Res 2004;10(7):2272–83
111. Gong Y, Symmans WF, Krishnamurthy S, Patel S, Sneige N. Optimal fixation conditions for immunocytochemical analysis of estrogen receptor in cytologic specimens of breast carcinoma. Cancer 2004;102(1):34–40
112. Hampton T. Breast cancer gene chip study under way: can new technology help predict treatment success? JAMA 2004;291(24):2927–30
113. Hao X, Sun B, Hu L, Lahdesmaki H, Dunmire V, Feng Y, et al. Differential gene and protein expression in primary breast malignancies and their lymph node metastases as revealed by combined cDNA microarray and tissue microarray analysis. Cancer 2004;100(6):1110–22
114. Jeffrey SS, Fero MJ, Borresen-Dale AL, Botstein D. Expression array technology in the diagnosis and treatment of breast cancer. Mol Interv 2002;2(2):101–9
115. Miller DV, Leontovich AA, Lingle WL, Suman VJ, Mertens ML, Lillie J, et al. Utilizing Nottingham Prognostic Index in microarray gene expression profiling of breast carcinomas. Mod Pathol 2004;17(7):756–64
116. Nagahata T, Onda M, Emi M, Nagai H, Tsumagari K, Fujimoto T, et al. Expression profiling to predict postoperative prognosis for estrogen receptor-negative breast cancers by analysis of 25,344 genes on a cDNA microarray. Cancer Sci 2004;95(3):218–25
117. Roh MS, Hong SH, Jeong JS, Kwon HC, Kim MC, Cho SH, et al. Gene expression profiling of breast cancers with emphasis of beta-catenin regulation. J Korean Med Sci 2004;19(2):275–82
118. Ross JS, Linette GP, Stec J, Clark E, Ayers M, Leschly N, et al. Breast cancer biomarkers and molecular medicine: part II. Expert Rev Mol Diagn 2004;4(2):169–88
119. Wajapeyee N, Somasundaram K. Pharmacogenomics in breast cancer: current trends and future directions. Curr Opin Mol Ther 2004;6(3):296–301
120. Weigelt B, Verduijn P, Bosma AJ, Rutgers EJ, Peterse HL, van't Veer LJ. Detection of metastases in sentinel lymph nodes of breast cancer patients by multiple mRNA markers. Br J Cancer 2004;90(8):1531–7
121. Wu W, Chaudhuri S, Brickley DR, Pang D, Karrison T, Conzen SD. Microarray analysis reveals glucocorticoid-regulated survival genes that are associated with inhibition of apoptosis in breast epithelial cells. Cancer Res 2004;64(5):1757–64

122. Yu K, Lee CH, Tan PH, Hong GS, Wee SB, Wong CY, et al. A molecular signature of the Nottingham prognostic index in breast cancer. Cancer Res 2004;64(9):2962–8
123. Zhang DH, Salto-Tellez M, Chiu LL, Shen L, Koay ES. Tissue microarray study for classification of breast tumours. Ann Acad Med Singapore 2003;32(5 Suppl):S75–6
124. Zhang D, Salto-Tellez M, Do E, Putti TC, Koay ES. Evaluation of HER-2/neu oncogene status in breast tumors on tissue microarrays. Hum Pathol 2003;34(4):362–8
125. Zhang D, Salto-Tellez M, Putti TC, Do E, Koay ES. Reliability of tissue microarrays in detecting protein expression and gene amplification in breast cancer. Mod Pathol 2003;16(1):79–84
126. Zhao H, Langerod A, Ji Y, Nowels KW, Nesland JM, Tibshirani R, et al. Different gene expression patterns in invasive lobular and ductal carcinomas of the breast. Mol Biol Cell 2004;15(6):2523–36
127. Davis RE, Staudt LM. Molecular diagnosis of lymphoid malignancies by gene expression profiling. Curr Opin Hematol 2002;9(4):333–8
128. Borovecki A, Kardum-Skelin I, Sustercic D, Hitrec V, Lasan R, Jaksic B. Chromosomal abnormalities and DNA image cytometry of haematological neoplasms in fine needle aspirates of lymph nodes. Cytopathology 2003;14(6):320–6
129. Safley AM, Buckley PJ, Creager AJ, Dash RC, Dodd LG, Goodman BK, et al. The value of fluorescence in situ hybridization and polymerase chain reaction in the diagnosis of B-cell non-Hodgkin lymphoma by fine-needle aspiration. Arch Pathol Lab Med 2004;128(12):1395–403
130. Bentz JS, Rowe LR, Anderson SR, Gupta PK, McGrath CM. Rapid detection of the t(11;14) translocation in mantle cell lymphoma by interphase fluorescence in situ hybridization on archival cytopathologic material. Cancer 2004;102(2):124–31
131. Salto-Tellez M, Zhang D, Chiu LL, Wang SC, Nilsson B, Koay ES. Immunocytochemistry versus molecular fingerprinting of metastases. Cytopathology 2003;14(4):186–90
132. Sneige N. Utility of cytologic specimens in the evaluation of prognostic and predictive factors of breast cancer: current issues and future directions. Diagn Cytopathol 2004;30(3):158–65
133. Nizzoli R, Bozzetti C, Crafa P, Naldi N, Guazzi A, Di Blasio B, et al. Immunocytochemical evaluation of HER-2/neu on fine-needle aspirates from primary breast carcinomas. Diagn Cytopathol 2003;28(3):142–6
134. Pellise M, Castells A, Gines A, Agrelo R, Sole M, Castellvi-Bel S, et al. Detection of lymph node micrometastases by gene promoter hypermethylation in samples obtained by endosonography- guided fine-needle aspiration biopsy. Clin Cancer Res 2004;10(13):4444–9
135. Bruijnesteijn Van Coppenraet ES, Lindeboom JA, Prins JM, Peeters MF, Claas EC, Kuijper EJ. Real-time PCR assay using fine-needle aspirates and tissue biopsy specimens for rapid diagnosis of mycobacterial lymphadenitis in children. J Clin Microbiol 2004;42(6):2644–50
136. Avidor B, Varon M, Marmor S, Lifschitz-Mercer B, Kletter Y, Ephros M, et al. DNA amplification for the diagnosis of cat-scratch disease in small-quantity clinical specimens. Am J Clin Pathol 2001;115(6):900–9
137. www.doh.gov.uk/chcguid1.htm

Chapter 3

Diagnostic interpretation of FNAC material

Contents

3.1 Slide Background 35
3.1.1 Cystic Background 39
3.1.2 Inflammatory Background 40
3.1.3 Necrotic Background 42
3.1.4 Myxoid and Mucinous Background 42
3.1.5 Lymphoid Background 43
3.1.6 Other Background Features 43

3.2 Cell Arrangement 44
3.2.1 Clusters 46
3.2.2 Sheets 46
3.2.3 Single Cells 47
3.2.4 Papillary Arrangement 47
3.2.5 Other Features 48

3.3 Cellular Features: the Nucleus 49
3.3.1 Nuclear Size 50
3.3.2 Nuclear Shape 51
3.3.3 Position of the Nucleus 52
3.3.4 Chromatin Pattern 53
3.3.5 Number of Nuclei 54
3.3.6 Nucleoli 54
3.3.7 Mitoses 55

3.4 Cellular Features: Cytoplasm 55
3.4.1 Relative Amount 55
3.4.2 Quality and Contents 55
3.4.3 Shape and Definition 56

3.5 Criteria of Malignancy 57

3.6 Cytology Report 57

References 58

This chapter gives the reader an introduction into the diagnostic principles involved in microscopic interpretation in diagnostic cytology. There are several relevant factors, all of which need to be considered when interpreting the FNAC slide. At the training stage this is done systematically, and subsequently, after gaining experience, it becomes instinctive. The relative importance of different factors in the diagnostic process may vary. Most commonly, it is their combination that contributes to the final diagnosis. From the outset, one should learn to appreciate that everything in the slide is important. It is by careful observation and looking for particular details that a diagnosis will emerge. Dual pathology may be spotted and unexpected findings may be revealed. Cytologists need to be meticulous in their scrutiny of the slide and objective in its interpretation. This way pitfalls will be avoided and a correct diagnosis reached.

3.1 Slide Background

The background material in the FNAC microscope slide reflects the environment that the cells were in before they were aspirated. It may represent an integral part of the lesion or it may reflect secondary changes, for example degeneration, necrosis or inflammation, which may be equally important. Inexperienced observers who turn their attention to the cellular detail too quickly often underestimate the slide background. The background on its own rarely reveals the diagnosis, but very often leads to it, as is shown in the examples given here. Different preparation, fixation and staining techniques may cause the background to be variably appreciated (Fig. 3.1). Thus, in cases where a particular feature in the background may be important for diagnosis, it is useful to make sure that the preparation technique is optimal.

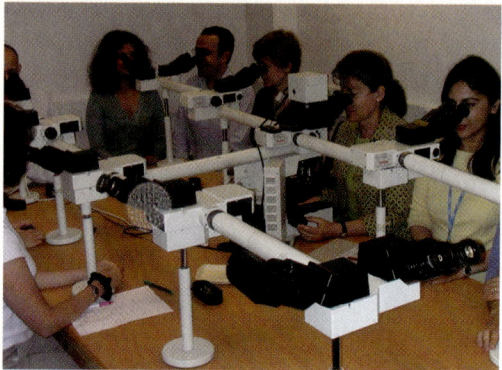

Fig. 3.1
Microscopic interpretation. Cytologists need to be meticulous in their scrutiny of the slide and objective in its interpretation. Shown here is a weekly discussion around the multi-head microscope, which contributes to cytology training

The slide background provides information about the origin of the sample and confirms that the sampled area is from the relevant anatomical site. For example, microcalcifications in the breast FNAC sample confirms that the sample is from the area of mammographic abnormality (Fig. 3.2). The background is often typical of certain conditions such as caseous necrosis in tuberculosis (TB; Fig. 3.3), mucinous in mucinous carcinoma of the breast (Figs. 3.4 and 3.5) or tigroid in seminoma testis (Fig. 3.6). The smear background sometimes provides clues beyond the cell morphology, for example the presence of psammoma bodies in papillary carcinoma of the thyroid (PTC), or serous adenocarcinoma of the ovary or meningioma (Figs. 3.7–3.9). The morphology as well as the amount of background material sometimes helps in the interpretation of cellular features. Inflammatory exudate in FNAC, for example, may serve as a safeguard against overestimating the cellular atypia associated with regenerative processes (Figs. 3.10 and 3.11). The presence of necrosis and cystic changes may provide clues as to the stage of disease, for example ductal carcinoma in situ of the breast (Fig. 3.12).

The composition of the cells in the background is sometimes as important as the main findings. The epithelium in lymphocytic thyroiditis not infrequently shows some cytological atypia associated with oncocytic change. Plasma cells and follicle centre cells in the background contribute to the diagnosis (Fig. 3.13). Medullary carcinoma of the breast has a prominent lymphoid cell population surrounding the epithelium (Fig. 3.14). The presence of colloid is often a very important factor in deciding the nature of thyroid lesions on FNAC. Abundant colloid is invariably associated with benign processes, whilst sparse or absent colloid suggests neoplasms (Fig. 3.15). Cellular and connective tissue elements in the background may contribute to a better definition of the lesion; fibroblasts, macrophages, endothelial cells or epithelioid cells all help to refine the diagnosis or point towards a narrower differential diagnosis (Fig. 3.16).

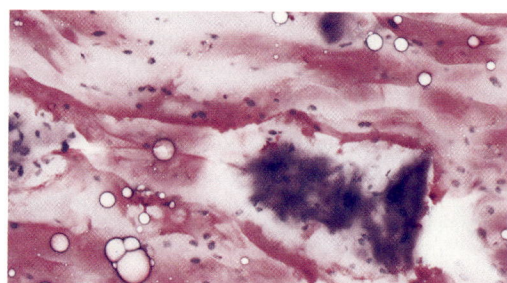

Fig. 3.2
Background. Fibrillary material in pleomorphic adenoma is almost diagnostic of this condition. It is better appreciated in air-dried, May Grünwald Giemsa (MGG)-stained smears

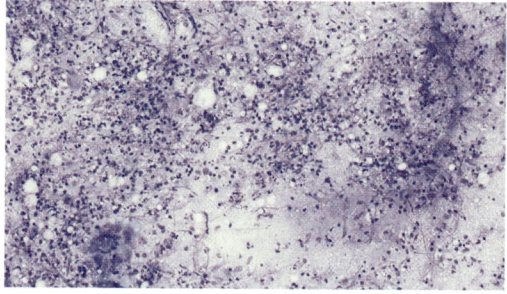

Fig. 3.3
Background. Caseous necrosis with inflammatory cells and epitheliod cells represents a background typical of mycobacterial infection in this case of lymph node FNAC

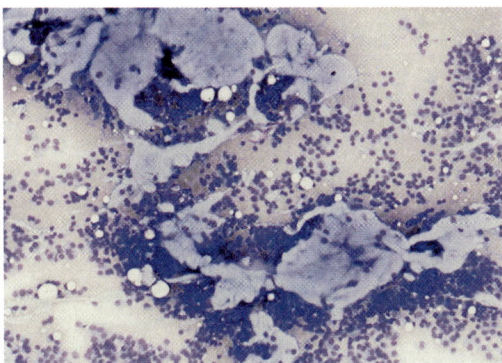

Fig. 3.4
Background. Mucinous background in mucinous carcinoma of the breast is often diagnostic of this lesion

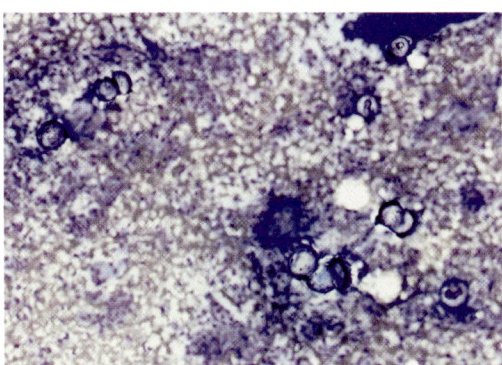

Fig. 3.7
Background. Psammoma bodies are a prominent features of the FNAC of meningioma

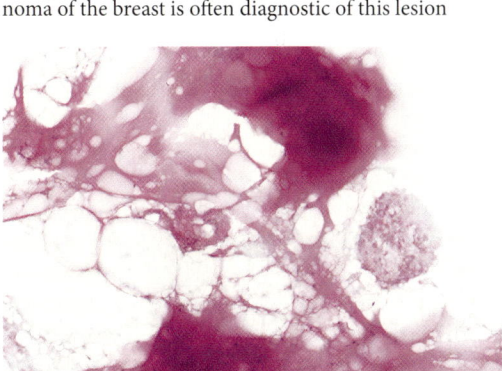

Fig. 3.5
Background. Same case as in Fig. 3.4. Mucinous carcinoma of the breast stained with PAS-d, shows prominent mucinous background

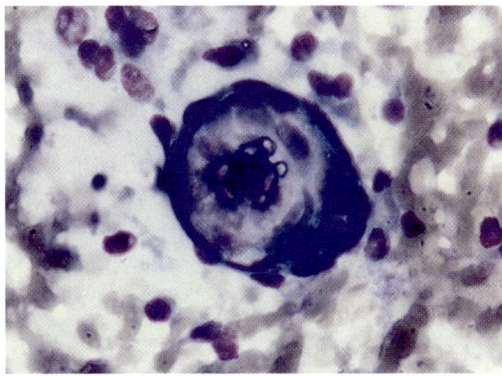

Fig. 3.8
Background. High-power view of the psammoma body shown in Fig. 3.7

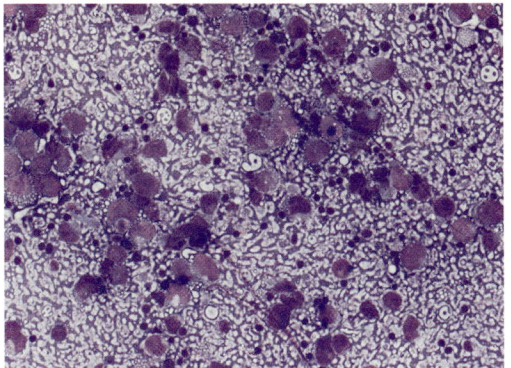

Fig. 3.6
Background. The tigroid background is typical of FNAC in testicular seminoma

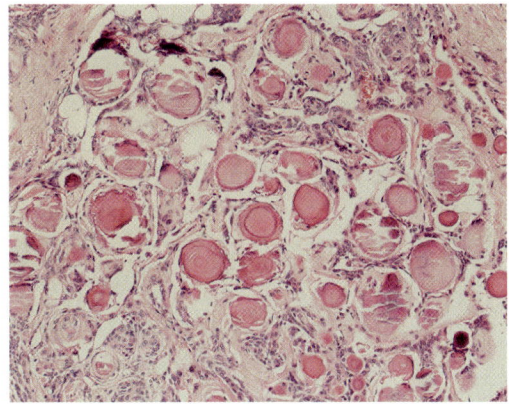

Fig. 3.9
Background. Meningioma with numerous psammoma bodies. Histology of the case shown in Figs. 3.8

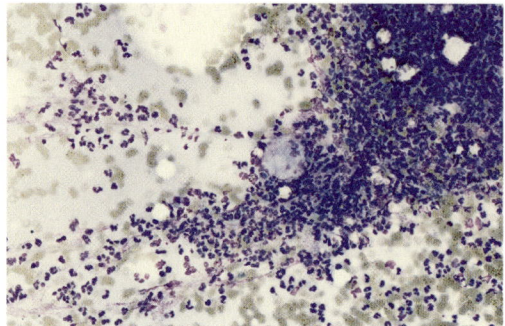

Fig. 3.10
Background. Inflammatory background with occasional flakes of keratin in a case of ruptured epidermoid cyst. Patient had a history of SqCC and metastasis was suspected

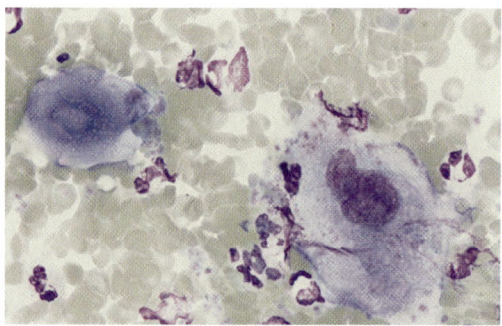

Fig. 3.11
Background. Same case as in Fig. 3.10. Atypical squamous cells may be misinterpreted as malignant if the background of the smear is not considered. This is a case of a ruptured epidermoid cyst

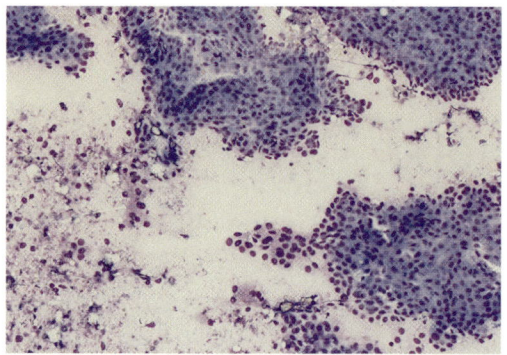

Fig. 3.12
Background necrosis. Necrotic background containing debris and macrophages is often found in cases of ductal carcinoma in situ of the breast, malignant cells floating in flat sheets

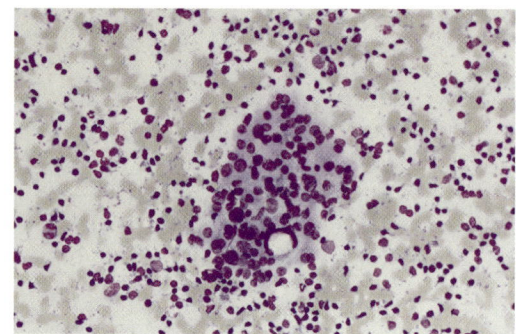

Fig. 3.13
Background. Epithelium in lymphocytic thyroiditis not infrequently shows some cytological atypia associated with oncocytic change. Plasma cells and follicle centre cells, seen in the background, contribute to the diagnosis

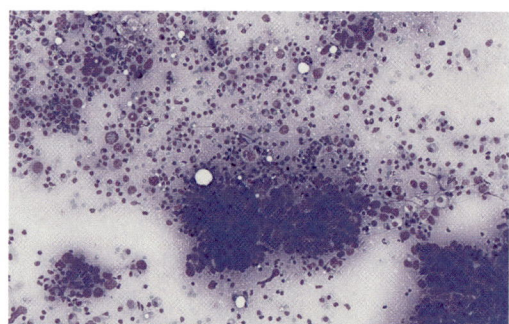

Fig. 3.14
Background lymphocytes. FNAC of medullary carcinoma of the breast contains a prominent lymphoid cell population in the background

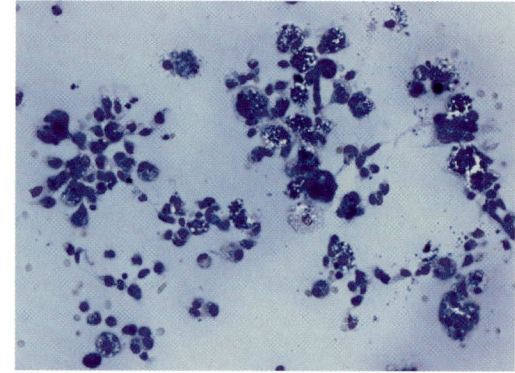

Fig. 3.15
Background colloid. FNAC thyroid shows abundance of colloid with haemosiderin-laden macrophages. The cell/colloid ratio is important in distinguishing between benign and malignant processes in the thyroid

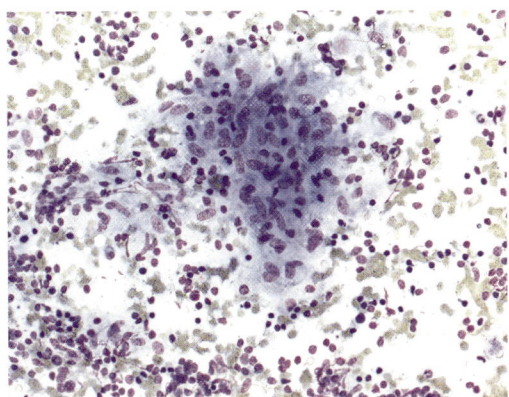

Fig. 3.16
Background. Epithelioid cells and lymphocytes in the background of this FNAC of the lymph node help refine the diagnosis or point towards a narrower differential diagnosis of granulomatous lymphadenitis

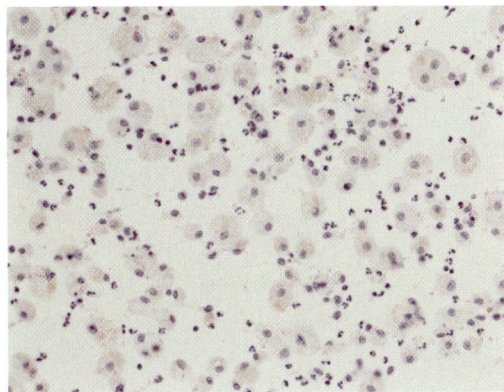

Fig. 3.17
Cystic background. FNAC of thyroglossal cyst shows numerous macrophages and inflammatory cells

3.1.1 Cystic Background

The cystic background refers to the fluid contents of the lesion presenting as a proteinaceous layer of variable thickness in which foamy macrophages and other cells may be present (Fig. 3.17). If there has been any bleeding, cholesterol crystals may be present. Fluid may be an integral part of the lesion, for example breast cysts, congenital cysts, odontogenic cysts or cystic tumours (e.g. Warthin's tumour or papillary cystic tumour of the pancreas), or it may be the result of degenerative changes within the lesion (e.g. cystic changes within fibroadenoma or benign nerve sheath tumour; Figs. 3.18 and 3.19). Cystic change is sometimes associated with necrosis and may be one of its manifestations in the FNAC slide (see 3.1.3). The differential diagnosis of various conditions that may show cystic change is discussed in Chap. 4.

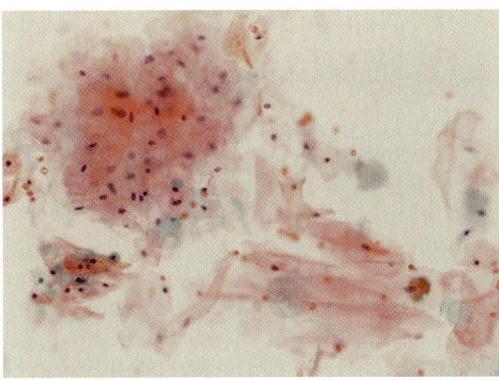

Fig. 3.18
Background. FNAC of an odontogenic keratocyst shows mature squamous epithelium, anucleate squamous cells and macrophages

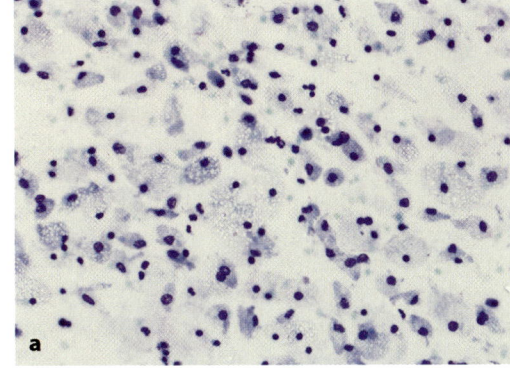

Fig. 3.19
Background. **a** FNA salivary gland shows numerous macrophages (MGG) **b** is following next page.

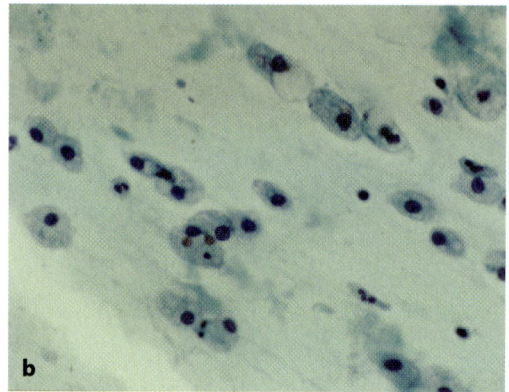

Fig. 3.19b
Macrophages in the background of mucin, typical of mucocoele.

3.1.2 Inflammatory Background

An inflammatory background may be representative of the main pathology or it may be secondary. Inflammatory exudates need to be assessed as to their predominant cell population: acute, chronic or mixed. Inflammatory lesions may have other components of the inflammatory reaction (e.g. suture granuloma or ruptured epidermoid cyst; Figs. 3.20 and 3.21). Inflammatory exudates may obscure cell detail and may explain changes seen in the surrounding epithelial cells. In the presence of inflammation, the diagnosis of malignancy has to be made with caution, for example EUS-FNAC of chronic pancreatitis vs. pancreatic carcinoma, or chronic sialadenitis vs. squamous cell carcinoma (SqCC; Fig. 3.22). Some tumours, like nasopharyngeal carcinoma, seminoma and thymoma, typically contain lymphoid cells (Fig. 3.23). Others, like acinic cell carcinoma (ACC), may occasionally contain an admixture of lymphoid cells. Lymphoid cells may represent an infiltration of a lymphoma in addition to the reactive cells, as in non-Hodgkin lymphoma in Hashimoto's thyroiditis. Acute inflammation and pus may explain a patient's symptoms of redness and tenderness, as seen with inflamed breast cyst/breast abscess or branchial cleft cyst (Fig. 3.24). Inflammatory cells in odd sites, like leukaemic infiltrates of the skin, need to be examined in detail to avoid pitfalls (Fig. 3.25). Specific inflammations, such as that associated with mycobacterial infection, contain epithelioid cells and giant cells in addition to the chronic inflammatory exudate (Fig. 3.26). With the help of special stains, specific organisms may be found in the inflammatory exudates. If receiving antiretroviral therapy, patients with HIV infection may have an altered immune response to infection and their FNAC aspirate may contain unusual inflammatory exudates (Fig. 3.27).

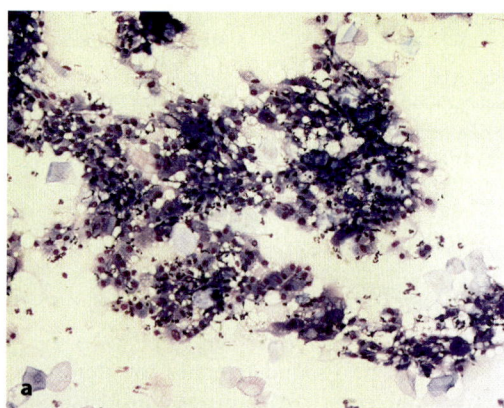

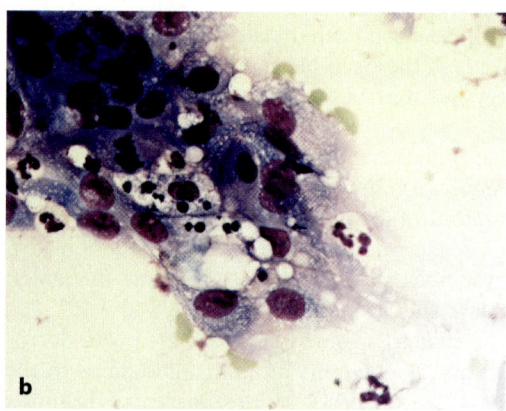

Fig. 3.20
Background. FNAC subcutaneous inguinal nodule in a patient with a history of transitional carcinoma of the bladder. **a** Macrophages and anucleate squamous cells reveal that the lesion is a ruptured epidermoid cyst. **b** High-power view revealing macrophages and inflammatory cells admixed with squamous cells

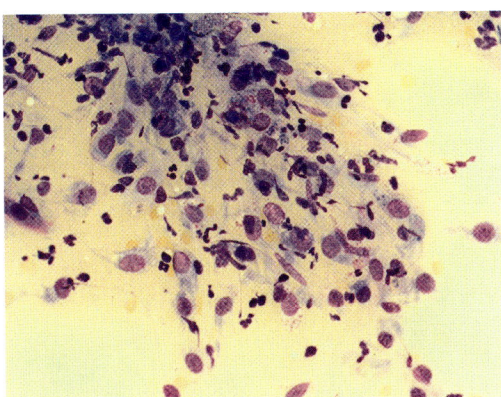

Fig. 3.21
Background. FNAC of the tooth granuloma shows granulation tissue cells: fibroblasts, hitiocytes, endothelial cells and inflammatory cells

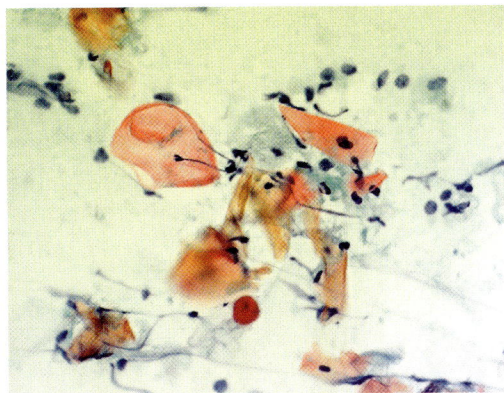

Fig. 3.24
Background. FNAC of an inflamed branchial cleft cyst shows polymorphs and benign squamous epithelium

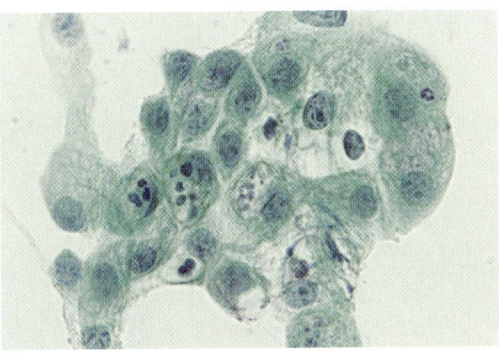

Fig. 3.22
Background. FNAC pancreas. Inflammatory cells within the epithelium may account for the regenerative changes with prominent nucleoli

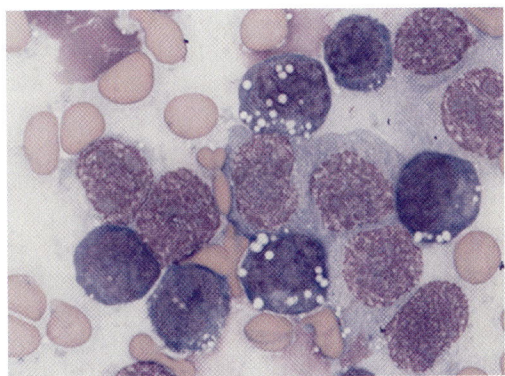

Fig. 3.25
Background. Cells from an NHL dominate the background

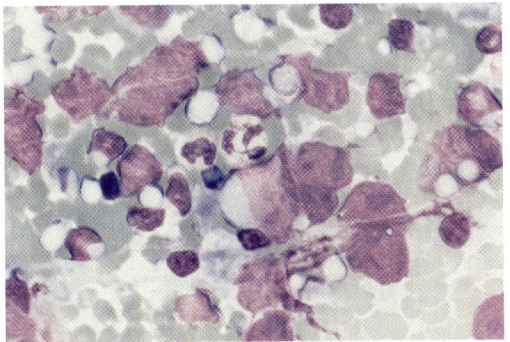

Fig. 3.23
Background. FNAC neck mass shows features of nasopharyngeal carcinoma. Some tumours typically contain lymphoid cells in the background

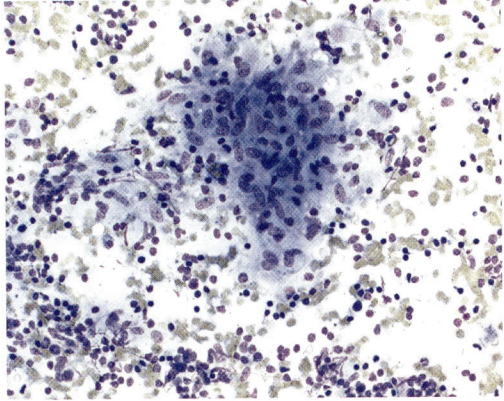

Fig. 3.26
Inflammatory background. Cluster of epitheliod cells suggests granulomatous inflammation

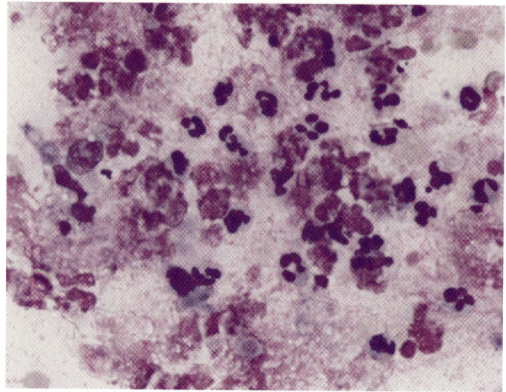

Fig. 3.27
Inflammatory background. FNAC of the neck node. Patients with HIV infection, if receiving antiretrovral therapy, may have an altered immune response to infection and contain unusual inflammatory exudates, as shown here in a patient with tuberculosis (see Fig. 3.29)

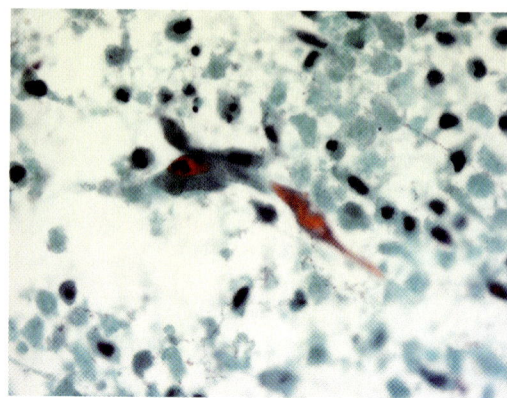

Fig. 3.28
Background. Inflammatory debris, stain deposit, crushed cells and other artefacts are not to be confused with necrosis. A necrotic background may sometimes obscure cells that are still viable. This is a case of SqCC cells that are barely visible amongst the debris and necrosis

3.1.3 Necrotic Background

A necrotic background represents evidence of cell death and is therefore always significant. It may be part of an inflammatory process (e.g. TB) or may accompany a neoplasm (e.g. SqCC). Inflammatory debris, stain deposit, crushed cells and other artefacts are not to be confused with necrosis. A necrotic background may sometimes obscure cells that are still viable (Fig. 3.28). It is important to make a note of this in the report rather than consider the sample insufficient for diagnosis. In the case of an abscess or caseous necrosis in TB, a necrotic background may be all that is seen on the slide. Special stains like the Ziehl Nielsen stain for acid-fast bacilli may be helpful in these cases (Fig. 3.29).

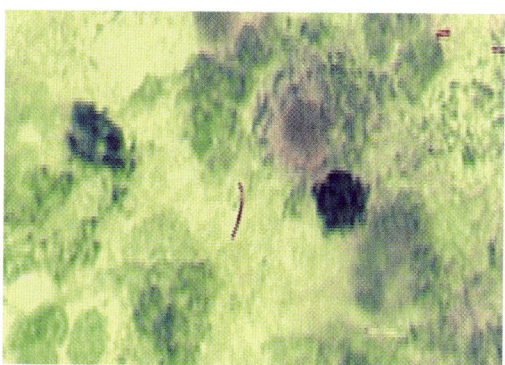

Fig. 3.29
Background. HIV-positive patient with an inflammatory background in which Ziehl Nielson staining reveals acid-fast bacilli

3.1.4 Myxoid and Mucinous Background

Myxoid and mucinous backgrounds are seen as by-products of some tumours or as a reflection of degenerative changes within tumours (e.g. pleomorphic adenoma, mucinous adenocarcinoma, mucoepidermoid carcinoma; Figs. 3.30 and 3.31). Special stains such as PAS-d can confirm the presence of mucin and thus its epithelial origin (Fig. 3.5). (see chapter 8.3 and 9.4)

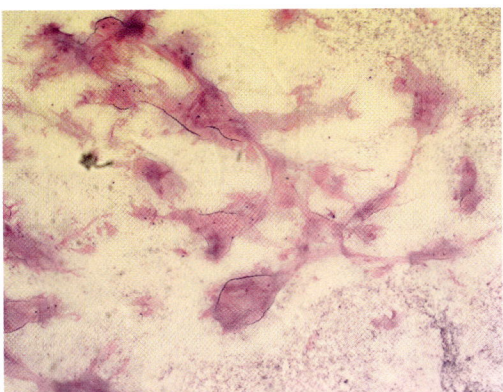

Fig. 3.30
Background. Mucinous background in an FNAC smear from mucinous cystadenoma of the pancreas. Epithelium is sparse (see Fig. 3.31)

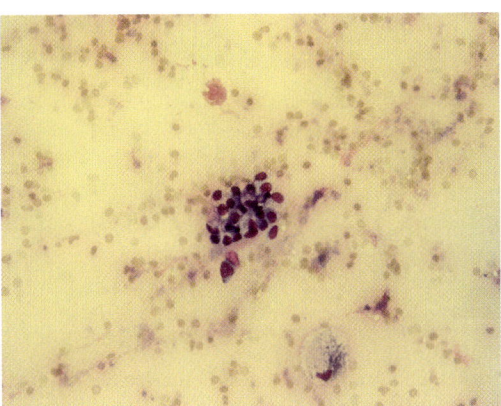

Fig. 3.31
Background. Mucinous. Epithelial cells in the FNAC of mucinous cystadenoma of pancreas are sparse and would not be sufficient for the diagnosis if the background was not mucinous

In some cases it is the lymphoid cells that define the entity and make allowance for the sometimes considerable epithelial atypia of, for example, Ashkenazy cells in Hashimoto's thyroiditis (Fig. 3.33).

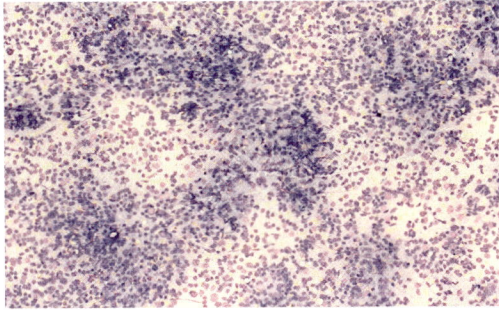

Fig. 3.32
Background. Lymphoid. Lymphoid background in the FNAC of a lymph node in the case of a low grade B-cell NHL (follicular). Further investigations are necessary to confirm the nature of the lymphoid cells

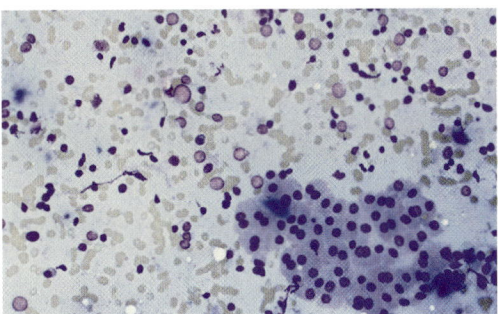

Fig. 3.33
Cytoplasm with apocrine changes. FNAC of lymphocytic thyroiditis shows lymphoid cells in the background and flat sheets of follicular epithelium showing apocrine changes

3.1.5 Lymphoid Background

Lymphoid cells usually represent a chronic inflammatory exudate or a lymphoma (Fig. 3.32). However, lymphoid cells in the background is a feature in some conditions, for example Warthin's tumour or seminoma (Fig. 3.6), nasopharyngeal carcinoma (Fig. 3.23), medullary carcinoma (Fig. 3.14), a variant of ACC, and others. In these cases, lymphoid cells may help define the entity.

3.1.6 Other Background Features

Colloid, various globules of material of stromal origin, for example collagenous spherulosis (Fig. 3.34), adenoid cystic carcinoma (Fig. 3.35), psammoma bodies (as found in, for example serous adenocarcinoma of the ovary, papillary thyroid carcinoma (PTC) and meningioma; Figs. 3.7–3.9), keratinous debris (e.g. epidermoid cyst;

Fig. 3.36), cartilage and soft-tissue fragments (Fig. 3.37) are all important in making the diagnosis and should be noted in the report.

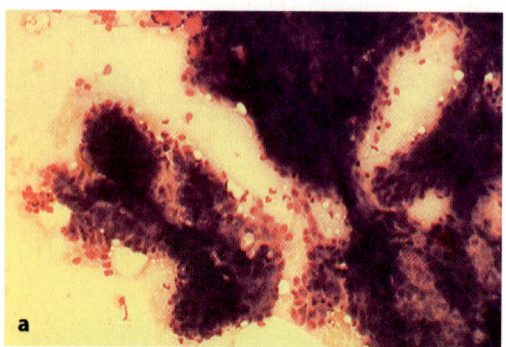

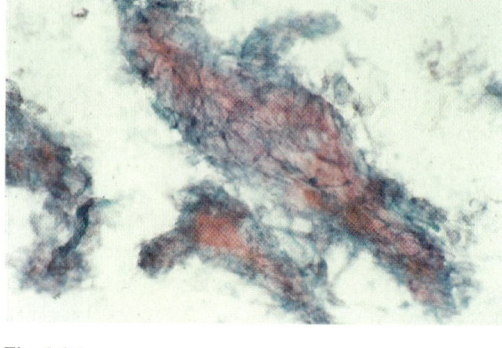

Fig. 3.36
Background. Keratinous debris in a case of epidermoid cyst of the neck. Patient had a history of surgical excision of neuroblastoma in this site

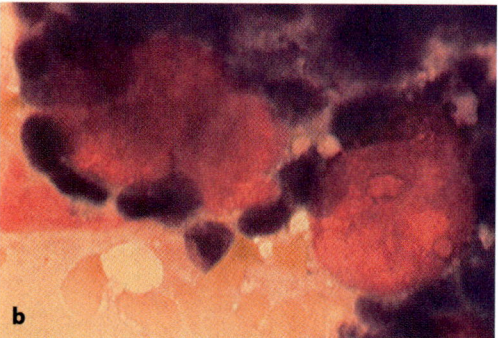

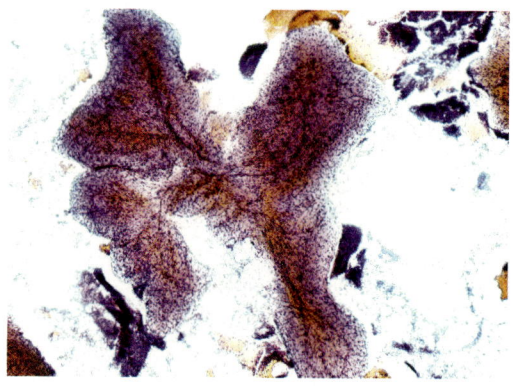

Fig. 3.34
Background. **a** Cellular preparation of breast epithelium with occasional pink globules. The epithelium may show marked proliferative changes. **b** High-power view of collagenous spherules in the FNAC breast, found in some cases of benign breast change, not to be confused with rare cases of adenoid cystic carcinoma of the breast

Fig. 3.37
Background. Stromal fragments in the shape of leaves may sometimes be seen in breast FNAC, suggesting a phyllodes tumour

3.2 Cell Arrangement

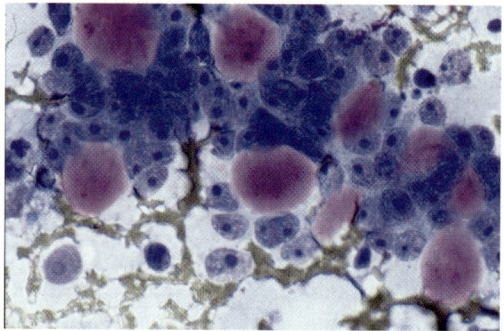

Fig. 3.35
Background. Eosinophillic globules surrounded by epithelium in a case of adenoid cystic carcinoma of the salivary gland

Although cytology relies primarily on the morphology of individual cells and not on the architectural features seen in histopathology, cell arrangement is almost equally important in some instances and reveals the microarchitecture the cells find themselves in (Fig. 3.38). At the same time, cell arrangement is the first impression the observer gets of the cytological preparation and as such is very important. The majority of the aspirated cells present themselves either singly or in aggregates (Fig. 3.39). The arrangement of the cells may be a first indication of their nature and origin (i.e. whether they are native to the site or alien, for example metastasis within a lymph node aspirate). Cell arrangement also reflects the relationships between different cells in the smear; overlapping and crowding, for example, may be a first indication of pathological behaviour in pancreatic FNAC (Fig. 3.40). Some cell arrangements are particular to certain tumours; the papillary arrangement is almost pathognomonic of papillary carcinomas in various sites, whereas others (e.g. acinar arrangements) usually indicate glandular differentiation (i.e. adenocarcinoma). The cell arrangement may reflect cell differentiation (e.g. keratinous pearls) or help to distinguish between malignant tumours of similar appearance (e.g. high-grade NHL and carcinoma). However, cell aggregates may sometimes be misleading if the cell morphology is not studied in detail (Figs. 3.41 and 3.42). The following are descriptions of some of the more commonly encountered types of cell arrangement.

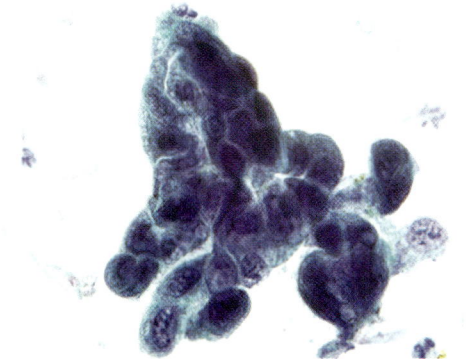

Fig. 3.40
Cell arrangement reflects the relationships between the different cells in the smear;. overlapping and crowding, for example, may be a first indication of pathological behaviour in pancreatic FNAC. The cells are from an adenocarcinoma of the pancreas

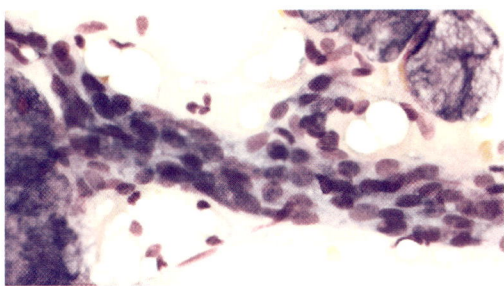

Fig. 3.38
Cell arrangement. FNAC of the normal salivary gland shows microarchitectural features of ductal epithelium surrounded by clusters of acinar epithelium

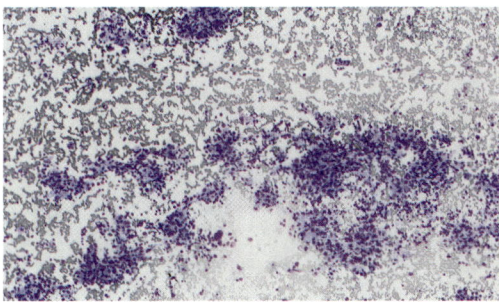

Fig. 3.41
Cell arrangement. Pseudoaggregates of cells in a case of diffuse large B-cell lymphoma (DLBL) may mislead the observer into thinking that this may be an epithelial lesion

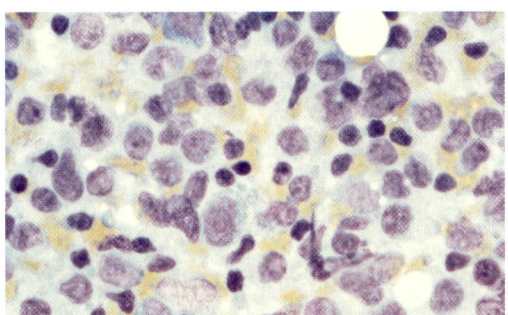

Fig. 3.39
Cell arrangement. Single cells in a case of NHL (follicular type)

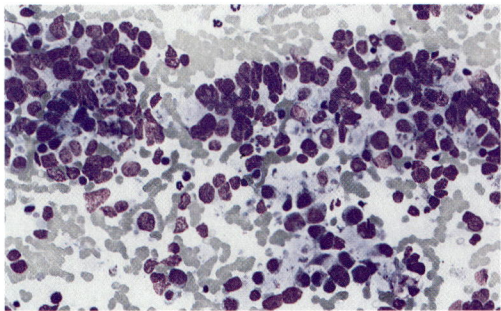

Fig. 3.42
High power of the case shown in Fig. 3.41 demonstrating that the pseudoaggregates are composed of a polymorphic population of cells, proved to be from a high-grade lymphoma

3.2.1 Clusters

Clusters is a generic term for cell aggregates seen with the aid of a microscope under low or medium power giving the first indication of the type of cell arrangement that is encountered (e.g. metastatic deposits in a sentinel lymph node; Fig. 3.43). Clusters are usually a feature of epithelial cells and are formed as a result of the cell adhesion mechanisms. However, cells from stromal tissues and some other tumours may also be arranged in clusters. Clusters are usually three dimensional, making it difficult to visualise the cells in the middle of the cluster (Fig. 3.44).

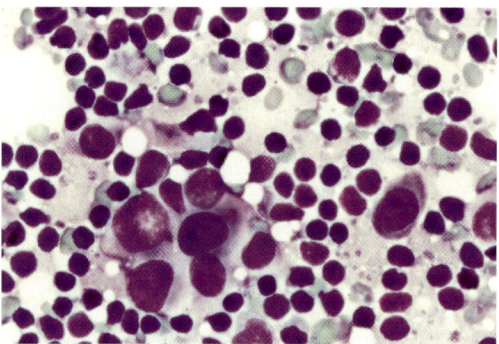

Fig. 3.43
Cell arrangement. Clusters is a generic term for cell aggregates seen under the microscope under the low or medium power giving the first indication of the type of cell arrangement that is encountered, in this case a metastatic deposit of a breast carcinoma in a sentinel lymph node

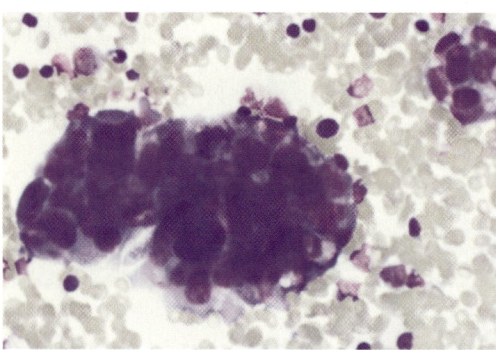

Fig. 3.44
Cell arrangement. Three-dimensional papillary clusters are typical of metastatic ovarian carcinoma in ascitic fluid

3.2.2 Sheets

Flat aggregates of cells are usually referred to as sheets. They are seen most commonly among epithelial cells. Because they are in a monolayer it is easier to appreciate both their architectural and cytological features (e.g. overlapping, crowding, anisonucleosis, mitotic figures; Fig. 3.45). Sheets of uniform cells are usually a reassuring sign of a benign lesion, although the whole slide should be examined before this feature is assumed to be dominant (e.g. fibroadenoma and ductal carcinoma in situ; Figs. 3.12 and 3.46).

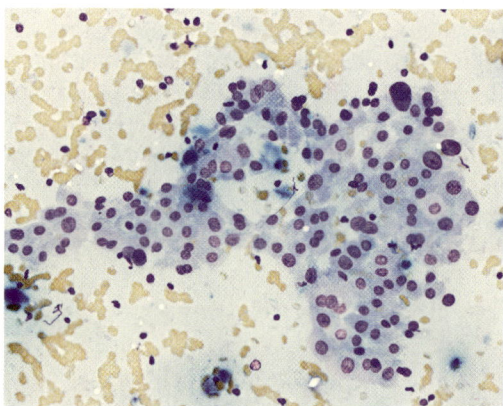

Fig. 3.45
Cell arrangement. Flat sheet of oncocytic type epithelium in a case of lymphocytic thyroiditis

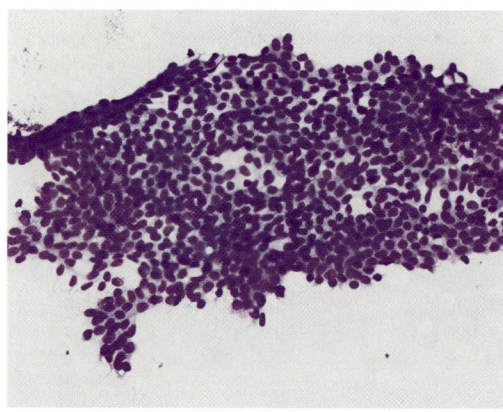

Fig. 3.46
Cell arrangement. FNAC breast shows ductal epithelium in flat sheets, typical of benign disease, in this case a fibroadenoma

3.2.3 Single Cells

Single cells in the slide may be due either to the nature of the lesion or to artificial separation as a result of the mode of cell preparation. Blood and haemopoietic cells usually appear singly in both benign and malignant conditions. Epithelial cells from benign conditions usually present in aggregates, either sheets or clusters. However, tumour cells from solid tumours show a tendency to dissociate, this becoming an important diagnostic feature in deciding the nature of the lesion (e.g. in breast carcinoma or melanoma; Fig. 3.47). Single cells may be seen in cases of a metastatic tumour even if this is not a feature of the primary tumour (Fig. 3.48). Single cells that are due to the pitfalls of cell preparation have to be distinguished from genuine dissociation in order not to make an erroneous conclusion. Fibroadenoma, for example, is the most frequent cause of false-positive breast FNAC, partly due to the wrong interpretation of poorly prepared slides causing the dissociation of epithelial cells (seen usually in breast carcinomas; see Chap. 9).

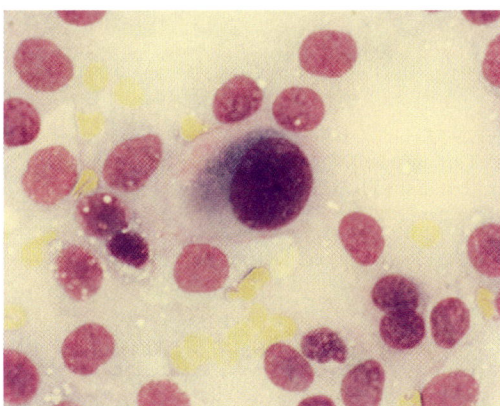

Fig. 3.47
Cell arrangement. Cells from solid tumours show a tendency towards dissociation. This is an important diagnostic feature in deciding the nature of the lesion, for example in this case of melanoma

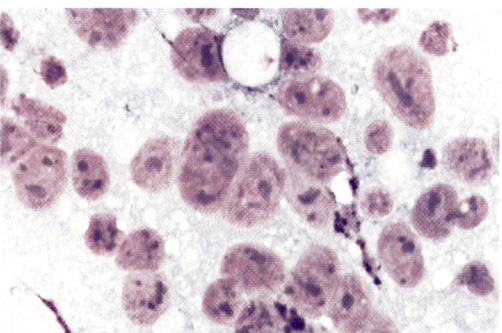

Fig. 3.48
Cell arrangement and nucleus. Single cells may be seen in cases of metastatic tumour even if this is not a feature of the primary tumour, as is the case in this breast carcinoma. Note the prominent irregular nucleoli

3.2.4 Papillary Arrangement

The papillary arrangement is usually seen as a helpful architectural detail in certain conditions (e.g. papillary proliferations or papillary tumours of the breast and PTC; Figs. 3.49 and 3.50). Cells within the cluster are difficult to see due to its thickness. It is usually not possible to see the stromal core of the papilla seen in histopathology. Similarly, the distinction between the myoepithelial cells and epithelial cells in benign breast lesions may be difficult. In cases of malignant tumours, papillary cell differentiation narrows the possibilities of the origin of the primary tumour; papillary carcinoma in ascites, for example, is most likely to be from an ovarian papillary adenocarcinoma. Similarly, the papillary arrangement of an unusual metastatic tumour in the lymph node of the head and neck is most likely to be from a thyroid primary (Fig. 3.51). Psammoma bodies are sometimes seen associated with papillary clusters and may be helpful in the diagnosis of conditions such as meningioma (Figs. 3.7–3.9), serous adenocarcinoma of the ovary and papillary thyroid carcinoma. In addition to papillary clusters, papillary tumours always have dissociated cells. In the case of breast tumours, this feature is important in distinguishing between benign and malignant lesions (Fig. 3.49).

3.2.5 Other Features

Cells tend to arrange themselves in a manner reminiscent of their pathogenesis, for example cells from an adenocarcinoma tend to arrange themselves in an acinar or follicular pattern, forming a lumen or "Indian file", in the case of lobular carcinoma of the breast (Fig. 3.52, 3.53). Cells from a benign nerve sheath tumour tend to be arranged in wavy bundles, and squamous cells sometimes form cell whorls and keratinised pearls (Figs. 3.54 and 3.55). Cell arrangement in these cases contributes to establishing cell differentiation. In the case of metastatic tumours, these features may be very helpful in suggesting a possible primary tumour site.

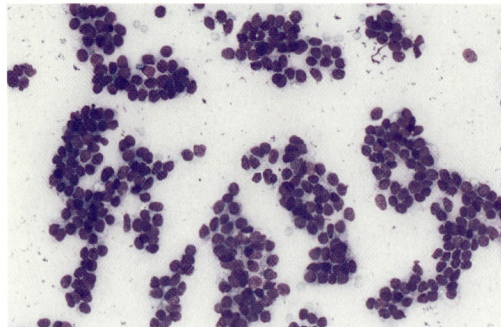

Fig. 3.49
Cell arrangement. Papillary clusters of monotonous-looking epithelium in a case of papillary carcinoma of the breast, similar to the appearances in the histological section (see Fig. 3.50)

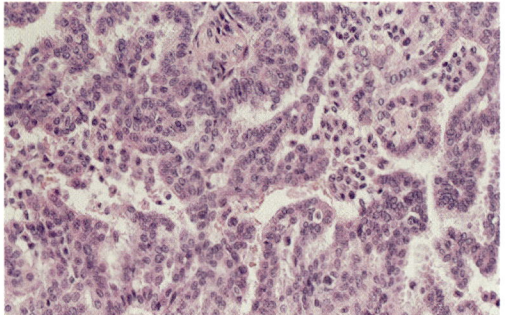

Fig. 3.50
Cell arrangement. Histological section of papillary carcinoma breast, corresponding to the FNAC of the similar appearances (see Fig. 3.49)

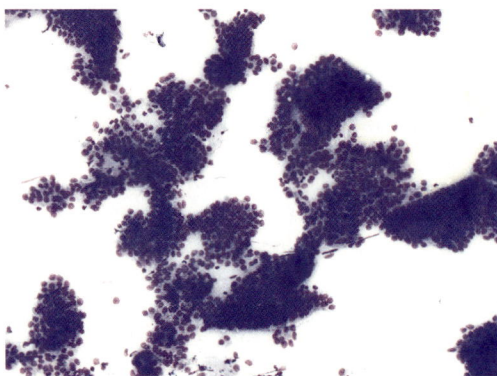

Fig. 3.51
Cell arrangement. Papillary arrangement of an unusual metastatic tumour in the lymph node of the head and neck is most likely to be from a papillary carcinoma of the thyroid.

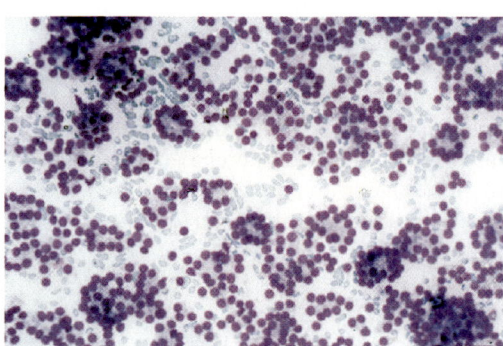

Fig. 3.52
Cell arrangement. Cells arranged in a microfollicular pattern in the FNAC thyroid in a case of follicular adenoma

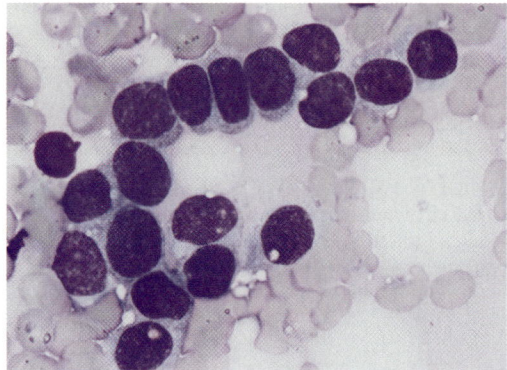

Fig. 3.53
Cell arrangement. This "Indian file" arrangement of epithelial cells is typical of lobular carcinoma of the breast

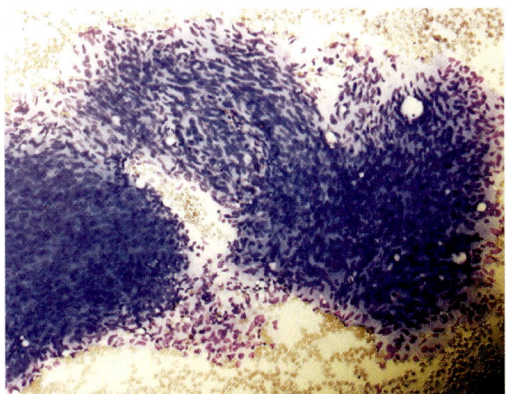

Fig. 3.54
Cell arrangement. Cells from a schwannoma tend to be arranged in wavy bundles immersed in metachromatic stroma

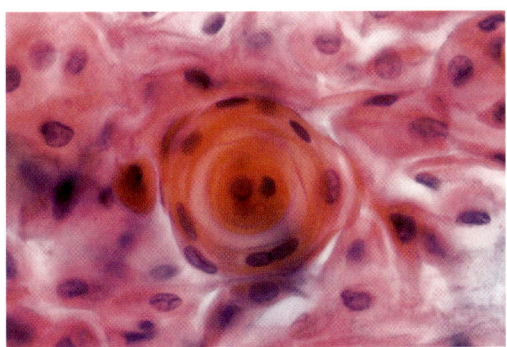

Fig. 3.55
Cell arrangement. Keratinised squamous cells are sometimes arranged in pearl-like structures

3.3 Cellular Features: the Nucleus

Having examined the cellularity of the smear, its background and the cell arrangement, the observer's eye is drawn to the individual cells. In most cases, these features hold the clue as to the nature of the lesion. The first consideration is if these cells are expected to be found in a particular site or if they are alien (e.g. malignant endothelial cells in a subcutaneous growth; Fig. 3.56). A good knowledge of normal cell constituents and possible contaminants is necessary to avoid mistakes (e.g. respiratory cells in thyroid aspirates due to contamination from the trachea, or gastric cells in EUS-FNAC material taken from the pancreas).

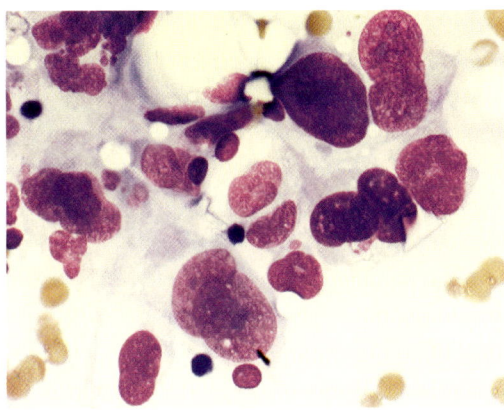

Fig. 3.56
Nucleus. Nuclear features in a case of angiosarcoma metastatic to the skin. The cells are alien to the subcutaneous tissue

In order to assess nuclear features, good preparation methods are essential. Slides that are poorly fixed or poorly prepared may have artefacts that are reflected particularly in the nuclear features. Air drying causes cells to explode, making the features fuzzy; alcohol fixation allows a better insight into the nuclear features (Figs. 3.57 and 3.58). Vigorous smearing or centrifugation may also cause cell distortion.

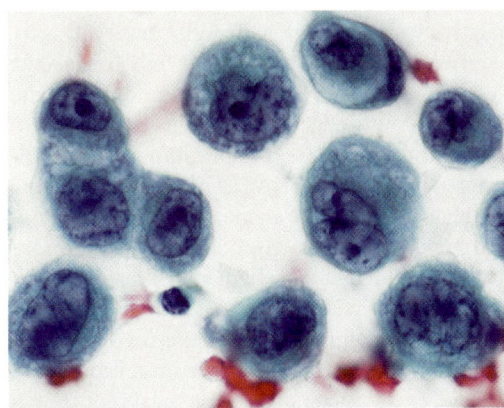

Fig. 3.57
Nucleus. Chromatin structure. Nuclear features in this case of multiple myeloma are seen clearly on alcohol-fixed preparations, although there is some cell shrinkage due to the fixative

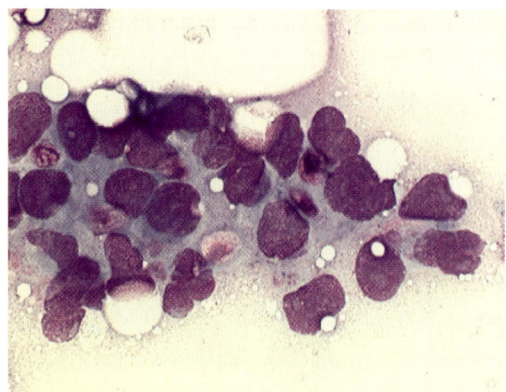

Fig. 3.58
Nucelus. Air-drying artefact. Nuclear features of, in this case, breast carcinoma are distorted by air drying

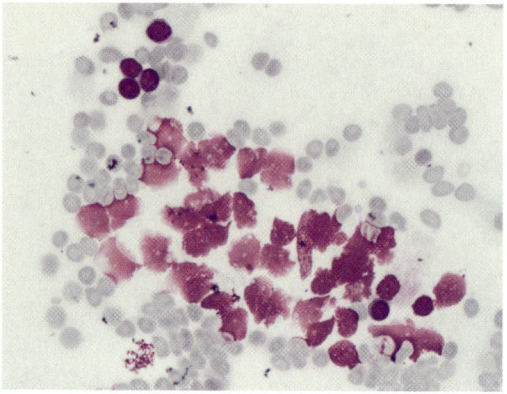

Fig. 3.59
Nucleus. Air-drying artefact prevents reliable assessment in this case of mediastinal FNAC. Histology showed a SCC of the lung

Although cellular features are assessed on the basis of individual cells, it is important to keep observing and comparing the features between different cells, to gain an overall impression. The uniformity of the features is commonly associated with benign conditions, whereas pleomorphism usually represents malignancy. In order to make this judgement, it is therefore essential to have a sufficient number of well-preserved cells. In some instances there are guidelines as to the optimal number of cells (e.g. the breast [1]). However, in the majority of cases it is not possible to quantify precisely the number of cells necessary for diagnosis. This can sometimes be made on a relatively small number of well-preserved cells, whilst at other times many more cells are needed. A judgment has to be made by an observer who has a full knowledge of the case, its clinical history and the management implications of cytological diagnosis. Since FNAC is not a screening, but a diagnostic test, the management implications are significant. When given, cytological opinions must be made only on adequately preserved material. Many medicolegal cases involving apparent FNAC malpractice are the result of a poorly prepared sample (Fig. 3.59). This fact is often either not mentioned in the cytological report or, if it is mentioned, is not reflected in the diagnostic conclusion. As a result, the referring clinician assumes that the conditions for making a reliable diagnosis were met.

3.3.1 Nuclear Size

Nuclear size may be expressed in absolute as well as in relative terms. Cytologists are interested in the relative nuclear size in relation to cell size and in comparison to other cells on the slide (Figs. 3.60–3.62). Relatively small cell nuclei (e.g. as observed in oat cell carcinoma of the lung) may occupy almost an entire cell, leaving a thin rim of cytoplasm that may not be noticeable at all, whereas the nuclei of apocrine epithelial cells are large but have abundant cytoplasm. The relative sizes of the nucleus and cytoplasm in a particular cell are reflected by the nucleo/cytopalsmic ratio (N/C) ratio. A raised N/C ratio is an important feature when considering the diagnosis of malignancy. The appreciation of a benign cell population at a given site is needed in order to avoid making a wrong judgment (e.g. in benign duct epithelium of the breast there may be relatively little cytoplasm and cells may appear to have a high N/C ratio). Most reactive inflammatory processes may have a slightly raised N/C ratio and yet be benign.

Diagnostic interpretation of FNAC material — Chapter 3

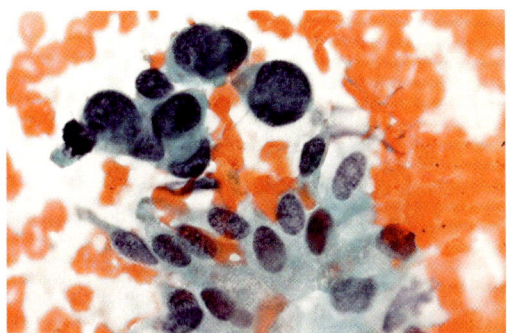

Fig. 3.60
Nuclear size. Cytologists are more interested in the relative nuclear size, its comparison with the normal cell population and with other cells within the slide. This is an example of cells from a cholangiocarcinoma, compared with normal biliary epithelium

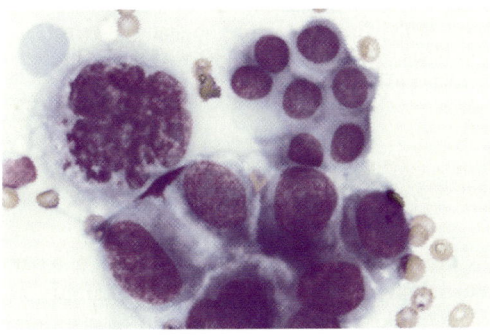

Fig. 3.61
Nucleus. High nucleo/cytoplasmic (N/C) ratio, mitotic figure and irregular shape of the nuclei of malignant cells from a cholangiocarcinoma, in contrast to the adjacent cluster of benign bile duct epithelium

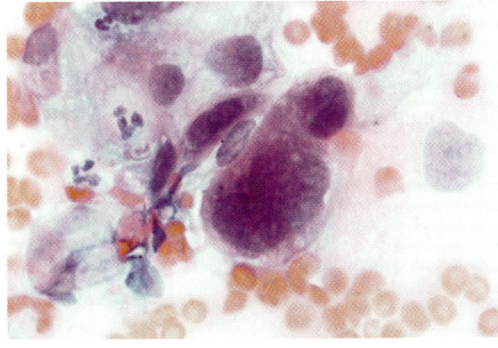

Fig. 3.62
Nucleus. Hish N/C ratio, anisonucleosis. High-power view of cholangiocarcinoma cells. Nuclei show a high N/C ratio and gross anisonucleosis

Anisonucleosis and anisocytosis are terms relating to the difference in nuclear and cell size amongst the cells on the same slide. Both reflect changes in size that may be important for interpretation. These changes may be either subtle or gross. Whilst an important feature, anisonucleosis is less important than the relative size of the nucleus, that is the N/C ratio (Fig. 3.63).

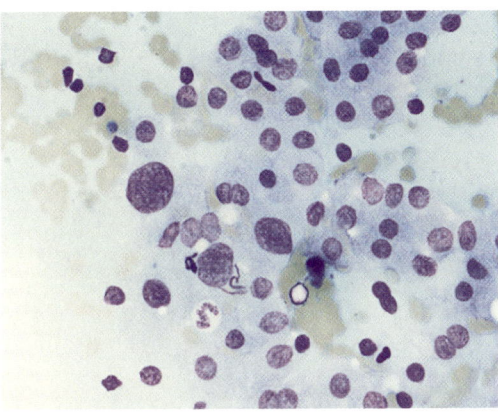

Fig. 3.63
Nucleus. Anisonucleosis may be seen in benign conditions, for example in this case of lymphocytic thyroiditis

3.3.2 Nuclear Shape

The nucleus is usually round or oval with a regular nuclear membrane. While many cytopathologists consider changes in nuclear shape like nuclear pleomorphism to be one of the main features of a malignancy, it is not the only one. Reactive conditions may show a degree of nuclear pleomorphism, usually with a preserved N/C ratio. The nuclear shape, as reflected in the nuclear contour or nuclear membrane, is generally better appreciated on the Pap than Romanowsky stains (Fig. 3.64). Minute details of nuclear membrane infoldings or protrusions can be seen as well as the membrane thickening and its irregularities. Some tumours (e.g. Langerhans' cell histiocytosis) have a characteristic nuclear shape that is pathognomonic of the condition. Others, like PTC, may have nuclear grooves and intranuclear cytoplasmic inclusions (Orphan Annie nuclei; Fig. 3.65). The consistency of nuclear shape within the cells of the same population usually indicates a good prognostic sign; carcinoid as a tumour of neuroendocrine origin, for example, has a remarkably bland cytological appearance with monotony of cell shapes as one of its major features (Fig. 3.66). Nuclear contour irregularity is a morphological feature that is sometimes taken as a parameter for morphological grading of tumours.

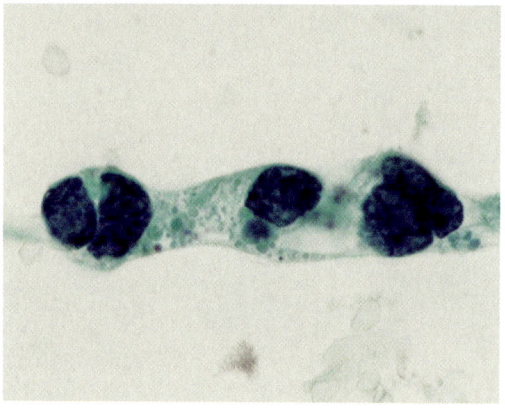

Fig. 3.64
Nucleus. The nuclear outline is irregular, binucleation, a high N/C ratio and irregular chromatin pattern are all indicative of malignancy in this case of a poorly differentiated SqCC of the lung

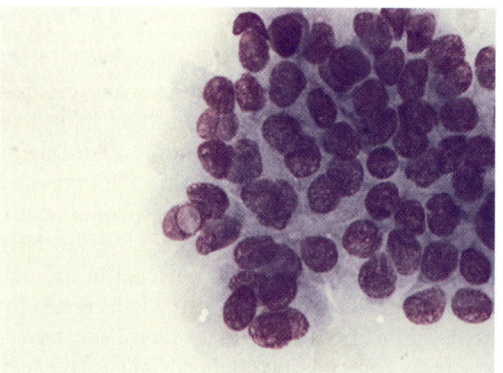

Fig. 3.65
Nucleus. Intranuclear inclusions. Papillary carcinoma of the thyroid may have nuclear grooves and intranuclear cytoplasmic inclusions (orphan Annie nuclei)

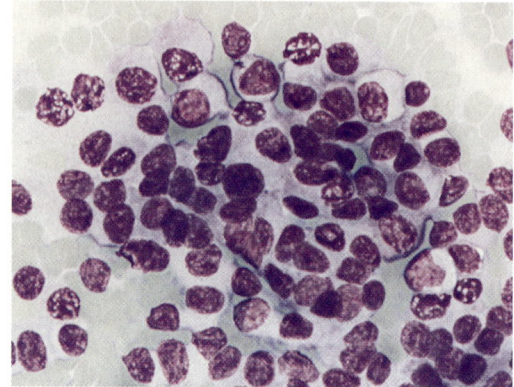

Fig. 3.66
Nucleus. The consistency of nuclear shape within the cells of the same population usually indicates a good prognostic sign as in this example of islet cell tumour of the pancreas in a patient with Zollinger Ellison syndrome. Cells of neuroendocrine origin have a remarkably bland cytological appearance with monotony of cell shapes as one of its major features

3.3.3 Position of the Nucleus

The position of the nucleus within a cell of a particular type is usually constant. For example, an eccentric position is usually a sign of glandular differentiation (respiratory or endocervical epithelium), but the nucleus usually holds a central position in squamous epithelium (Fig. 3.67). Whilst the position of the nucleus does not usually contribute to the decision about the nature of the pathological process, it may contribute to the decision about the possible cell origin (Fig. 3.68). This feature is commonly used when trying to establish the primary site of a metastatic tumour and, together with cytoplasmic features, may narrow the search.

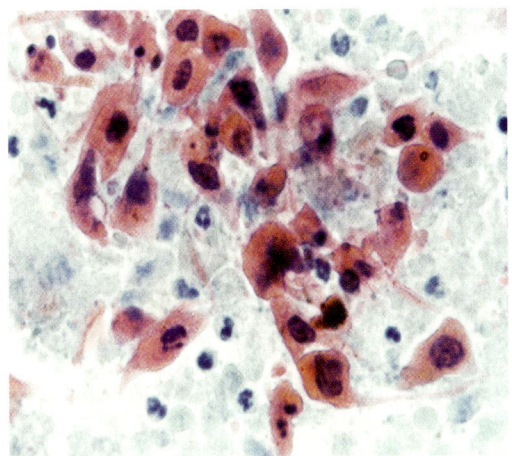

Fig. 3.67
Cytoplasm. Keratinisation and centrally placed nuclei in the case of FNAC lung containing SqCC cells

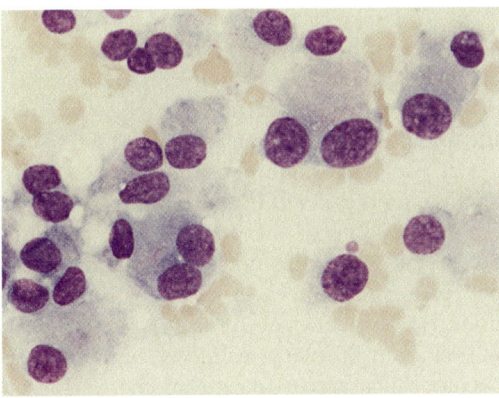

Fig. 3.68
Nucleus. The position of the nucleus may be significant in assessing tumour type. This is a case of medullary carcinoma of the thyroid with typically eccentrically placed nuclei

3.3.4 Chromatin Pattern

The chromatin pattern is a crude morphological expression of the DNA content of the nucleus. As such, in addition to the N/C ratio, the chromatin pattern is probably the single most important feature when determining the nature of the pathological process. In order to accurately assess the chromatin pattern, it is essential to have good staining and fixation of the material (Figs. 3.69 and 3.70). Chromatin may be appreciated best on the microscope high-power view (×40, ×60, ×100). With traditional staining, as described in Chap. 2, the chromatin pattern of the normal cell presents a dormant nucleus with smooth, even staining throughout. In the case of increased cell activity, either reactive or neoplastic, the chromatin pattern undergoes changes, becoming more apparent. It is variably described as reticular, granular, coarse, clumped and, most importantly, regular or irregular. An irregular chromatin pattern is one of the stronger indications that the cell is malignant (Fig. 3.64).

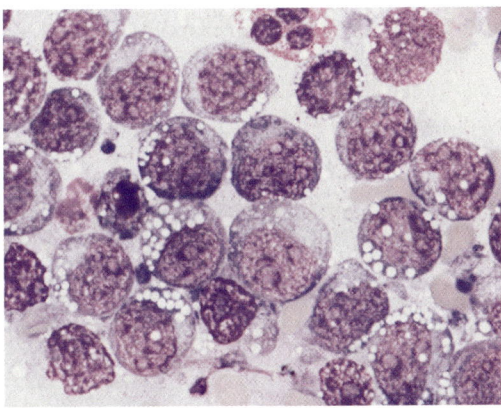

Fig. 3.69
Nucleus. Chromatin structure of lymphoid cells as seen in this case of non-Hodgkin's DLBL

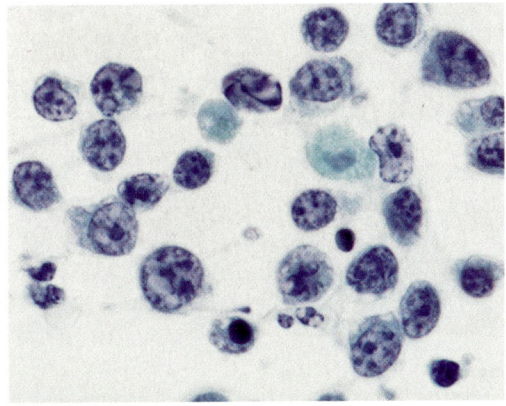

Fig. 3.70
Nucleus. Chromatin structure may be appreciated better on alcohol-fixed preparations from the FNAC in the case of non-Hodgkin's DLBL shown in Fig. 3.69

3.3.5 Number of Nuclei

The number of nuclei may vary within the cell under physiological conditions. This is often a reflection of a reactive change to infection or a foreign body (e.g. a foreign-body reaction to starch or silicone, TB, Wegener's granuloma, herpes or the measles virus; Fig. 3.71). Nuclei have to be assessed as described under the headings given above; their size, shape and chromatin pattern have to be regular in order to be considered as reactive. However, different tumours may have multinucleate cells such as reactive histiocytes (e.g. breast carcinoma or PTC) or tumour giant cells (e.g. Reed Sternberg cells, cells of ALCL or malignant nerve sheath tumour; Fig. 3.72). Recognition of these features may be helpful in making a diagnosis, although multinucleation alone is not a deciding factor.

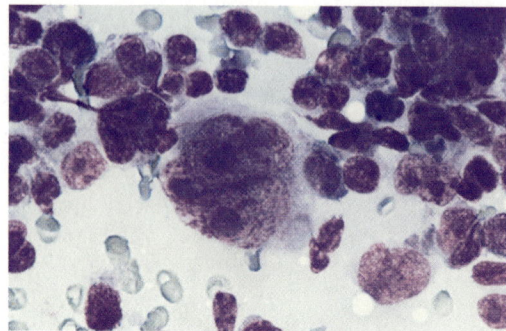

Fig. 3.72
Nucleus. Bizarre nuclear features, including multinuclear giant cells with prominent nucleoli, are seen here in a case of anaplastic large-cell lymphoma

3.3.6 Nucleoli

Nucleoli may be visible to a variable extent in the normal, dormant cells stained with routine cytological stains (e.g. bronchial epithelial cells and squamous cells). The intensity of the staining under physiological conditions reflects the activity of RNA synthesis within the cell. It is therefore not surprising that the nucleoli become more prominent when cells undergo regenerative/repair processes, as seen in inflammatory conditions. However, nucleoli are also characteristically prominent in many malignant tumours (e.g. hepatocellular carcinoma, melanoma, anaplastic carcinoma of the lung and thyroid, Hodgkin lymphoma and many other tumours; Fig. 3.73).

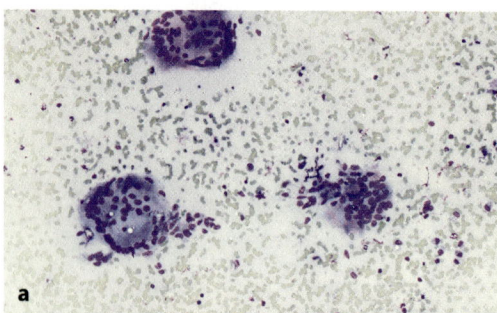

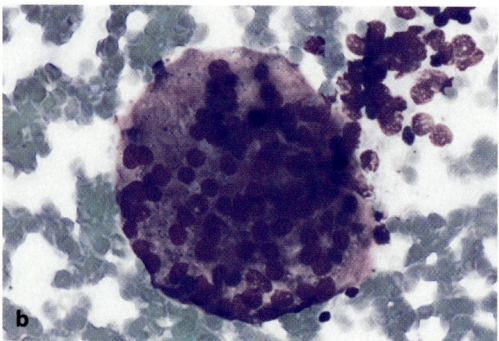

Fig. 3.71
Nucleus. **a** Multinucleation is a common occurence amongst cells and can be seen in all types of cells, both in benign and malignant conditions. These are multinucleate histiocytes of the foreign-body type in a case of subacute thyroiditis. **b** High-power view of the same case show multinucleation

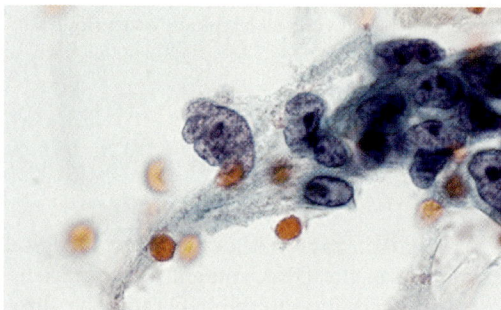

Fig. 3.73
Nucleus. Nucleoli are often better seen on alcohol fixed slides. They are large, irregularly shaped and multiple in this case of cholangiocarcinoma

Nucleoli are characterised not only by their prominence (i.e. size and staining pattern) but also by their shape and number (e.g. a poorly differentiated SqCC is more likely to have multiple irregular nucleoli than adenocarcinoma, which tends to have one or two prominent nucleoli). Nucleoli in Reed Sternberg cells have a particularly prominent blue rim, making their contour stand out.

3.3.7 Mitoses

Mitotic figures may be seen in normal cells undergoing division. However, in FNAC practice, this is relatively rare. Mitoses seen in normal cells are few and they appear regular. Mitoses seen in malignant tumours are also relatively rare in FNAC material compared to histology samples, and may appear either regular or irregular (Fig. 3.74). In cytology, the presence of mitotic figures is noted in the report. Mitotic count, a semi-quantitative assessment of some tumours used in histopathology, is not directly applicable to cytology because of the variability of the material preparation. Rather than being interested in the number of mitotic figures, cytologists concern themselves with their presence and shape (Fig. 3.75).

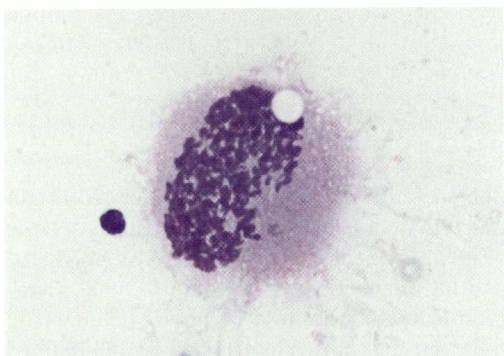

Fig. 3.74
Nucleus. Mitotic figures do not always signify malignancy. They may be present in benign conditions where there is a high degree of cell proliferation (e.g. reparative processes). This is an example of a mitotic figure in a benign mesothelium

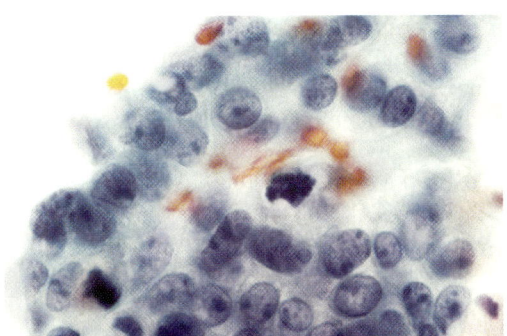

Fig. 3.75
Nucleus. Mitoses are present in a case of pancreatic adenocarcinoma

3.4 Cellular Features: Cytoplasm

3.4.1 Relative Amount

The amount of cytoplasm is a function of the cell type and its quantity is more or less constant (e.g. salivary gland epithelium, lymphoid cells). There are physiological situations where the amount of cytoplasm becomes appreciably larger than usual (e.g. apocrine or oncocytic change; Fig. 3.45). Rather than the absolute amount, the relative amount or N/C ratio, as explained in 3.3.1, is important. The reduction of cytoplasm due to the expansion of the nucleus is usually an important feature of malignancy and, if observed, is significant. Cytoplasmic boundaries are sometimes not sharp enough to allow judgment of the N/C ratio. In this case, other features have to be considered in order to make the diagnosis.

3.4.2 Quality and Contents

The quality of the cytoplasm reflects cell differentiation (e.g. keratinised cells, mucin-producing cells, endothelial cells; Figs. 3.76–3.79). Sometimes this is visible with routine staining and sometimes it needs special stains (e.g. amyloid-producing cells of medullary carcinoma, melanin-producing cells of a melanoma, c-kit-positive cells from a gastrointestinal stromal tumour). Cytoplasm may have fine vacuoles or granules, contain pigment and be dense or clear (e.g. hepatocellular carcinoma and clear-cell carcinoma kidney or ovary; Fig. 3.80).

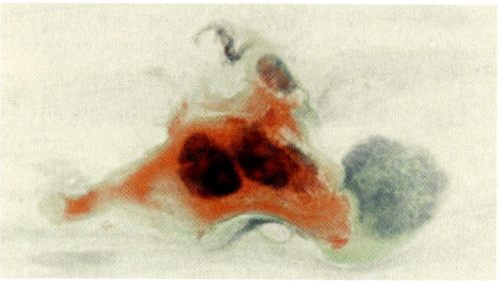

Fig. 3.76
Cytoplasm. The orange colour signifies keratinisation, in this case of adenosquamous carcinoma of the pancreas

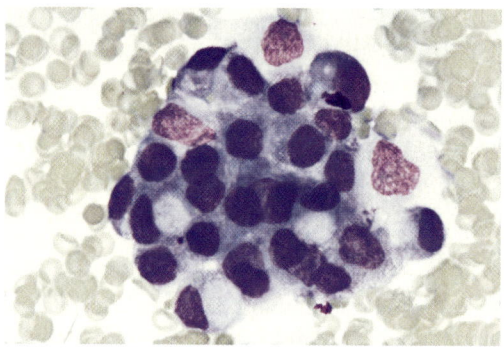

Fig. 3.77
Cytoplasm. Cytoplasmic vaculation is found typically in the case of lobular carcinoma of the breast

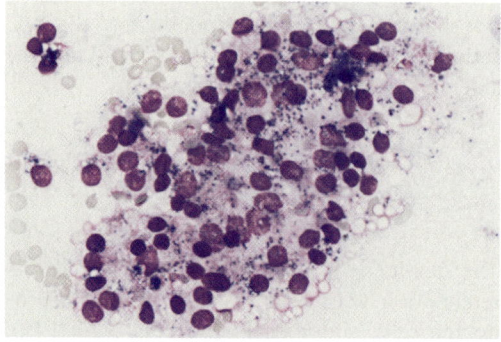

Fig. 3.78
Cytoplasm. Granules of haemosiderin in the case of cystic colloid goitre with evidence of old haemorrhage

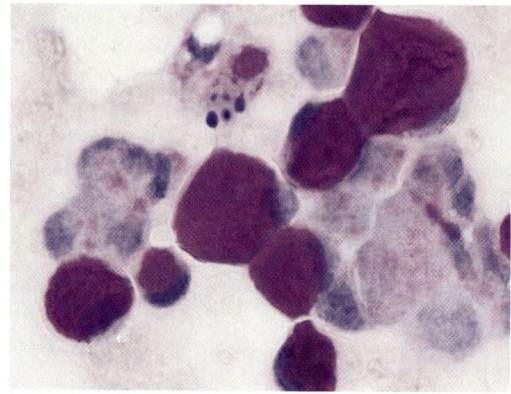

Fig. 3.79
Cytoplasm. PAS-d staining of cytoplasmic mucin in a case of signet-ring adenocarcinoma

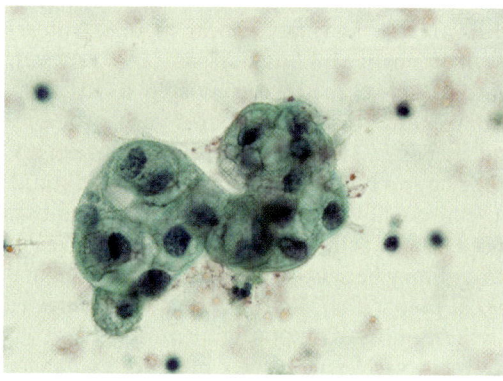

Fig. 3.80
Cytoplasm. Vacuolated cytoplasm in cells from a metastatic clear-cell carcinoma of the ovary

3.4.3 Shape and Definition

The shape of the cytoplasm reflects cell origin and function. Soft-tissue cells are usually spindle shaped, epithelial cells are round or polygonal and haemopoietic cell are round or oval. Cytoplasmic boundaries may be poorly defined (e.g. follicular cells in a colloid goitre) or well-defined by routine staining (e.g. PTC; Fig. 3.81). The definition of the cytoplasmic boundaries may vary with staining and fixation so if cytoplasmic outlines are important for diagnosis it is advisable to have both Pap- and Romanowsky-stained material with good fixation for both (Fig. 3.82).

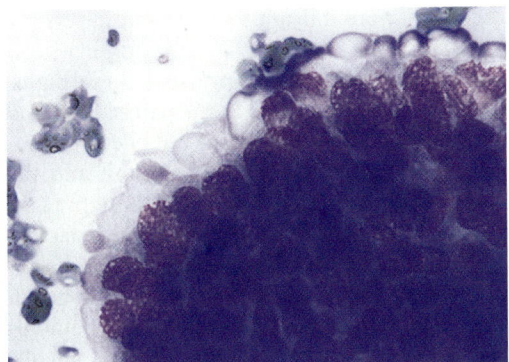

Fig. 3.81
Cytoplasm. Cytoplasmic outline may be important for diagnosis. Scalloping of the well-outlined cytoplasm in this case of FNAC thyroid is typical of papillary carcinoma

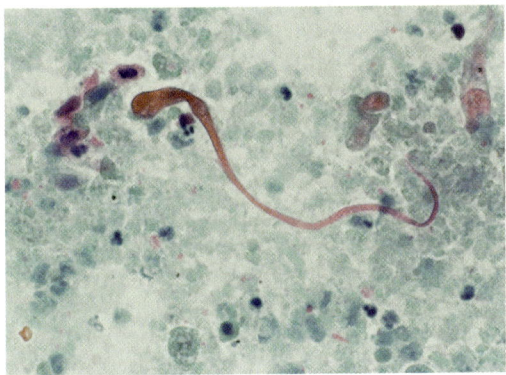

Fig. 3.82
Cytoplasm. The tadpole shape of this mummified squamous cell is typical of bizarre shapes found in SqCC

3.5 Criteria of Malignancy

"Criteria of malignancy" is a phrase that is often used when justifying a diagnosis of a malignant tumour. Unfortunately, there are no morphological features that can be used universally and consistently, in a mathematical algorithm, in order to make a diagnosis of malignancy. Instead, criteria of malignancy constitutes the composite finding of abnormal features in any individual case. A good knowledge of underlying pathological processes and variations of the normal morphology is a prerequisite for a diagnosis of malignancy. The same morphological criteria cannot be applied throughout all systems: each system has its own specific features that, when present, add up to the diagnosis. However, some of the features mentioned earlier are more important than others. These include: a high N/C ratio, nuclear pleomorphism, an irregular chromatin pattern, anisonucleosis, prominent and/or irregular nucleoli and mitoses. Cytoplasmic differentiation, whilst not a criterion of malignancy, may be important when considering the site of the lesion.

3.6 Cytology Report

The FNAC report is a reflection of the complete process within the cytology laboratory, from receiving the specimen to making the final diagnosis. The cytology report should include the following parts: patient identification details, clinical history, dates of obtaining and receiving specimens, macroscopic description, microscopic description, conclusion, recommendation for further management, signature of the pathologist, date of the report and diagnostic code. The cytology report is a legal document and can be used as evidence in a particular case. It is therefore important that attention is paid to every part of the report since misunderstandings due to omissions are difficult to rectify later.

Patient identification data include: the hospital number, the patient's name and date of birth and a laboratory number. Ideally, it should also include the patient's address (home address or ward), type (inpatient, outpatient, National Health Service, private), referring clinician and address where the report should be sent. Material lacking the minimum identification data should not be processed but should be kept until the identity of the patient is confirmed. This can be done either in person, by the originator of the sample, or by telephone. In both cases, this process should be carefully documented, noting the names of the participants and dates the information was obtained.

The clinical history needs to be an integral part of the report. If it includes drawings, these may need to be scanned into the final report. Otherwise they need to be transcribed carefully to reflect the drawing. If there are no clinical data or if they are incomplete, this needs to be recorded (e.g. "FNAC breast. Side not stated.").

The macroscopic description of the material received needs to be clear and precise. The date, type and origin of the specimen must be clearly noted. This is usually a description of either the slides received or the diagnostic material (e.g. fluid) or, in case the procedure was performed by a cytopathologist, a description of the procedure including the consistency of the lesion, its mobility and detailed anatomical position. Sometimes a photograph of the site(s) of aspiration may be needed. If there is a delay in specimen delivery this should be noted too.

The main body of the report contains the microscopic description, which may be more or less descriptive, depending on the local preferences. Generally, all descriptions should convey relevant morphological information. Words like atypical, suspicious, probable, suggestive, in-keeping with and consistent with, should be kept to a minimum and reserved for a conclusion. The conclusion should be as unambiguous as possible. If the diagnosis is less than certain, this should be expressed clearly, with a request for further investigation. The conclusion is usually a one-line sentence, based on the features described in the body of the report. The conclusion cannot be at variance with the description. For example, if the main description described malignant cells from a metastatic carcinoma, the conclusion should also be that of malignancy and not suggestive or suspicious thereof. In cases where it is not possible to make a one-line conclusion, this needs to be stated and the reader should be referred to the main body of the text. In addition to a conclusion, most FNAC reports also include management advice for further investigation or patient follow-up. The diagnosis is sometimes followed by a numerical grade (e.g. C1–C5 in FNAC breast, according to the national guidelines; see Chap. 4 [1]).

Most centres use diagnostic coding systems for easy retrieval of diagnostic material and auditing. The codes for both topography and pathology should be used carefully since incorrect digits are more difficult to spot than the wrong spelling. Some computer systems automatically generate diagnoses by converting these digits. This may not be obvious to the pathologist who is signing the report but does not check the coding. The signature of the pathologist and the date are also an essential part of the report. In some centres, pathologists operate a system of electronic signatures. It is important that the appropriate systems are in place to avoid abuse of this system. By signing the report, the pathologist assumes full responsibility for its contents. It is therefore important that the signature on the report belongs to the person who made the diagnosis.

The cytology report is an important vehicle of communication between the clinician and the cytopathologist. Given that other lines of communications are often difficult and sometimes impossible, the cytology report needs to convey all of the information available from the cytology specimen in clear terms, preferably adhering to the reporting guidelines for that particular area. At the same time, in some cases it needs to advise as to the course of further diagnostic action (e.g. in cases of non-Hodgkin lymphoma, although it is perfectly possible to diagnose it cytologically, most centres still perform a lymph node tissue biopsy to be performed as a baseline investigation before treatment). Many clinicians may not be clear about the role of FNAC in management, hence the management advice should be part of a report, where appropriate. A breakdown in communication is probably the most common cause of errors in clinical medicine and a very frequent cause of medicolegal disputes. We should therefore ensure that the content and format of the cytology report is as accurate and clear as possible.

References

1. NHSBSP. Guidelines to Cytology Procedures and Reporting in Breast Cancer Screen
2. Orell S, Sterret GF, Walters MN, Whitaker D. Fine Needle Aspiration Cytology. Churchill Livingstone. ISBN 0443-04239-X Second edition 1996.
3. Young JA. Fine Needle Aspiration Cytopathology. Blackwell ISBN 0-632-02393-7, 1993.

Chapter 4

Diagnostic Dilemmas in FNAC Practice: Cystic Lesions

Contents

4.1	Cysts in the Neck	59
4.1.1	Thyroglossal Duct Carcinoma	60
4.1.2	Branchial Cleft Cysts	61
4.1.3	Salivary Gland Lesions	62
4.1.4	Lymphoepithelial Cysts	63
4.1.5	Cystadenolymphoma	64
4.1.6	Acinic Cell Carcinoma	66
4.1.7	Pleomorphic Adenoma	67
4.1.8	Dermoid Cyst	68
4.1.9	Thyroid Cysts	68
4.1.10	The Lymph Nodes	70
4.1.11	Parathyroid Cysts	71
4.1.12	Cysts of the Jaw	72
4.1.13	Teratoid Cyst	72
4.2	Cysts in the Abdomen	73
4.2.1	Cystic Lesions of the Pancreas	73
4.2.2	Cystic Lesions of the Liver	77
4.2.3	Adrenal and Renal Cystic Lesions	78
4.2.4	Cystic Lesions of the Peritoneum	79
4.3	Thoracic Cysts	79
4.4	Breast Cysts	80
4.5	Other Cysts and Artefacts	82
References		85

Lesions containing fluid are a relatively common indication for FNAC, sometimes for diagnostic and sometimes for therapeutic reasons. In addition to cytology, the collected material may be sent to be cultured for microbiology analysis. Fluid is processed as described in Chap. 1. It is essential that the material is prepared without delay since the cells in the fluid may already have partly degenerated so that any further delay in processing may exacerbate deterioration in their morphological preservation.

The term cyst comes from the Greek word, kystis, meaning a sac or bladder. It usually implies epithelial lining. Pseudocyst is a term used for all other lesions that contain fluid but are not lined with epithelium. This term is sometimes used loosely and it is worth remembering instances where the presence or absence of epithelium may be important for management (e.g. pancreatic cysts and pseudocysts).

4.1 Cysts in the Neck

FNAC can effectively distinguish between benign and malignant cystic lesions of the head and neck. However, in some instances it may be difficult to arrive at a definite diagnosis due to limited cellularity, reactive changes and cellular degeneration. Dejmek reviewed the frequency of cystic lesions of the head and neck region (excluding the thyroid gland) and their diagnosis by FNAC to be 10% of the total head and neck material. Furthermore, 23% of cysts were in parotid gland aspirates and 3% in lymph node aspirates; 82% of cystic lymph node lesions were malignant. A histologically correct diagnosis of benign or malignant was rendered by cytology in 85% of the cystic cases, with 4% false negatives and 2% false positives [1].

Cystic lesions in the neck may be either congenital or acquired. Congenital cysts of the neck most commonly encountered in FNAC practice are branchial cleft and thyroglossal cysts (Fig. 4.1, Case history 4.1). Although branchial cysts may present as asymptomatic swellings, about one-third present acutely due to inflammation [2]. A branchial cleft cyst, although containing lymphoid cells in its wall, almost never contains lymphoid cells in the FNAC sample, which is usually taken from the centre of the lesion. Thyroglossal cysts do not commonly contain any epithelium in the FNAC sample, but contain macrophages and cholesterol crystals, and sometimes inflammatory cells and squamous metaplasia (Fig. 4.2a,b). They are recognised clinically by their midline position and clinical history of a long-standing midline neck swelling of variable size.

> **Case history 4.1:** A 28-year-old male presented with a 4-cm-diameter swelling in the anterior triangle. FNAC yielded 15 ml of yellow turbid fluid. Cyst markedly reduced in size after the FNAC. Microscopy showed numerous mature squamous cells, anucleate squamous cells and polymorphs. No lymphoid cells were seen. FNAC diagnosis: branchial cleft cyst (Fig. 4.1).

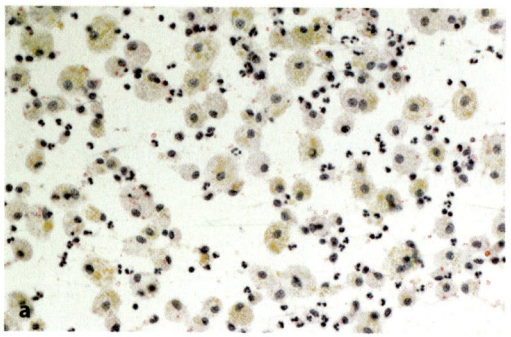

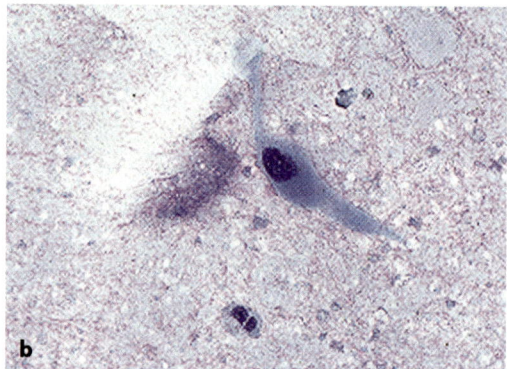

Fig. 4.2
a Thyroglossal cysts do not commonly contain any epithelium in the FNAC sample, but contain macrophages, cholesterol crystals and sometimes inflammatory cells.
b Thyroglossal cysts occasionally contain cells with features of squamous metaplasia

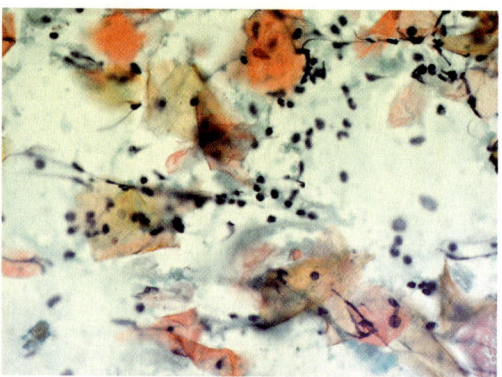

Fig. 4.1
Branchial cleft cyst. Cytological preparations contain mature squamous epithelium and anucleate squamous cells. There is frequently an acute inflammatory exudate present

4.1.1 Thyroglossal Duct Carcinoma

Approximately 150 cases of thyroglossal duct carcinoma, predominantly of the papillary type, have been reported, but the preoperative FNAC diagnosis of such neoplasms has rarely been cited. Histologically, these are diagnosed as papillary and squamous thyroglossal duct carcinomas, although Hurthle cell carcinomas have also been described [3]. Familiarity with the FNAC findings of thyroglossal duct carcinoma is limited by its rarity. The presence of large, atypical squamous cells, or psammoma bodies, in the FNAC material of a midline anterior cystic neck mass should suggest papillary thyroglossal duct carcinoma [3].

4.1.2 Branchial Cleft Cysts

A diagnostic dilemma in diagnosing branchial cleft cysts occurs in distinguishing it from a metastasis of a well-differentiated carcinoma with an unknown primary (Fig. 4.3, Case history 4.2). Gourin and Johnson sought to identify the incidence of solitary cystic SqCC metastasis in 121 adult patients who presented with an initial diagnosis of lateral cervical cyst and had no known malignancy. Metastatic SqCC was found in 9.9% of these patients [4]. The development of an invasive SqCC within a lateral cervical cyst as a result of malignant transformation of the epithelium is considered a rare circumstance, the principal diagnostic criterion for lateral cervical cyst carcinoma being the histological demonstration of transition from benign epithelium into invasive SqCC [5–8]. Khafif et al. made a critical analysis of 67 cases reported in the English literature, which showed that 14 patients had incontrovertible evidence of branchiogenic carcinoma, as evidenced by a branchial cyst with histological evidence of epithelial dysplasia progressing to SqCC within the cyst wall [9].

Case history 4.2: Male 47 years old with painless neck swelling of 2 months duration. No relevant clinical history. FNAC yielded well-differentiated squamous epithelium with very little cytological atypia (Fig. 4.3). The question arose as to whether the lesion was a metastatic SqCC or an inflamed branchial cleft cyst. In the case of the former, a radical neck dissection would be needed and in the case of the latter, excision may be local and would not be urgent. Cytologically, this distinction is very difficult to make in the absence of clear features of malignancy. In this case a report was issued leaving the possibility of either lesion open. The case was discussed at a multidisciplinary meeting. The patient submitted to examination of the oropharynx and an ulcerated tumour of the tonsil was found and biopsied. Histology showed a SqCC. The patient underwent a radical neck dissection.

A careful clinical history, the patient's age, history of smoking, clinical examination and appropriate cell fixation at the time of FNAC (alcohol fixation is usually better for the detection of keratin and nuclear detail) and careful microscopic scrutiny for evidence of immature cells, dyskaryotic nuclei, pleomorphism and necrosis, should clarify the distinction in most cases. However, solitary cystic SqCC metastases may be difficult to distinguish clinically from a benign cervical cyst. The incidence of solitary cystic SqCC metastasis in patients presenting with apparently benign cervical cysts is significantly greater in patients over 40 years of age (23.5%, P<0.0001) [4].

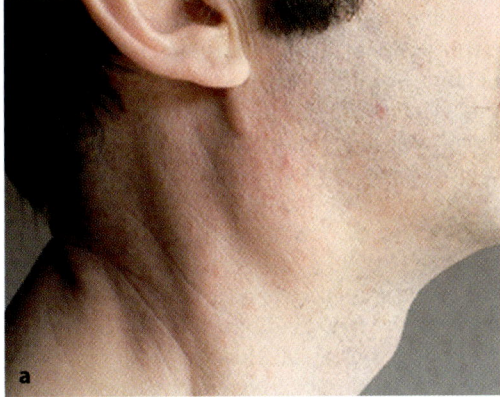

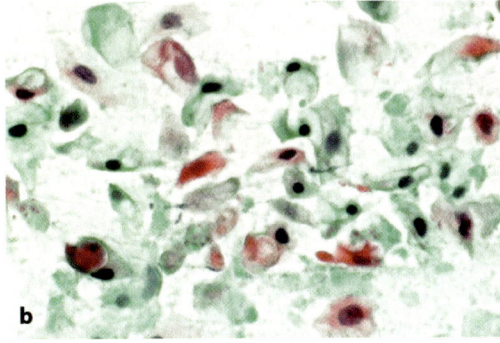

Fig. 4.3
SqCC. **a** Diagnostic dilemma in diagnosing branchial cleft cysts occurs in distinguishing it from a metastasis of a well-differentiated carcinoma with an unknown primary. **b** A careful clinical history, the patient's age, history of smoking, clinical examination and appropriate cell fixation at the time of FNAC (alcohol fixation is usually better for the detection of keratin and nuclear detail) and a careful microscopic scrutiny for evidence of immature cells, dyskaryotic nuclei, pleomorphism and necrosis, should clarify the distinction in most cases

Panendoscopy with directed biopsy sampling often reveals an occult primary in the base of tongue, tonsil and nasopharynx. Pitfalls that might be seen in FNAC of SqCC of the head and neck include: cystic changes, well-differentiated SqCC, spindle SqCC and SqCC with foreign-body giant cells, keratin plaques and ghost cells [10]. Nasuti et al. examined the usefulness of six cytological features including the presence or prevalence of nuclear atypia, anucleated cells, tissue fragments, necrosis and background inflammation in distinguishing between benign and malignant cystic lesions of the head and neck and found that an increased number of tissue fragments ($P<0.001$), a greater degree of nuclear atypia ($P<0.001$) and background necrosis ($P<0.001$) were more frequent in cystically degenerating SqCC as compared to benign squamous cystic lesions. They found no significant difference in the number of single cells, anucleate cells, the amount of background inflammation or p53 levels in aspirates of benign vs. malignant cystic squamous lesions [11].

Since branchial cleft cysts are usually excised surgically, it may appear that the distinction between the two conditions on FNAC material is not very important. However, the importance in making a correct preoperative diagnosis is in staging and therefore managing appropriately a patient with metastatic SqCC. The clinician will usually search for the primary site and perform a radical lymph node neck dissection, even when this is not found. Nordemar et al. successfully used image cytometry DNA analysis of nuclear ploidy to help in the distinction between benign and malignant cystic lesions [12, 13].

Acquired cysts in the head and neck may present due to degenerative processes, inflammation or neoplasms that are either cystic or have undergone cystic change. An appreciation of the local anatomy and knowledge of underlying pathological processes is essential in order to avoid pitfalls (Fig. 4.4).

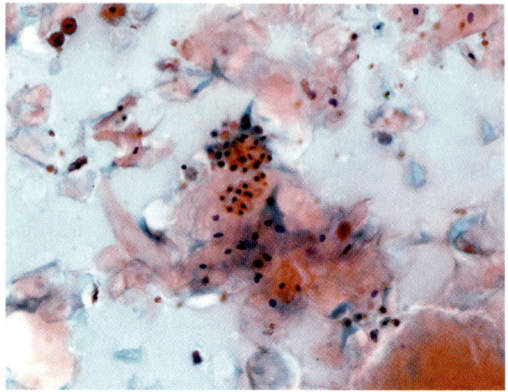

Fig. 4.4
Odontogenic keratocysts are cysts that occur in the jaw containing keratinised squamous cells and flakes of keratin. It is usually diagnosed radiologically and clinically as a cyst of the jaw. The morphological appearance may otherwise be mistaken for one of the other neck cysts or with a well-differentiated squamous cell carcinoma

4.1.3 Salivary Gland Lesions

Salivary gland lesions that can be cystic, either as a primary or a secondary phenomenon, are: mucocoele, salivary gland retention cysts/chronic sialadenitis, lymphoepithelial cyst, Warthin's tumour, pleomorphic adenoma, cystic mucoepidermoid carcinoma, adenoid cystic carcinoma, a variant of ACC, papillary adenocarcinoma and metastatic tumours, in particular, melanoma. FNAC is a valuable tool in the primary diagnosis and management of cystic parotid gland lesions, approximately 20% of which turn out to be malignant [11]. The diagnostic accuracy of FNAC can be significantly improved by acquiring a detailed clinical history, obtaining an adequate cellular specimen and having knowledge of the variety and frequencies of possible diagnostic entities that may present as cystic parotid gland lesions [11].

4.1.4 Lymphoepithelial Cysts

Bilateral and multiple lymphoepithelial cysts (cystic benign lymphoepithelial lesions) of the major salivary glands, in particular of parotid glands, are quite rare with an incidence of about 3–6%. These lesions represent an early manifestation of HIV infection and are rarely found in patients with advanced acquired immunodeficiency syndrome. They are usually a reflection of an underlying lymphadenopathy. Patients are usually young and have a short clinical history of painless swelling (Figs. 4.5 and 4.6). The diagnosis is not difficult if all components are present (i.e. lymphoid cells, epithelial cells and macrophages). In my experience this is rare. Usually, the lymphoid component and cellular debris dominate whilst the epithelium is sparse and attenuated. It is often difficult to decide whether the squamous cells in the fluid are not a contaminant from the skin (Case history 4.3). Similarly, if lymphoid cells dominate and are represented by a florid proliferation of centroblasts, features may appear alarming and an erroneous diagnosis of a follicular B-cell NHL may be made. If, on the other hand, cystic components with macrophages, debris and epithelium dominate, the lesion may be dismissed as a banal salivary gland retention cyst (Fig. 4.7). Chronic sialadenitis/salivary gland retention cysts may show prominent squamous metaplasia of the ductal epithelium of the salivary gland (Fig. 4.8).

> **Case history 4.3:** A 23-year-old patient with a history of HIV infection presented with a 2 month history of unilateral fluctuant, painless parotid swelling. FNAC yielded 5 ml of slightly turbid, colourless fluid. Microscopy showed numerous lymphoid cells, including follicle centre cells, macrophages and very few epithelial cells against much background debris. No acute inflammation or normal salivary gland epithelium was seen. Lymphoid cells looked alarming because of the prominence of their centroblasts. FNAC diagnosis: lymphoepithelial cyst (Figs. 4.5 and 4.6).

FNAC could represent both a diagnostic and a therapeutic tool for parotid lymphoepithelial cysts. In some cases smears showed numerous crystalloids identical to those described as crystallised amylase [14]. Sometimes, numerous multinucleated giant cells without the epithelial component are seen.

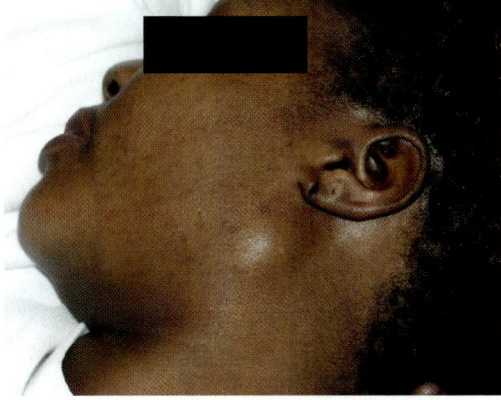

Fig. 4.5
Lymphoepithelial cysts represent an early manifestation of HIV infection and are rarely found in patients with advanced acquired immunodeficiency syndrome. They are usually a reflection of an underlying lymphadenopathy. Patients are usually young and have a short clinical history of painless swelling

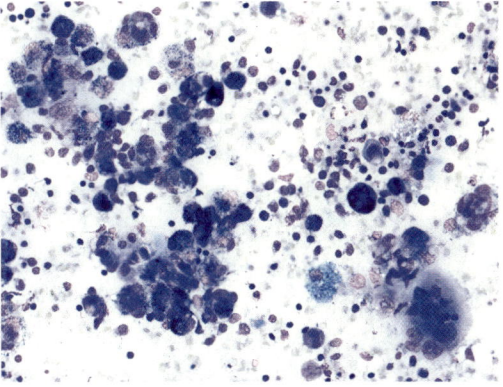

Fig. 4.6
On FNAC smears, lymphoepithelial cysts exhibit a cystic component with macrophages, debris and epithelium; the lesion is similar to the salivary gland retention cyst (see Fig. 4.7). In some cases smears show numerous crystalloids identical to those described as crystallised amylase, associated with numerous multinucleated giant cells. Differential diagnosis in the setting of HIV infection includes TB

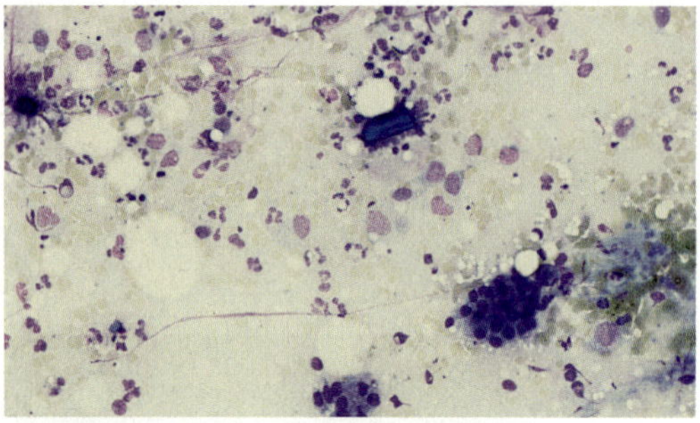

Fig. 4.7
The salivary gland retention cyst is in many ways similar to the lymphoepithelial cyst seen in HIV patients. The background usually contains acute as well as chronic inflammatory exudates and amylase crystals; ductal epithelium showing squamous metaplasia may also be seen

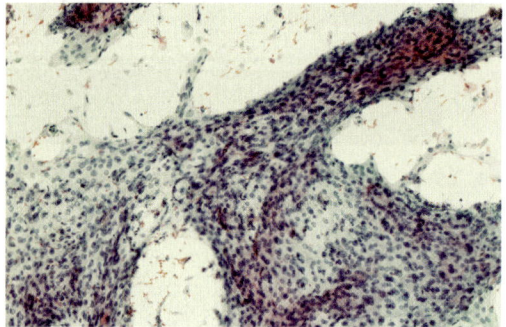

Fig. 4.8
Chronic sialadenitis/salivary gland retention cysts may exhibit prominent squamous metaplasia of the ductal epithelium, which should not be mistaken for metastatic squamous cell carcinoma, particularly in cases where there is a clinical history of neck irradiation

Similarly to the nasopharyngeal (adenoid and tonsil) lymphoid tissue of HIV-positive patients, intense immunoexpression of S-100 and p24 (HIV-1) protein is present in multinucleate giant cells. Vicandi et al. suggest that the diagnosis of HIV-associated lymphoepithelial cyst should always be considered if a parotid cystic lesion presents with numerous multinucleate giant cells [15]. Surgical therapy is not usually required for these lesions, and aspiration of cystic fluid with FNAC is therapeutic, although evidence of further relapses does exist. Surgical excision may become necessary when pain occurs because of persistent and progressive swelling of the parotid gland [16].

4.1.5 Cystadenolymphoma

Cystadenolymphoma (Warthin's tumour, named after Aldred Scott Warthin, MD, PhD 1866–1931) is a relatively common salivary gland tumour in patients presenting with a neck mass. Although usually found in the parotid or, less frequently, in the submandibular gland, it can be found in the ectopic salivary gland tissue in the neck. Surgery is recommended for most salivary gland tumours because of progressive enlargement and the risk of malignant transformation. This behaviour is unusual with Warthin's tumour and surgery is usually advocated for pathological confirmation. A highly accurate diagnosis by FNAC may justify conservative management for the asymptomatic patient [17]. The classical features of a mixture of apocrine-type cells, macrophages and lymphocytes do not usually create diagnostic problems. A regular apocrine epithelium is characteristically spread in flat sheets, sometimes with prominent mast cells (Figs. 4.9 and 4.10). However, a variable quantity of its component cells on an FNAC slide may mislead the observer. Dominance of the epithelium, particularly when present as dissociated single cells, may be interpreted as an SqCC, and its absence as an inflammatory process or a lymphoma (Fig. 4.8).

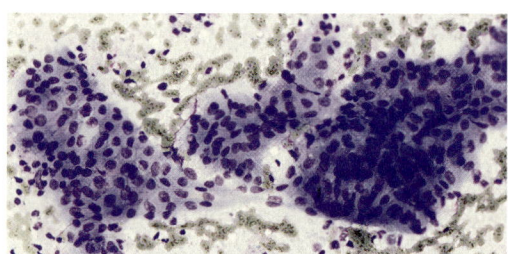

Fig. 4.9
Warthin's tumour. Classical features with a mixture of apocrine type cells, macrophages and lymphocytes usually do not create diagnostic problems. A regular apocrine epithelium is characteristically spread in flat sheets, sometimes with prominent mast cells (Fig. 4.10). However, the variable quantity of its component cells on an FNAC slide may mislead the observer. The dominance of epithelium, particularly when present as dissociated single cells, may be interpreted as a squamous cell carcinoma or mucoepidermoid carcinoma, and its absence as an inflammatory process or a lymphoma

Papillary adenocarcinoma and mucoepidermoid carcinoma both may have a similar background as Warthin's tumour. Infarcted Warthin's tumour after FNAC may, on histology, sometimes mimic mucoepidermoid carcinoma. Cystic mucoepidermoid carcinoma may be interpreted as a benign cystic lesion (Case history 4.4).

> **Case history 4.4:** A 64-year-old patient had a history of neck swelling. FNAC yielded turbid fluid that, on microscopy, appeared to be thick and amorphous and contained necrotic debris. Very few epithelial nests were noted, but these were too poorly preserved for assessment. A report was issued suggesting an inflammatory salivary gland lesion. Excision biopsy showed a low-grade, predominantly cystic mucoepidermoid carcinoma (Figs. 4.11 and 4.12).

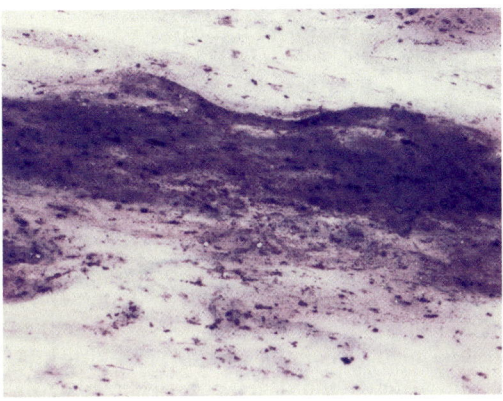

Fig. 4.11
Mucoepidermoid carcinoma. Cystic mucoepidermoid carcinoma may be interpreted as a benign cystic/inflammatory lesion if the epithelial component is not prominent and the mucoid content of the fluid is not appreciated

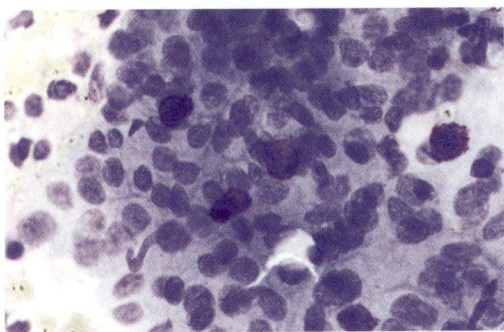

Fig. 4.10
Warthin's tumour. The apocrine, oncocytic epithelium in Warthin's tumour often has mast cells associated with it. These can be very helpful when trying to establish the diagnosis in doubtful cases. Mast cells are best appreciated on air-dried, MGG-stained slides

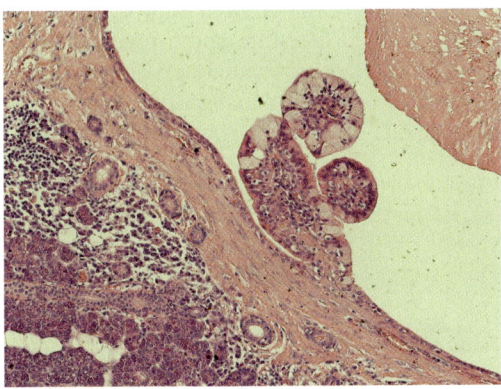

Fig. 4.12
Mucoepidermoid carcinoma. Excision biopsy of the case in Fig. 4.11. Histology shows a mainly cystic mucoepidermoid tumour with only minimal papillary epithelial growth of tumour cells in the cyst wall

In separate studies, Sheahan et al. and Postema et al. showed that in the case of a carcinomatous mass when an adequate sample had been obtained, the most common cause for a false-negative result was a cystic neoplasm [18, 19]. Importantly, a close association between epithelium and lymphoid cells in Warthin's tumour is not to be confused with metastasis of a well-differentiated carcinoma (e.g. PTC) [20]. In order to avoid a false-positive diagnosis, immunocytochemistry for thyroglobulin and a radioiodine uptake scan may be advised. Results have to be interpreted critically because background debris and macrophages in Warthin's may show non-specific uptake of the antibody, which may look like colloid positivity, whereas the epithelium remains negative. Radioactive isotope uptake may also show false-positive findings [21]. In my experience, such cases are rare and usually arise when the anatomical site of the FNAC is not clearly defined.

4.1.6 Acinic Cell Carcinoma

ACC, papillary-cystic variant, often presents a diagnostic dilemma in salivary gland aspiration, resulting in a relatively high rate of false-negative diagnoses of this rare tumour. Morphological characteristics of this variant of acinic carcinoma in FNAC include tightly cohesive fragments of neoplastic epithelium, seen as monolayered sheets or with a prominent papillary architecture, a high N/C ratio, ductal-type epithelium, cystic material and degenerated cellular debris, histiocytes, cells with squamoid and metaplastic oncocytic changes, vacuolated and pigmented histiocyte-like tumour cells and lack of a predominantly single-cell component or naked neoplastic cell nuclei [22] (Figs. 4.13 and 4.14). An erroneous interpretation may occur due to lack of experience of this tumour subtype, the rarity of published literature and a predominantly cystic, somewhat variegated appearance mimicking other benign and malignant salivary gland lesions [22].

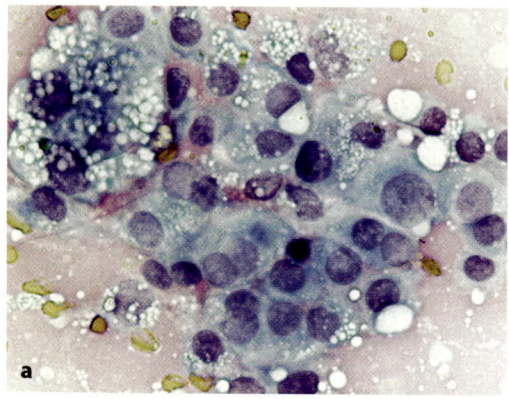

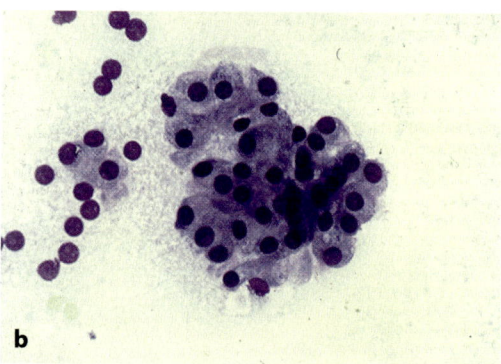

Fig. 4.14
Acinic cell carcinoma, **a** papillary-cystic variant; a higher-power view of the case shown in Fig. 4.13. The morphological characteristics of this variant of acinic carcinoma in FNAC include tightly cohesive fragments of neoplastic epithelium seen as monolayered sheets or with a prominent papillary architecture, a high N/C ratio, ductal-type epithelium, cystic material, degenerated cellular debris, histiocytes, cells with squamoid and metaplastic oncocytic changes, vacuolated and pigmented histiocyte-like tumour cells and lack of a predominantly single-cell component or naked neoplastic cell nuclei **b** Classic variant of acinic cell caricoma

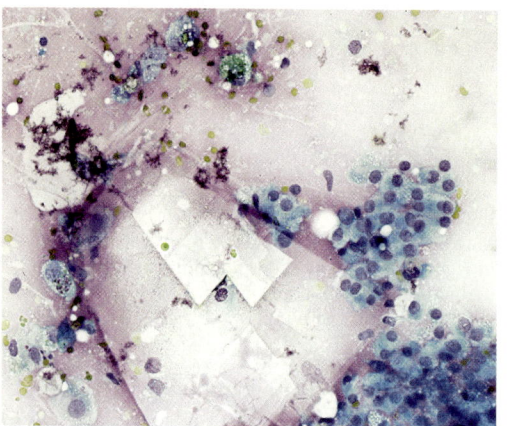

Fig. 4.13
Acinic-cell carcinoma, a papillary-cystic variant, often presents a diagnostic dilemma, the salivary gland aspiration resulting in a relatively high rate of false-negative diagnoses of this rare tumour. For a detailed view see Fig. 4.14. An erroneous interpretation may occur due to lack of experience of this tumour subtype, the rarity of published literature and a predominantly cystic, somewhat variegated appearance mimicking other benign and malignant salivary gland lesions

4.1.7 Pleomorphic Adenoma

Pleomorphic adenoma may, on occasion, also be cystic due to degeneration and/or haemorrhage within the tumour making the imaging diagnosis less accurate [23]. Cellular atypia (20.6%), cystic transformation (7%) and the presence of a cylindromatous pattern (5%) resembling adenoid cystic carcinoma are the most common cytological variations of pleomorphic adenoma that sometime cause diagnostic difficulties [24] (Figs. 4.15–4.17). FNAC of a low-grade papillary adenocarcinoma of minor salivary gland origin exhibits geographic sheets and papillary groups of epithelial cells (Figs. 4.18 and 4.19). Individual cells are medium sized, with scant cytoplasm, finely clumped chromatin and occasional prominent nucleoli. Pleomorphism is conspicuously absent. Differential diagnosis includes pleomorphic adenoma, basal cell adenoma, basal cell adenocarcinoma, low-grade mucoepidermoid carcinoma and metastatic papillary carcinoma [25].

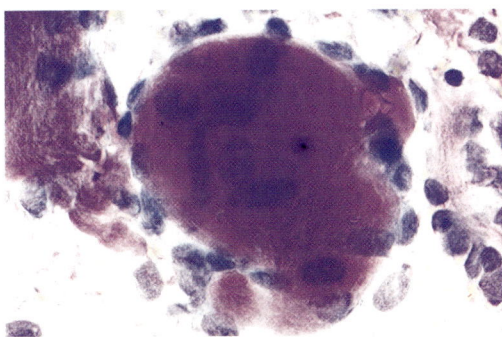

Fig. 4.16
Pleomorphic adenoma; the focal presence of a cylindromatous pattern may be observed. In this case, excision was advised and the histology revealed a pleomorphic adenoma (Fig. 4.17)

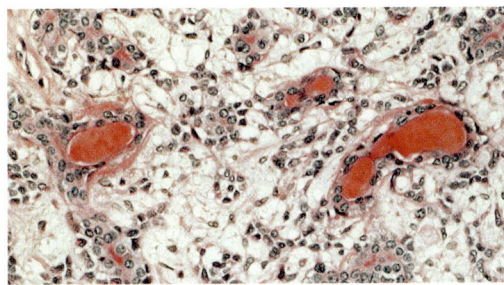

Fig. 4.17
Pleomorphic adenoma. Histological section of a case from Fig. 4.16 showing focal cylidromatous pattern in a pleomorphic adenoma. This feature does not imply different behaviour

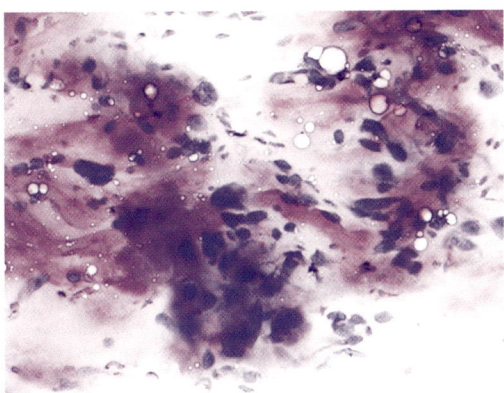

Fig. 4.15
Pleomorphic adenoma may on occasion exhibit cellular atypia, cystic transformation and the presence of a cylindromatous pattern, resembling that seen in adenoid cystic carcinoma, sometimes causing diagnostic difficulties

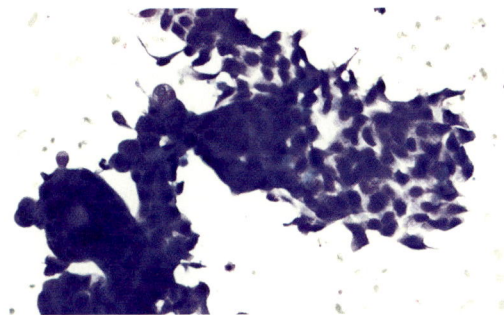

Fig. 4.18
Low-grade papillary adenocarcinoma of minor salivary gland origin exhibiting geographic sheets and papillary groups of epithelial cells. Differential diagnosis includes pleomorphic adenoma, basal cell adenoma, basal cell adenocarcinoma, low-grade mucoepidermoid carcinoma and metastatic papillary carcinoma. See Fig. 4.19 for details of the cellular features

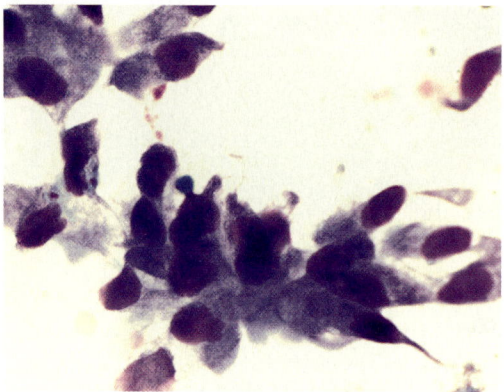

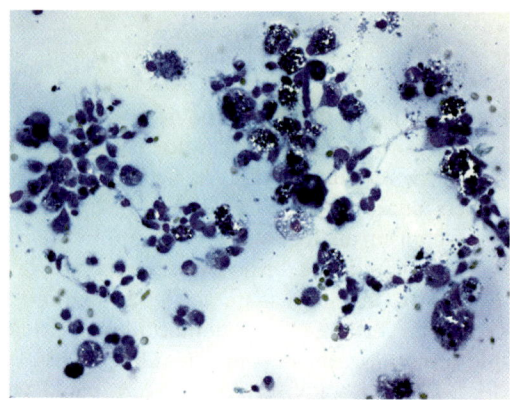

Fig. 4.19
Low-grade papillary adenocarcinoma of minor salivary gland origin. Higher magnification of cells from the case shown in Fig. 4.18 showing that the individual cells are medium sized, with scant cytoplasm, finely clumped chromatin and occasional prominent nucleoli. Pleomorphism is conspicuously absent

Fig. 4.20
Thyroid cyst. Thyroid gland FNAC most commonly contains cyst fluid as part of the degenerative process in colloid goitre. Fluid is usually haemorrhagic and contains sparse follicular epithelium

4.1.8 Dermoid Cyst

The cytological features of dermoid cyst of the parotid gland and the value of preoperative diagnosis by FNAC have been described by Baschinsky [26]. Dermoid cysts are freely mobile, painless parotid masses that appear cystic on a CT scan. FNAC shows anucleated and nucleated squamous epithelium and keratin debris. The clinical features and cytological findings are consistent with a dermoid cyst.

4.1.9 Thyroid Cysts

Thyroid cysts usually do not create diagnostic problems, except if found outside the normal anatomical confines of the gland (e.g. in the anterior or posterior triangle). In these cases, metastasis from a well-differentiated thyroid carcinoma has to be considered. Thyroid gland FNAC most commonly contains cyst fluid as part of the degenerative process in colloid goitre. Fluid is usually haemorrhagic and contains sparse follicular epithelium (Fig. 4.20).

Squamous metaplasia of thyroid follicular epithelium is known to occur in a variety of non-neoplastic lesions as well as in thyroid neoplasms, notably PTC (Fig. 4.21). It is rare in follicular thyroid tumours. FNAC from the cystic areas may yield only necrotic material and squamous cells that, being mostly of immature type, may not be recognised as squamous in the cytological smears. If the needle misses the solid (neoplastic) component of the lesion, the cytological picture may be considered equivocal [27].

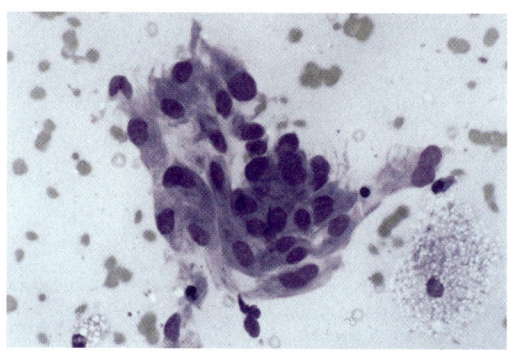

Fig. 4.21
Thyroid cyst. Squamous metaplasia of thyroid follicular epithelium is known to occur in a variety of non-neoplastic lesions as well as in thyroid neoplasms, notably papillary carcinoma

PTC may also present as a cystic lesion that contains growth within its walls, which on ultrasound may sometimes be seen as a complex cyst. The appearance of follicular epithelium floating in the fluid may be deceptively different from those found in the solid type (Fig. 4.22). Three-dimensional cell groups as well as scalloping of the cytoplasm are helpful if nuclear features (e.g. nuclear grooves and intracytoplasmic nuclear inclusions) are not seen. Cystic papillary carcinoma may present as a neck metastasis, in which case distinction needs to be made from Warthin's tumour, as discussed previously (see Fig. 4.9). Immunocytochemistry for thyroglobulin may prove helpful (Fig. 4.23)

Case history 4.5: A 27-year-old patient with a history of mantle-zone irradiation for Hodgkin's disease (HD) 15 years ago, presented with a lump in the neck, which on FNAC proved to be cystic. Cytology showed macrophages and sparse bland follicular epithelium (Fig. 4.24). FNAC of the thyroid gland showed no evidence of malignancy. The diagnostic and management dilemma was whether or not the patient had a metastatic PTC. To date, no histology from the neck is available and the clinicians adopted a watch and see policy to monitor the patient.

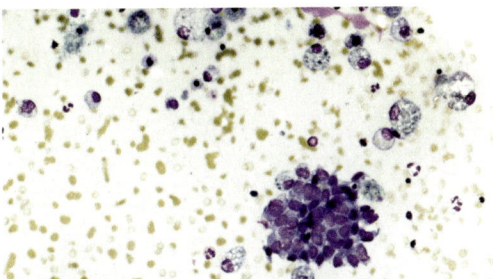

Fig. 4.22
Papillary carcinoma. Papillary carcinoma of the thyroid may also present as a cystic lesion that contains growth within its wall, which sometimes may be seen as a complex cyst on the ultrasound. The appearances of follicular epithelium floating in the fluid may be deceptively different from those found in the solid type

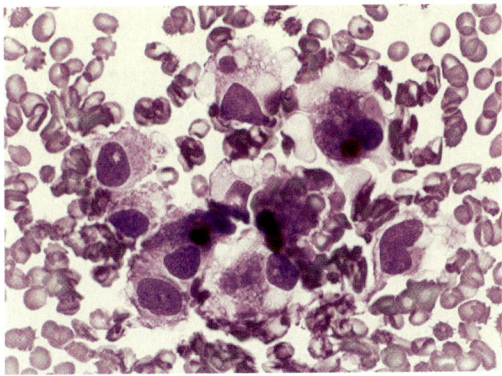

Fig. 4.24
FNAC neck node distant from the thyroid. Macrophages and colloid are present, suggesting a metastasis from a papillary carcinoma. No epithelium is seen

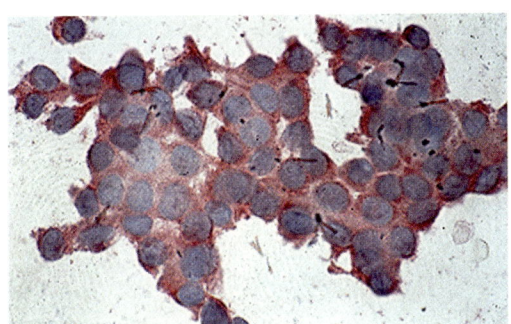

Fig. 4.23
Papillary carcinoma, metastasis, antithyroglobulin staining. Cystic papillary carcinoma may present as a neck metastasis, in which case distinction needs to be made from Warthin's tumour. Immunocytochemistry for thyroglobulin may prove helpful

Seven et al. showed that nearly one out of every ten lateral cervical cysts in young adult patients represents lymphatic metastases from occult thyroid carcinoma. They suggested that in these cases an excisional biopsy for definitive diagnosis should be undertaken without prolonged delay, even if FNAC does not reveal malignancy [28]. Even when using ultrasound-guided FNAC, Lin and Huang diagnosed (only) 4 out of the 19 patients with cystic papillary thyroid carcinoma [29]. Papotti et al. report that galectin-3 immunostaining can be used as a valid preoperative adjunct in those cases where a very poor number of epithelial cells may lead to a cytological misdiagnosis (Fig. 4.25). They suggest the use of the antibody in poorly cellular FNAC samples of simple or complex thyroid cysts, galectin-3 expression by epithelial cells being consistent with a cystic carcinoma [30]. However, despite the low rate of accurate diagnoses for the cystic malignancy, clinical staging and the survival rates are not statistically different when cystic papillary carcinoma is compared with the other groups [29].

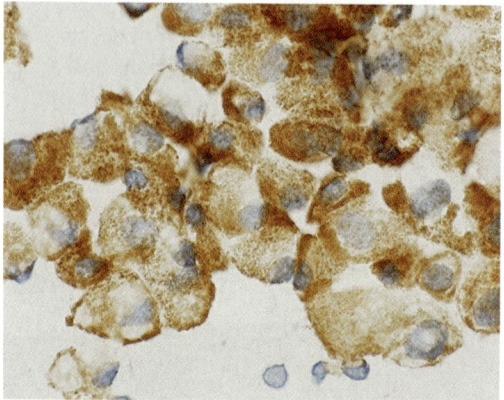

Fig. 4.25
Papillary carcinoma. Positive galectin 3 positivity may help diagnose this tumour when it presents in an unusual site

4.1.10 The Lymph Nodes

Lymph nodes in the neck may undergo cystic degeneration (e.g. in the case of specific infections). Fluid obtained is usually thick and yellow. A culture needs to be sent for microbiology analysis (Fig. 4.26). FNAC diagnosis of toxoplasma lymphadenitis with demonstration of a cyst containing bradyzoites can be made. Smears show features of reactive lymphoid hyperplasia, including tingible body macrophages and groups of epithelioid histiocytes. Bradyzoites may be demonstrated in a Pap-stained smear. Serology reveals a high titre of IgG and the presence of IgM-specific antibodies to Toxoplasma gondii, indicating active/recent disease [31].

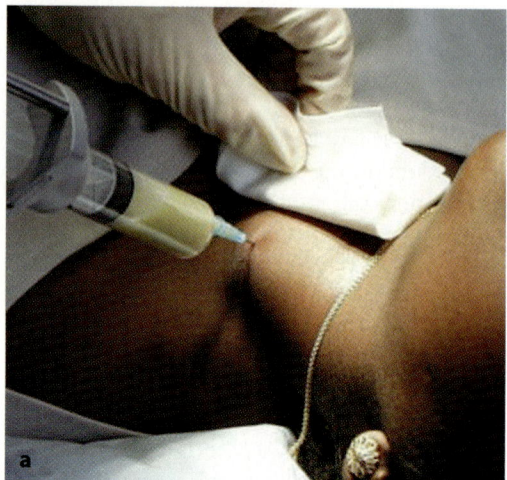
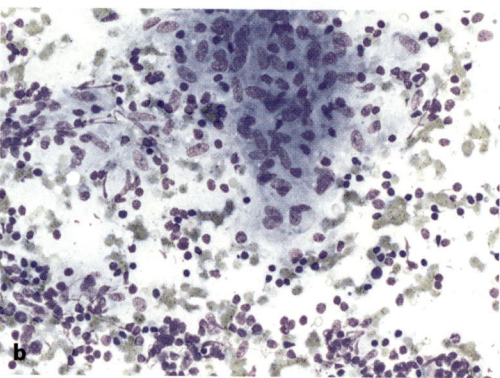
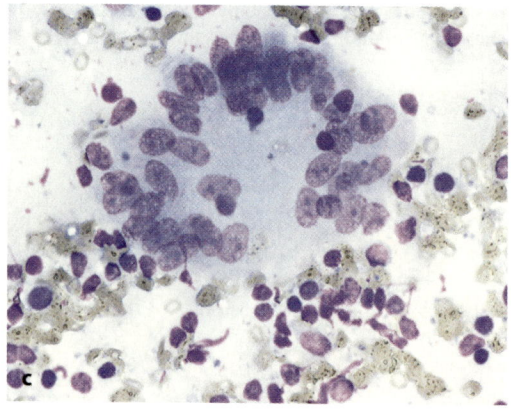

Fig. 4.26
Tuberculous lymphadenitis. **a** FNAC of a neck mass yielded thick yellow fluid. **b** Smears contain aggregates of epithelioid cells forming granulmata. **c** Langhans-type giant cells are present. Necrosis was seen in other parts of the smear

Lymph-node metastases may undergo degeneration and necrosis and appear cystic, as described earlier for SqCC, papillary carcinoma and melanoma.

> **Case history 4.6:** A 23-year-old HIV-positive male patient presented with a bilateral painless parotid swelling of several weeks duration. Clinically, it did not fluctuate in size and was soft and ill-defined. This was suspected non-Hodgkin lymphoma or specific infection. FNAC yielded 15 ml of turbid fluid. Cytospin preparations showed a mixture of lymphoid cells, with prominence of centroblasts, macrophages and attenuated epithelial cells. Lymphoepithelial cyst was diagnosed. There was no evidence of lymphoma or specific infection (Fig. 4.27).

4.1.11 Parathyroid Cysts

Parathyroid cysts are rare. Only about 200 cases have been reported to date. They arise from remnants of the pharyngeal pouch or as a result of cystic degeneration of a parathyroid adenoma. Two types of parathyroid cysts have been recognised: the non-functioning or essential forms, which occur more frequently, and the adenomatous or functioning parathyroid cysts, which are rarer and cause hyperparathyroidism. The diagnosis of a parathyroid cyst is difficult, particularly in its differentiation from thyroid cyst (Fig. 4.28). It has clinical significance because parathyroid cysts can mimic a thyroid mass and can be associated with hyperparathyroidism. The FNAC of the five parathyroid cysts described by Absher et al. yielded virtually acellular fluid with a characteristic water-clear appearance [32]. The preoperative diagnosis is best done by assaying parathyroid hormone levels in the cystic fluid, obtained by FNAC, and correlating these values with serum levels of the hormone [33, 24]. Parathyroid cysts should be in the differential diagnosis in any patient initially seen with an anterior cystic neck mass. Radiological imaging and FNAC can be used to accurately diagnose parathyroid cysts. Surgical excision may be needed for cysts that recur after FNAC [35, 36].

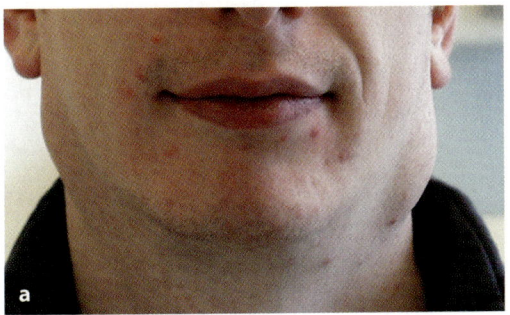

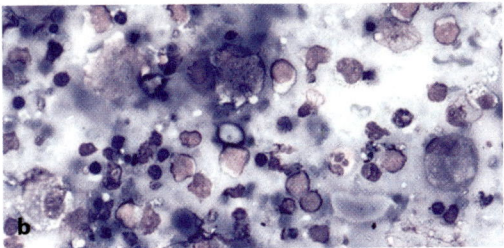

Fig. 4.27
a Lymphoepithelial cyst. A 23-year-old HIV-positive male patient presented with a bilateral painless parotid swelling of several weeks duration. Clinically, it did not fluctuate in size, and was soft and ill-defined. Clinically, the suspicion was that of a NHL or specific infection. FNAC yielded 15 ml of turbid fluid b Cytospin preparations show a mixture of lymphoid cells, with prominence of centroblasts, macrophages and attenuated epithelial cells. There is no evidence of lymphoma or specific infection

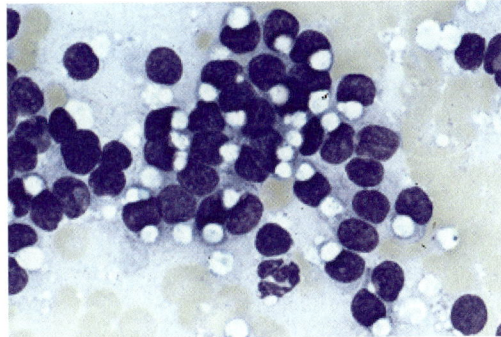

Fig. 4.28
Parathyroid cyst. The diagnosis of a parathyroid cyst is difficult, particularly in its differentiation from thyroid cysts. Cells are monotonous with cytoplasmic vacuolation

4.1.12 Cysts of the Jaw

FNAC material from the cysts of the jaw is seen infrequently, most lesions being managed surgically, based on the imaging. Of all odontogenic cysts in the jaw, the radicular cyst is the most common (Fig. 4.29), followed by dentigerous cysts and keratocysts (Fig. 3.18). Although it is a rare event, odontogenic tumours such as ameloblastoma, ameloblastic fibroma, ameloblastic fibro-odontoma, and odontoma have been reported associated with calcifying odontogenic cyst [37] (Fig. 4.30). Goldenberg et al. have found only nine malignant odontogenic tumours in 22 years: four cases of malignant ameloblastomas, two cases of ameloblastic carcinoma, one case of malignant Pindborg tumour (calcifying epithelial odontogenic tumour), one case of odontogenic ghost cell carcinoma and one case of SqCC arising in an odontogenic keratocyst [38]. Potentially aggressive lesions such as odontogenic keratocysts and cystic ameloblastomas need special diagnostic consideration [39]. Immunohistochemical staining may be necessary to distinguish the odontogenic keratocyst entity from other cystic lesions of the jaw, and aggressive surgical management is required [40]. Differences between the immunohistochemical expression of tenascin, fibronectin and collagen IV might indicate a more aggressive biological behaviour of some keratocysts [41]. Glandular odontogenic cyst is a separate entity that should be separated from the other types of odontogenic cyst and central mucoepidermoid tumours of salivary gland origin [42].

4.1.13 Teratoid Cyst

The term teratoid cyst was first used by Meyer in his classification of dysontogenetic cysts of the cervicofacial region, which was based on the type of germinative layers included in the cyst wall. Sublingual location of a dermoid cyst is not common, with an incidence of 1.6%. The teratoid cyst is the least common, accounting for 1.8% of sublingual dermoid cysts. FNAC shows sheets

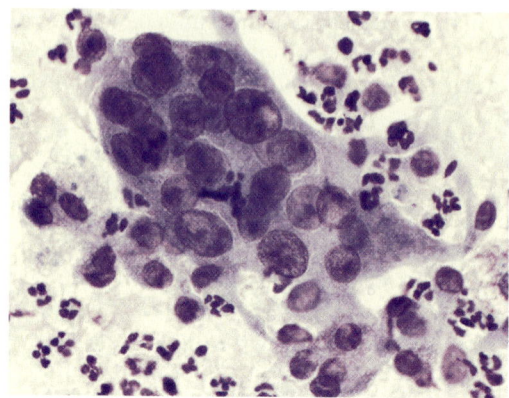

Fig. 4.29
Radicular cyst. Numerous polymporphs, histiocytes and osteoclast-type giant cells are present. No epithelium is seen

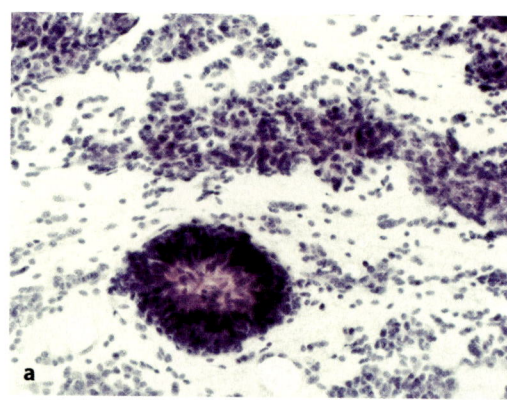

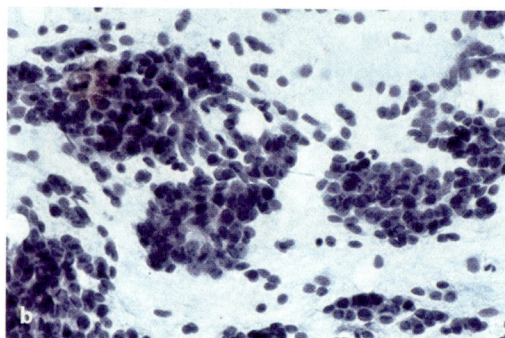

Fig. 4.30
Ameloblastoma. a Potentially aggressive lesions such as odontogenic keratocysts and cystic ameloblastomas need special diagnostic consideration. Immunohistochemical staining may be necessary to distinguish the odontogenic keratocyst entity from other cystic lesions of the jaw, and aggressive surgical management is required
b High power view of ameloblastoma cells.

of large, benign-appearing, anucleated and nucleated squamous cells, several neutrophils and no atypical cells [43]. Histopathological examination shows the presence of skin appendages along with mature cartilage and respiratory epithelium, confirming the diagnosis of a teratoid cyst. FNAC might be valuable for the diagnosis of lesions occurring in this anatomical location. Other lesions that may present as cysts in the head and neck are schwannoma (benign nerve sheath tumour), haemangioma, lymphangioma and lipoma (Fig. 4.31) [44]. Cavernous haemangioma is a benign congenital vascular malformation that occasionally affects the thyroid [45]. Juvenile haemangioendothelioma, mimicking a spindle-cell neoplasm of the parotid has been described in a 4-month-old child [46]. FNAC of lymphangioma consists predominantly of a uniform population of small and round lymphocytes, centrocytes, centroblasts and histiocytes. The lesion is clearly circumscribed with a multilocular cystic appearance, yielding abundant yellowish liquid on FNAC. It very rarely occurs within the parotid gland [47–49].

4.2 Cysts in the Abdomen

Cystic lesions in the abdomen have always presented a diagnostic challenge for radiologists. With the increasing use of EUS-FNAC, cytopathologists are sharing some of the diagnostic difficulties associated with these lesions. Here, we shall discuss cystic lesions of the pancreas, liver, kidneys, adrenal glands and peritoneum.

4.2.1 Cystic Lesions of the Pancreas

Cystic tumours and tumour-like lesions of the pancreas are rare, but have attracted a great deal of attention because they are easily recognised with the new imaging methods. In contrast to ductal adenocarcinoma, they can usually be cured surgically. The increasing resection rate in recent years has also increased our knowledge of cystic pancreatic tumours by conspicuously enlarging their morphological spectrum. Known entities have been better characterised (i.e. solid pseudopapillary neoplasm – SPN, intraductal papillary mucinous neoplasm – IPMN) and new ones described (serous oligocystic adenoma, mucinous non-neoplastic cyst, acinar cell cystadenoma and cystic hamartoma) [50]. Apart from cystic pancreatic tumours and pseudocysts, cystic lesions of the pancreas also include congenital cysts, acquired cysts, extrapancreatic cysts and cystic degeneration of solid tumours (Fig. 4.32). The classification of cystic pancreatic lesions proposed by Kosmahl distinguishes between neoplastic and non-neoplastic lesions, with further subdivisions into epithelial (adenomas, borderline neoplasms and carcinomas) and non-epithelial tumours [51].

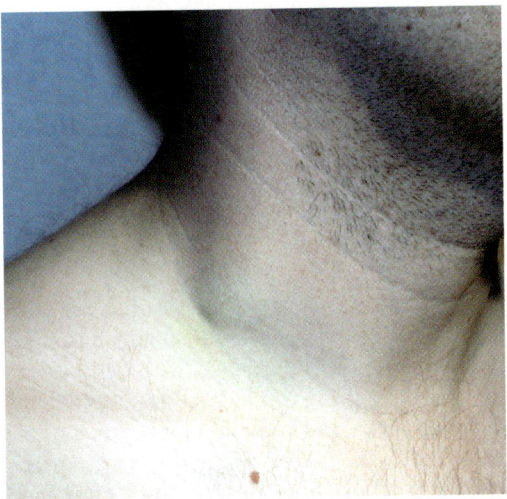

Fig. 4.31
Haemangioma. Careful examination of the patient revealed a bluish nodule. The patient had a history of changes in the size and colour of the lesion. FNAC yielded blood and very few endothelial cells

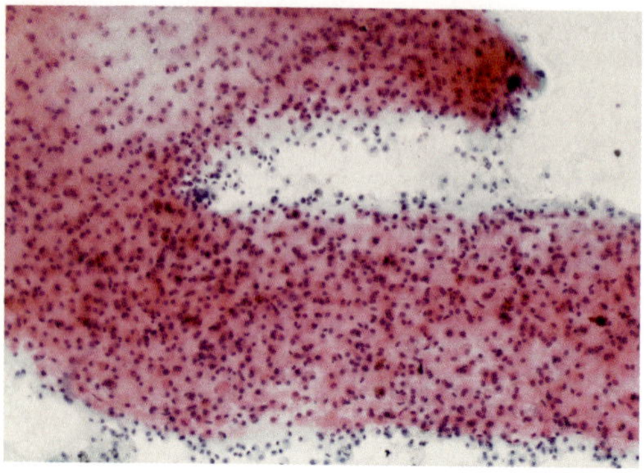

Fig. 4.32
Pseudocyst of the pancreas. Cyst fluid consists entirely of macrophages. It may also contain inflammatory cells. A finding of necrosis and inflammation should raise the suspicion of an underlying tumour

EUS imaging criteria of an indolent pancreatic cystic lesion include a clear thin wall, smooth contour, round or oval shape, no septum or nodules, asymptomatic clinical presentation and no findings of chronic pancreatitis [52]. However, the sensitivity, specificity, positive predictive value and negative predictive value of EUS imaging compared with the EUS-FNAC method to indicate whether a lesion needed further surgery were 71 and 97%, 30 and 100%, 49 and 100%, and 40 and 95%, respectively [53]. This confirms that the information gathered from clinical history and EUS, complemented by fluid analysis after EUS-FNAC, predicts neoplastic pancreatic cysts and assists in decision-making for the medical or surgical approach [54].

EUS-FNAC is particularly useful in the preoperative cytodiagnosis of pancreatic tumours of low malignant potential. It extends the indication for organ-preserving pancreatic resections and avoids the unnecessary sacrifice of adjacent organs [55]. Clinical signs are not really useful in the clinical work-up since most patients have no symptoms. FNAC and anthracitic fluid tumour marker levels are very useful despite the pitfalls. Good cooperation between surgeons, pathologists, radiologists and gastroenterologists is mandatory to increase the chances of making a proper diagnosis. Age, sex, clinical history, location of the tumour and radiological features are all important in order to avoid the mistake of treating a cystic neoplasm as a benign lesion or as a pseudocyst. Surgical treatment differs with the diagnosis and may be avoided in some cases. The role of diagnosis is central in the treatment of these tumours because the surgery could be curative when complete resection is possible [56].

Cystic tumours of the pancreas are classified into two different types: benign (with glycogen-rich, serous cells) and mucinous cystic neoplasms (with overt and latent malignancy). Serous cystadenomas, mucinous cystadenoma, cystadenocarcinoma, solid/cystic papillary neoplasm, intraductal papillary mucinous tumour, mucinous adenocarcinoma and neuroendocrine tumours are all, or can be, at least partly cystic [56–58].

Mucinous varieties of cystic pancreatic tumours (mucinous cystic neoplasms and intraductal papillary mucinous tumours) are pre-malignant or malignant, and surgical resection is generally recommended in good operative candidates (Figs. 4.33 and 4.34). In contrast, non-mucinous tumours include serous cystadenomas with a very low malignant potential, or pseudocysts, which are always benign. As a result, non-mucinous cystic lesions are generally resected only when inducing symptoms or complications. Management decisions are usually based on the combined results of laboratory, imaging and clinical findings [59]. When comparing the results of EUS, cyst fluid cytology, and cyst fluid tumour markers (carcinoembryonic antigen – CEA, CA 72-4, CA 125, CA 19-9 and CA 15-3), Brugge et al. concluded that the accuracy of cyst fluid CEA (79%) makes it the best test available for differentiating between mucinous and non-mucinous lesions of the pancreas [60]. Values for CA 125 are high in all malignant cysts, low in pseudocysts and variable in mucinous cystic neoplasms and serous cystadenomas. Levels of CA 19-9 are non-discriminatory. Cyst fluid amylase and lipase content are variable but are generally high in pseudocysts and low in cystic tumours. Amylase isoenzyme analysis is useful to differentiate pseudocysts from cystic tumours. Measurement of the relative viscosity in cyst fluid showed high (>serum viscosity) values in 89% of mucinous tumours and low values (<serum) in all pseudocysts and serous cystadenomas [61].

Diagnostic Dilemmas in FNAC Practice: Cystic Lesions   Chapter 4   75

The combination of viscosity, CEA, CA 125 and FNAC can reliably distinguish malignant cystic tumours and potentially pre-malignant mucinous cystic neoplasms from pseudocysts and serous cystadenomas. Amylase content with isoenzyme analysis is useful for the identification of pseudocysts [61].

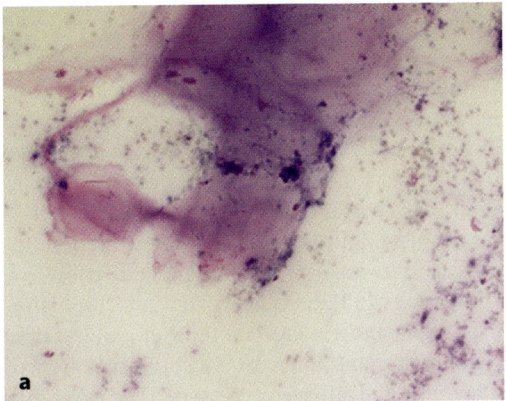

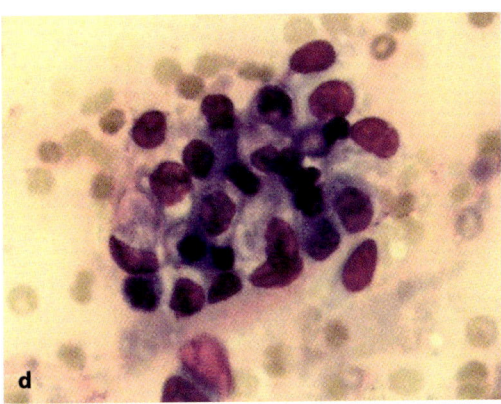

Fig. 4.33
FNAC pancreas. Mucinous cystadenoma. **a** Low-power view revealing pools of eosinophilic material with sparse macrophages present. **b** Pap staining does not show the background material so well, but shows crisper cellular detail of epithelial clusters. **c** Higher-power view of the bland, monotonous, mucin-secreting epithelium. **d** Pas-d staining confirms the presence of mucin

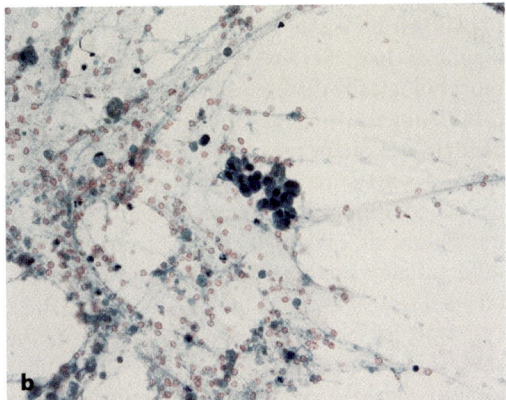

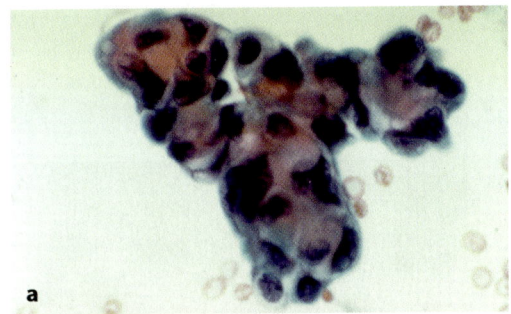

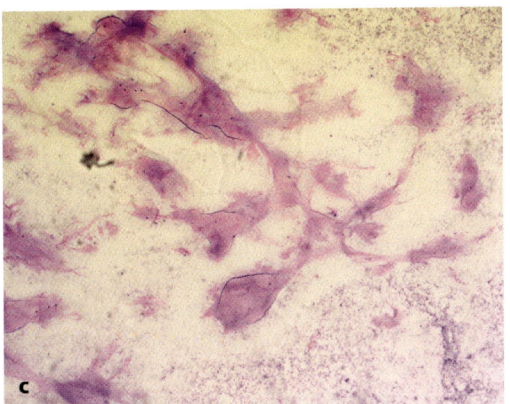

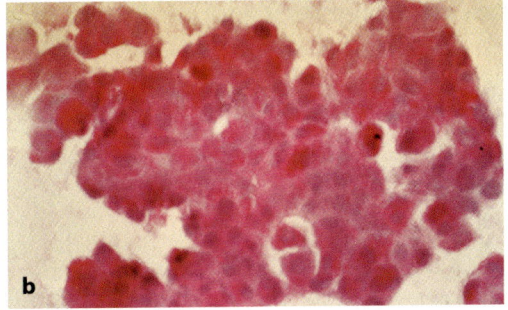

Fig. 4.34
FNAC pancreas. Mucinous carcinoma. **a** Cell clusters are sparse and usually found in a pool of mucinous and necrotic background with macrophages (MGG) **b** PAS-d staining demonstrates the presence of intracytoplasmic mucin and confirms the epithelial nature of the cells

Case history 4.7: FNAC performed on a young woman who presented with a mass in the left hypochondrium yielded fluid. Smears and Cytospin preparations of the fluid showed good cellularity, consisting of relatively monomorphic cells forming a perivascular papillary pattern. FNAC thus suggested a diagnosis of papillary cystic neoplasm of the pancreas. Surgical removal of the pancreatic tumour and detailed histological study confirmed the cytological diagnosis (Fig. 4.35) [62].

Fig. 4.35
FNAC pancreas. Papillary solid and cystic carcinoma. **a** Variable numbers of branching fragments with central capillaries and myxoid stroma. **b** Higher-power view demonstrating epithelial cells with a relatively bland appearance, eccentic nuclei with nuclear grooves and a well defined cytoplasm. Extensive necrosis may be present and mitotic figures may be seen. **c** Resection specimen reveals a cystic tumour with central necrosis and haemorrhage

Serous cystic neoplasms of the pancreas include serous microcystic adenoma, serous oligocystic ill-demarcated adenoma, solid serous adenoma, von Hippel-Lindau-associated cystic neoplasm and serous cystadenocarcinoma. These neoplasms are histologically similar but differ in their localisation, gross appearance, gender distribution, and biology [63]. Serous microcystic cystadenoma of the pancreas is a rare tumour and has little or no malignant potential. Most patients are women with a mean age of 59 years. The cysts may cause symptoms and may need to be resected. FNAC can be useful for making a preoperative diagnosis [64]. Serous cystadenoma is usually morphologically distinguishable from mucinous cystadenoma, which requires resection because of their malignant potential. A macrocystic variant of serous cystadenoma has recently been described, rendering this important distinction more difficult. Helpful EUS characteristics that differentiate mucinous cystadenoma from macrocystic serous cystadenoma include a thick cyst wall in the former and microcysts in the latter [65]. Neuron-specific enolase (NSE) alpha-inhibin and MUC6, are being described as new markers for serous cystic neoplasms [63].

Tumours of the pancreas associated with extracellular mucin production include mucin-producing ductal adenocarcinoma, mucinous cystic neoplasms and IPMN. FNAC findings for mucinous ductal adenocarcinoma include moderate to high cellularity, mild to moderate background mucin, three-dimensional clusters, a high N/C ratio and mild to moderate nuclear membrane irregularities (Fig. 4.34). Cytological features of low-grade mucinous tumours include mild to moderate cellularity, abundant background mucin, small clusters and flat sheets of relatively bland glandular cells (Fig. 4.33). IPMN

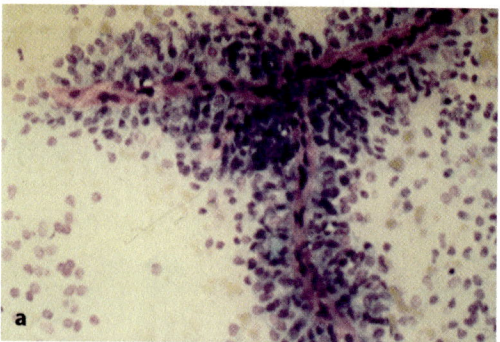
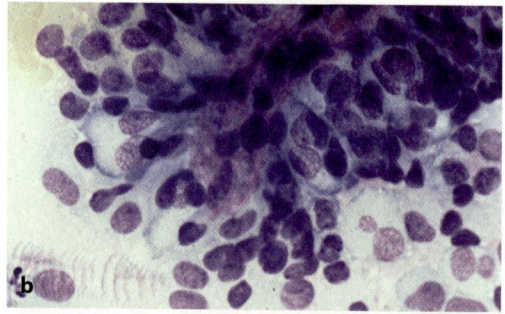
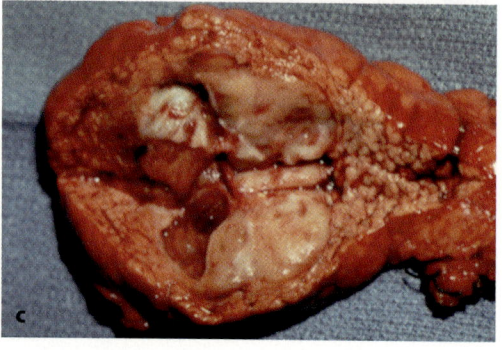

represents a new type of cystic tumour that has been described in detail in recent years. It typically grows for a long time within the ducts, before approximately 50% of them eventually become invasive, a feature that distinguishes IPMNs from ductal adenocarcinomas. IPMNs are currently the most commonly resected cystic tumour of the pancreas. Recent studies have shown that IPMNs may be distinguished into different types that exhibit a different biology according to their mucin pattern [66]. FNAC findings of IPMNs include moderate to high cellularity, abundant background mucin and prominent papillary arrangement of tall columnar cells with mild to moderate nuclear atypia. Recine et al. consider that IPMN and low-grade mucinous neoplasms possess distinctive cytological features that can be used to diagnose them correctly and distinguish them from one another and from other cystic tumours [67]. Duplication cysts closely mimic low-grade mucinous tumours, which may lead to false-positive diagnoses. Because of the substantial overlap in cytological features, mucin-producing ductal adenocarcinomas are difficult to distinguish cytologically from mucinous cystadenocarcinomas [67].

SPNs of the pancreas represent a special tumour entity, both morphologically and biologically. They form large solitary tumours that occur predominantly in young women. Histologically, they show solid, pseudopapillary and pseudocystic patterns. FNAC shows variable numbers of branching fragments with central capillaries and myxoid stroma (Fig. 4.35). The cells have bland nuclear features and rare grooves. Extensive necrosis may be present and mitotic figures may be seen. The tumour shows immunoreactivity for vimentin and focal weak keratin reactivity and is strongly positive for NSE, alpha1-antitrypsin and alpha1-antichymotrypsin stains [68–70]. Complete resection cures the tumour in about 90% of cases. However, because recurrences and even metastases may occur in a small number of cases, it is classified as a low-grade malignant tumour. The most important differential diagnosis to consider is neuroendocrine tumour of the pancreas [71]. Mucinous non-neoplastic cyst, acinar cell cystadenoma and cystic hamartoma are also newly described rare pancreatic lesions that may represent differential diagnoses of cystic lesions [72–75]. To date, the cytological features of these lesions have not been described.

Lymphoepithelial cyst of the pancreas is an extremely rare benign entity. It is a rare, true cyst of uncertain histogenesis that may clinically and radiologically mimic a pseudocyst or cystic neoplasm. FNAC yields paste-like yellow/grey material. Cytology includes a mixture of squamous epithelial cells, anucleate squames and keratinous debris. Unlike a similar cyst of the head and neck region, only rare lymphocytes and histiocytes are present, including multinucleated histiocytes. The histology shows a multiloculated cystic lesion with a stratified squamous epithelial lining surrounded by well-formed lymphoid tissue. The differential diagnosis includes other pancreatic pseudocysts, dermoid cyst, mucinous cystic neoplasms, adenosquamous carcinoma and metastatic SqCC [76–80].

Soft-tissue tumours occurring in the pancreas may also present as cystic lesions. Benign tumours comprise lymphangiomas, haemangiomas, schwannomas, solitary fibrous tumours, adenomatoid tumours, clear-cell tumours and hamartomas. Malignant mesenchymal tumours include leiomyosarcomas, malignant peripheral nerve sheath tumours, liposarcomas, malignant fibrous histiocytomas, Ewing's sarcomas and primitive neuroectodermal tumours, all of which may undergo central necrosis [81].

4.2.2 Cystic Lesions of the Liver

FNAC is only moderately successful in preoperatively separating neoplastic from non-neoplastic (inflammatory and congenital) liver cysts (sensitivity of 66%, specificity of 100%). CEA measurements on the supernatant gave a sensitivity of 100% and a specificity of 94%, thus enhancing the sensitivity of FNAC for the detection of malignancy in cystic liver lesions [82–83]. Shariff et al., practicing in India, found that cystic lesions in the liver were being diagnosed as either abscesses, hydatid cysts or congenital cysts. The physical appearance of the cyst fluid proved to be of diagnostic value in many cases [84]. FNAC assisted by cell-block examination is also useful for distinguishing between primary benign and malignant liver masses and for confirmation of tumours metastatic to the liver, all of which may be partly cystic [85]. Selection of EUS-FNAC over percutaneous biopsy is usually based on a decreased risk of bleeding (coagulopathy, cirrhosis, ascites, aspirin intake), the presence of small liver tumours (<2 cm) or liver lesions found incidentally [86].

Das et al. aspirated eight cases of hydatid cysts (the Greek word *hydatid* meaning a drop of water) in the liver, kidney, lung and mediastinum. FNAC yielded clear or turbid fluid containing a laminated cyst wall, scolices and hooklets in various ratios (Fig. 4.36). Laminated cyst walls exhibit a positive PAS reaction. An inflammatory and granulomatous cell reaction was also noted in some cases. There were no untoward allergic reactions following FNAC [87, 88].

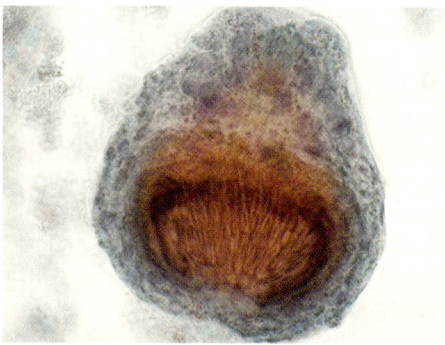

Fig. 4.36
FNAC liver. Hydatid cyst. Scolex (head) of *Echinococcus granulosus* has a distinctive structure with four sucking discs and a circle of hooklets. Hydatid sand found in the cyst fluid consists of scolices from ruptured brood capsules

4.2.3 Adrenal and Renal Cystic Lesions

Adrenal vascular cysts are rare lesions that might be considered in the differential diagnosis of adrenal tumours. Touch imprints of excised lesions show groups of spindle cells with elongated nuclei, without atypia. Histologically, the lesion is well-delineated by a fibrous capsule that contains numerous cystic spaces and is lined by endothelial cells and filled with erythrocytes, fibrin thrombi and necrotic debris. Immunohistochemical analysis shows strong positivity for factor VIII-RA, CD31 and CD34 [89]. Haemorrhagic adrenal pseudocysts are uncommon non-neoplastic lesions that have been reported as secondary to intraparenchymal haemorrhage or, alternatively, related to endothelial (vascular) cysts. Ultrastructural and immunohistochemical evidence in support of the latter have been presented, but the exact nature of haemorrhagic adrenal pseudocysts remains poorly defined. FNAC of adrenal haemorrhagic pseudocysts may be bloodstained and inconclusive. There may be a history of FNAC prior to a diagnosis of adrenal pseudocyst on surgical resection. The presence of papillary endothelial hyperplasia and immunohistochemical findings support the theory that adrenal pseudocysts are post-haemorrhagic and derive from vascular disruption. Furthermore, FNAC or other interventional studies may be associated with papillary endothelial hyperplasia in haemorrhagic adrenal pseudocysts [90]. Metastatic tumours of the adrenal gland may present as cystic lesions.

The fluid from the benign renal cysts shows macrophages, epithelial cells from the cyst lining, tubular cells, neutrophils and Liesegang rings. Fluid from the acquired cystic kidney and the cystic renal cell carcinoma may show features similar to those of benign cysts. Atypical epithelial cell clusters may be seen in low-grade renal cell carcinomas and a simple benign cyst with many tubular cells. Cytologically malignant lesions include cystic renal cell carcinomas with abundant tumour cells, partially clear cytoplasm and atypical nuclei admixed with abundant macrophages and lymphocytes. Simple cysts remain the most frequently aspirated renal lesions, but complex cystic lesions are being increasingly recognised. Since many renal cysts are composed of independent loculi, a non-representative sample is a potential problem, and radiological correlation becomes mandatory [91]. Brierly et al. recommend FNAC of renal masses particularly for the diagnosis of small (<5 cm) tumours or renal cysts. The sensitivity is reported to be 89% for large (<5 cm) solid masses, 64% for small (<5 cm) solid masses and 50% for complex cysts

[92]. Differential diagnosis of benign renal cysts includes acquired cystic kidney and cystic renal-cell carcinoma. Other rare lesions with characteristic FNAC that can be distinguished from benign cysts and renal-cell carcinoma include angiomyolipoma, multilocular cystic nephroma, adult polycystic kidneys, acquired cystic kidney and cystic papillary renal-cell carcinoma. Apart from the renal-cell carcinoma, other malignant lesions seen in FNAC kidney include transitional-cell carcinoma, lymphoma, small-cell undifferentiated carcinoma and metastatic carcinoma. As mentioned earlier, for the diagnosis of cystic lesions, cytological-radiographic correlation is needed to avoid misinterpretation [93].

Cystic papillary renal cell carcinoma may contain abundant intracytoplasmic haemosiderin in both histiocytes and neoplastic cells and therefore present as a diagnostic pitfall in FNAC and its distinction from a haemorrhagic cyst and benign tubular epithelium, which may also contain haemosiderin. Cystic papillary renal-cell carcinoma is usually a low-grade neoplasm and is associated with cystic degeneration, haemorrhage and presence of abundant haemosiderin-laden macrophages. Papillary epithelial cell features should be helpful, but differentiation of haemosiderin-laden macrophages from neoplastic cells with massive intracytoplasmic haemosiderin may be difficult, especially when epithelial fragments are scanty [94].

4.2.4 Cystic Lesions of the Peritoneum

Benign cystic mesothelioma is an uncommon lesion of the peritoneum that occurs predominantly in women of reproductive age. Abdominal ultrasonography and CT show a well-defined cystic mass with a solid papillary projection in its lumen. FNAC specimens show a monomorphous population of mesothelial cells without cytological atypia, arranged in three patterns: monolayered sheets, single cells and two-cell-thick strands of mesothelial cells with little or no intervening stroma. The background is clean and without necrotic debris or abundant inflammatory cells. Mesothelial cells are not arranged in prominent papillary formations; mitotic figures are not found. The mesothelial cells are positive for cytokeratin, calretinin and vimentin, and negative for CEA and factor VIII. The FNAC findings should be distinguished from those of a variety of other abdominal lesions, including cystic lymphangioma, ovarian and primary peritoneal epithelial tumours, necrotic tumours with cystic degeneration, developmental cysts and infectious cysts [95]. Patients remain well and symptom-free after surgery [96–100].

Foregut duplication cysts may be diagnosed using EUS-FNAC. Microscopic examination of the cyst content reveals mucinous material and cellular debris, and may also show detached ciliary tufts. Electron microscopy may reveal both in routine cytological preparations and with EUS-FNAC. Thanks to EUS-FNAC-confirmed diagnoses of foregut duplication cysts, these patients do not need to undergo surgical resection [101].

4.3 Thoracic Cysts

Benign mediastinal cysts, which account for approximately 20% of mediastinal masses, may present a diagnostic challenge. Information regarding the use of EUS and EUS-FNAC in this setting is limited. Wildi et al. described 20 patients who underwent examinations for suspected mediastinal cysts, either as a follow-up of a known cyst or for a mediastinal mass of unknown origin. They conclude that EUS-FNAC provides a minimally invasive approach to the diagnosis of benign mediastinal cysts [102].

Multiloculated thymic cysts are uncommon lesions that can be either acquired or associated with malignancies. Primary thymic mucosa-associated lymphoid tissue lymphoma (MALT) should be considered as one of the differential diagnoses of anterior mediastinal tumours having multilocular cysts that arise in patients with immunological abnormalities (Fig. 4.37) [103]. Silverman reported a mediastinal seminoma with prominent cystic change [104]. FNAC revealed clusters of malignant oval- to polygonal-shaped cells with large oval nuclei possessing prominent nucleoli set in a pale-to-eosinophilic cytoplasm. These cells were surrounded by a dense lymphoid infiltrate along with a few non-caseating granulomas. The large malignant seminoma cells stained positive for placental alkaline phosphatase (PLAP) and negative for both low- and high-molecular-weight cytokeratin. Other germ cell tumours in the mediastinum may also present as cystic lesions due to the tumour necrosis (Fig. 4.38).

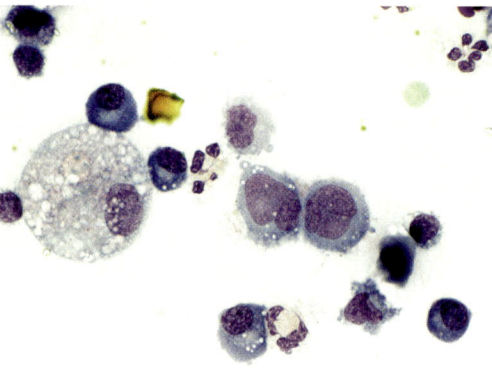

Fig. 4.37
FNAC mediastinum. Mucosa-associated lymphoid tissue (MALT) lymphoma. Primary thymic MALT lymphoma should be considered as one of the differential diagnoses of anterior mediastinal tumours having multilocular cysts that arise in patients with immunological abnormalities

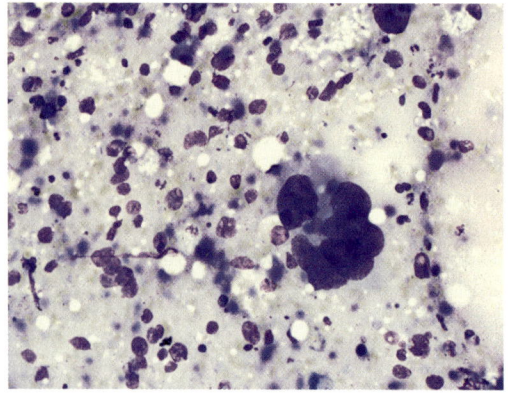

Fig. 4.38
FNAC mediastinum. Germ-cell tumour. Other germ cell tumours in the mediastinum may also present as a cystic lesion due to the tumour necrosis. Bizarrely shaped malignant cells are seen here against a background of necrosis, inflammation and cystic change

Solid and cystic thymoma with a high CA 125 content (35,532 μl/ml, as measured by enzyme immunoassay in the cyst fluid) may be diagnosed by FNAC (Fig. 4.39). The initial smears may contain scanty foam cells, lymphocytes and benign epithelial cells. In view of the discrepancy between the cytological diagnosis, a suspicious radiological appearance and high fluid CA 125 levels, FNAC of the solid portion of the mass may be performed. Smears/cell-block examination shows large, cohesive clusters of benign, spindle-shaped epithelial cells (keratin positive) admixed with mature lymphocytes diagnostic of thymoma. Pinto et al. point out the importance of sampling solid areas of solid/cystic tumours, rapid assessment of FNAC material and appropriate clinical and radiological correlation [105].

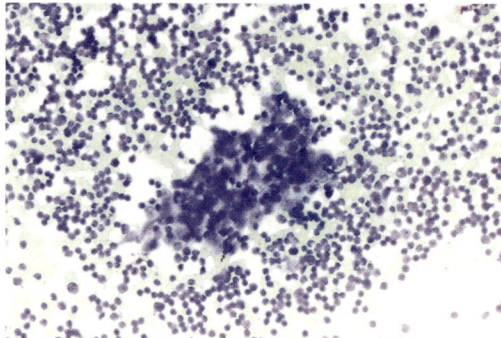

Fig. 4.39
Thymoma. Numerous lymphocytes surrounding an island of epithelial cells. The latter are difficult to visualise. Immunocytochemistry revealed the epithelial island to be positive for cytokeratin

FNAC of suspected mediastinal cysts should be undertaken with caution because of the risk of infection. EUS-FNAC is a safe and minimally invasive diagnostic technique for the analysis of mediastinal lesions. However, rare complications include mediastinitis and haemorrhage into the cyst [106, 107].

4.4 Breast Cysts

Analysis of the cells from breast cyst fluid is a very common cytological investigation in symptomatic breast patients. Current surgical practice favours discarding any clear fluid after drainage of the cyst. Cytological examination is usually requested only of those cysts that are macroscopically cloudy, turbid or bloodstained [108]. Cytological findings in benign breast change (fibrocystic disease) vary from macrophages only to apocrine cells, inflammatory cells and haemosiderin (Fig. 4.40). Epithelium is usually sparse and presents in flat sheets. Three-dimensional clusters may suggest the presence of an intracystic papillary lesion (Fig. 4.41).

Intracystic papillary lesions pose a diagnostic dilemma since they may be either benign or malignant. Intracystic papillary carcinoma (IPC) tends to present as a larger tumour in older women (average 65 years). Papilloma, however, tends to present as a smaller tumour (average, 1.5 cm) in younger women (average, 43 years; Fig. 4.42). Both lesions yield highly cellular aspirates with complex vascular papillae and single columnar cells [109]. Macrophages are a constant feature of IPC and may be present in papilloma. Although cellular atypia is not a prominent feature in either IPC or papilloma, moderate atypia may be noted, particularly in papilloma. IPC tends to be more cellular and contain single intact cells (Fig. 4.43). However, no single feature or group of findings is consistently reliable in distinguishing IPC from papilloma. In the absence of overt cytological malignancy, distinguishing between benign and malignant papillary breast lesions is difficult, if not impossible [110] (see section 4.6.).

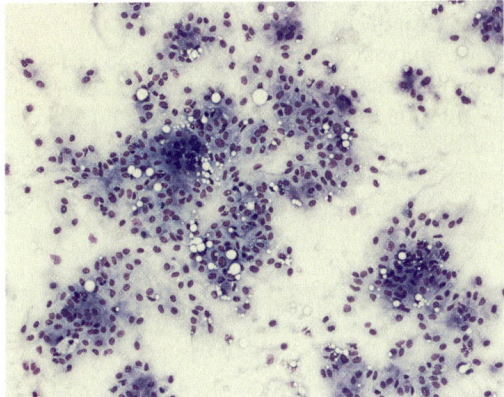

Fig. 4.40
FNAC breast. Cytological findings in benign breast change (fibrocystic disease) vary from macrophages only to apocrine cells, inflammatory cells and haemosiderin

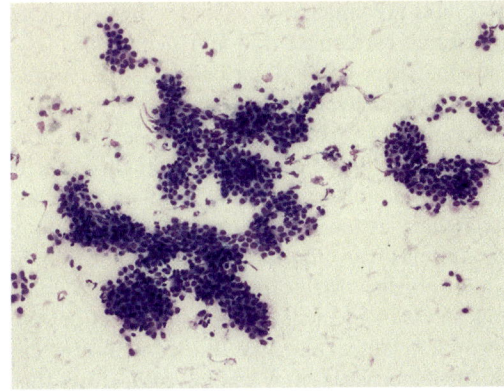

Fig. 4.42
FNAC breast. Intraduct papilloma. Intracystic papillary lesions pose a diagnostic dilemma since they may be either benign or malignant. Both papilloma and papillary carcinoma yield highly cellular aspirates with complex vascular papillae and single columnar cells. No single feature or group of findings is consistently reliable in distinguishing intracystic papillary carcinoma (IPC) from papilloma

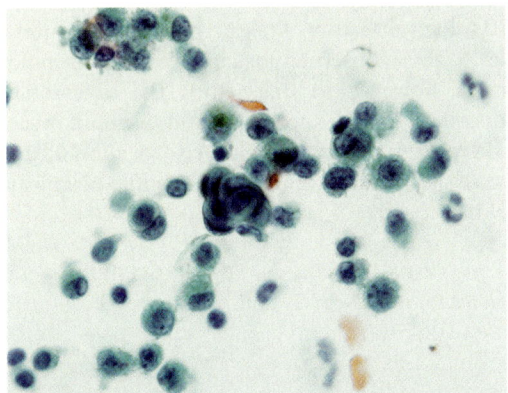

Fig. 4.41
FNAC breast. Three-dimensional clusters may suggest the presence of an intracystic papillary lesion

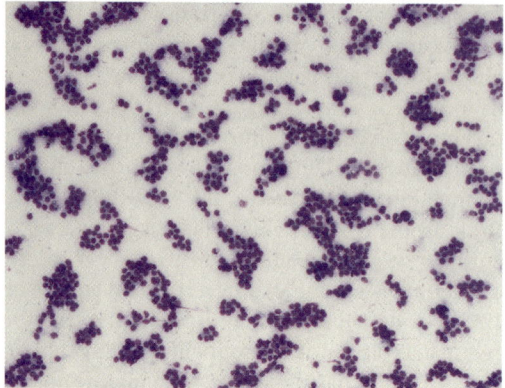

Fig. 4.43
FNAC breast. intracystic papilarry carcinoma. Cellular atypia is not a prominent feature in either IPC or papilloma. Moderate atypia may be noted, particularly in papilloma. IPC tends to be more cellular and contain single intact cells. In the absence of overt cytological malignancy, distinguishing between benign and malignant papillary breast lesions is difficult

Another group of breast lesions that may present as cystic are mucinous lesions. These include mucinous carcinoma and mucocoele-like lesions, the latter being described as either simple or with ductal hyperplasia (typical or atypical see chapter 9.4). Simple mucocoele-like lesions show scant cellularity, no or rare intact single epithelial cells, a monolayered arrangement and absence of nuclear atypia. In contrast, most mucinous carcinomas show higher cellularity, more single tumour cells, three-dimensional clusters, and mild to marked nuclear atypia (see section 4.6; Fig. 4.23). Mucocoele-like lesions with atypical ductal hyperplasia show cytological features that overlap with those of mucinous carcinoma. Mucocoele-like lesions have a non-specific mammographic appearance and appear cystic on ultrasonography. Mucinous carcinomas appear as solid masses on ultrasonography and as distinct nodules on mammography. Based on the combination of FNAC and imaging findings, a benign mucocoele lesion may be correctly distinguished from mucinous carcinoma before surgery [111]. Excisional biopsy is advised for all hypocellular cases for further separation into benign and malignant mucocoele-like lesion and to rule out the possibility of hypocellular mucinous carcinoma [112].

Sarcomatoid/metaplastic carcinoma of the breast is a rare breast malignancy that shows a variety of cytological features in FNAC. These poorly differentiated invasive carcinomas contain both ductal and mesenchymal elements, with transitional forms displaying spindle, squamous, chondroid or osseous differentiation. They may also show cystic changes, although this is unusual [113]. Cystic adenomyoepithelioma and atypical haemangioma of the breast are examples of other rare breast tumours that may present as a cyst [114]. The FNAC of atypical haemangioma may show the presence of numerous atypical single spindle cells scattered throughout a haemorrhagic background. The degree of cytological atypia may suggest a malignant process, and an excision biopsy should be advised. Differential diagnosis includes angiosarcoma and other benign and malignant spindle-cell lesions of the breast [115]. (see chapter 9.7.5.)

4.5 Other Cysts and Artefacts

Epidermoid cysts may be found in many locations including the testis, and may be diagnosed using FNAC. The macroscopic and cytological features are a creamy aspirate, squamous cells, keratinous debris, anucleate squames and fragments of granulomatous tissue (Fig. 4.44). Cytological features are fairly typical and similar to those observed for cutaneous epidermoid cysts; however, in this setting the differential diagnosis includes teratoma and dermoid cysts. The patient's age and the precise location of the mass are paramount in the differential diagnosis [116].

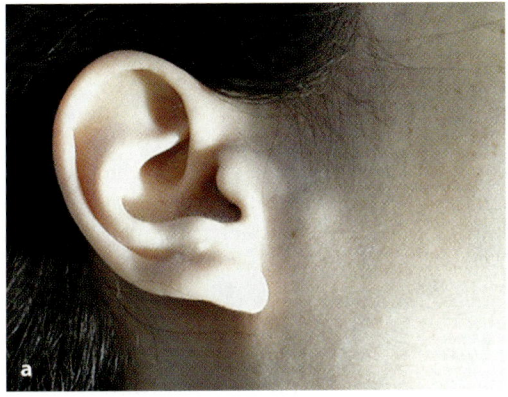

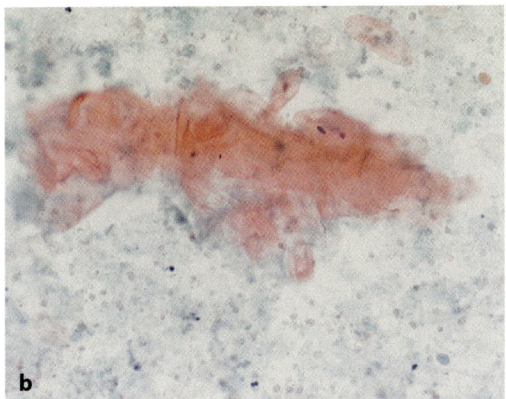

Fig. 4.44
FNAC skin nodule. Epidermoid cyst. **a** Patient presented with a preauricular nodule thought to be either a lymph node or a benign salivary gland tumour. **b** The macroscopic and cytological features are a creamy aspirate containing squamous cells, keratinous debris and anucleate squames

Colloid cyst of the brain is a rare, non-neoplastic lesion that is thought to arise from misplaced endodermal tissue in the anterosuperior portion of the third ventricle. Stereotactic FNAC shows a characteristic sticky and viscous quality on macroscopic examination. Cytological features include abundant, amorphous, proteinaceous material with staining qualities similar to the colloid aspirated from thyroid tissue. This includes a purplish, film-like coating of the slide with occasional cracking artefact, thick, globular, eosinophilic fragments and granular, rope-like, and somewhat viscous, mucinous material. Pathognomonic radiating hyphae-like structures may not be seen. The cellular components vary from isolated cuboidal/columnar cells to large tissue fragments of glandular-type epithelium with a focal ciliated border. Goblet cells are frequently identifiable, as are fragments of the collagenous cyst wall [117].

Ganglion cyst is a relatively common lesion resulting from mucoid, cystic degeneration of the soft tissues adjacent to a joint space. Aspiration of cyst contents has been increasingly advocated as a diagnostic and, in some instances, therapeutic modality. FNAC usually yields a thick, gelatinous fluid and a smear comprises rare histiocytes embedded in a mucoid matrix. Although these findings are non-specific, in the appropriate clinical setting, the diagnosis of ganglion cyst can be made with confidence using FNAC [118] (Fig. 4.45).

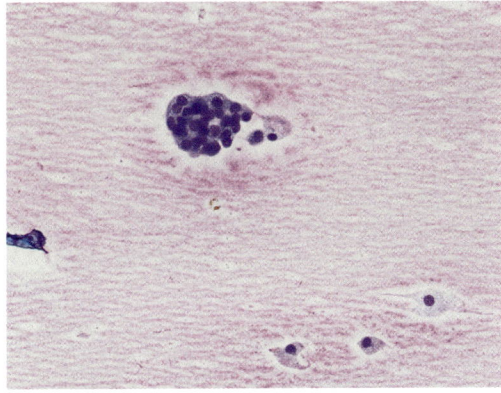

Fig. 4.45
FNAC nodule in the wrist. A smear comprises rare histiocytes embedded in a mucoid matrix. Although these findings are non-specific, in the appropriate clinical setting, the diagnosis of ganglion cyst can be made with confidence by FNAC

FNAC of ovarian cysts is performed rarely. Occasional FNAC samples include follicular cysts, endometriotic cysts, paraovarian/paratubal cysts and neoplasms. Although the specificity of FNAC for most non-follicular cystic ovarian lesions approaches 100%, the sensitivity ranges from 36% for endometriotic cysts to 83% for proliferating/malignant serous tumours (Figs. 4.46–4.50). Prior to FNAC of the ovary in an individual patient, consideration should be given to the likely diagnosis, the limitations of the technique and the high false-negative rate for non-follicular cystic lesions [119].

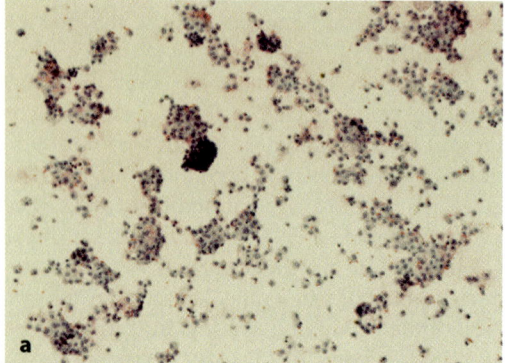

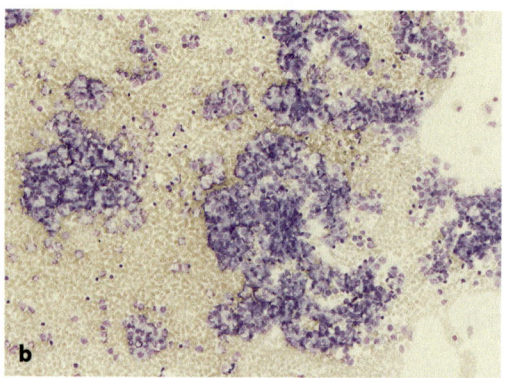

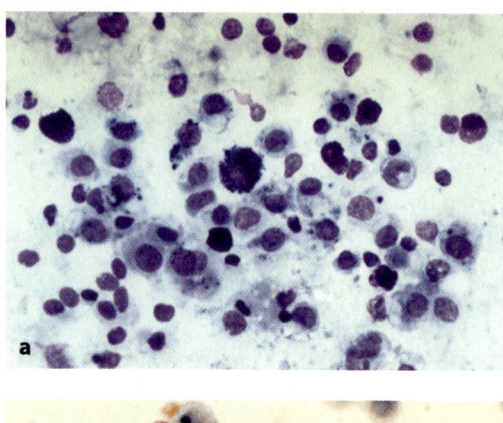

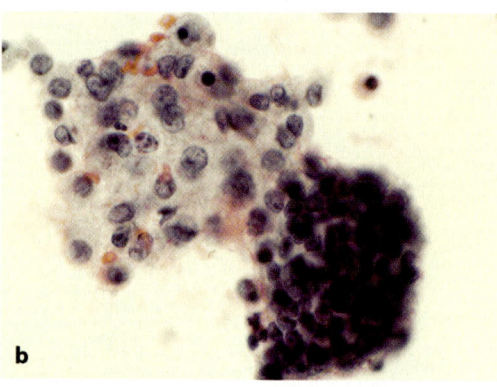

Fig. 4.47
FNAC ovary. Endometriotic cyst. **a** The background of the endometriotic cyst is usually haemorrhagic with numerous haemosiderin-laden macrophages. **b** The epithelium is relatively sparse, if present at all

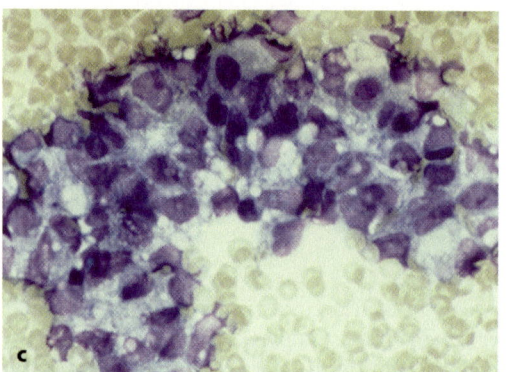

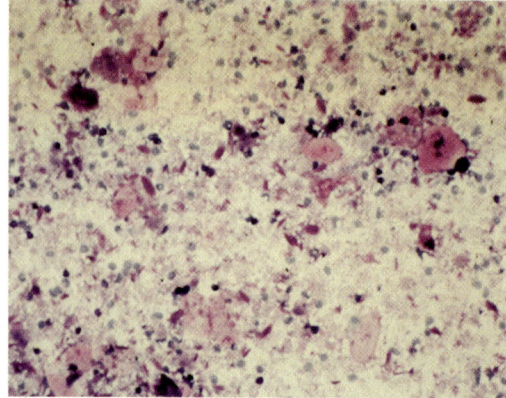

Fig. 4.46
FNAC ovary. Functional cysts. **a** Follicular cyst. **b, c** Corpus luteum cyst. Functional cysts are commonly aspirated in patients who are receiving hormonal stimulation for fertility treatment. Caution should be excercised to avoid misinterpreting the cellularity in functional cysts as neoplastic

Fig. 4.48
FNAC ovary. Dermoid cyst. Aspirates from dermoid cysts usually contain sebaceous material macroscopically. Slides contain keratinous debris and macrophages

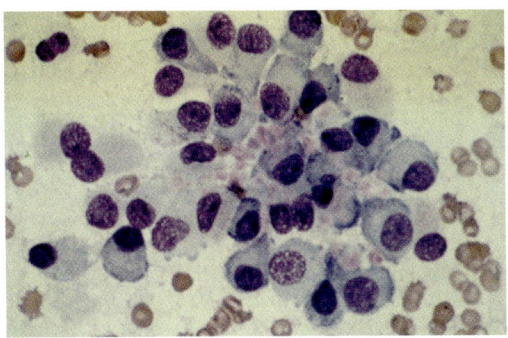

Fig. 4.49
FNAC ovary. Serous cystadenoma. Bland epithelial cells from a benign tumour. Attention needs to be paid to nuclear detail. An important decision is that the cells are epithelial, in which case excision is performed and the tissue is examined for signs for stromal invasion

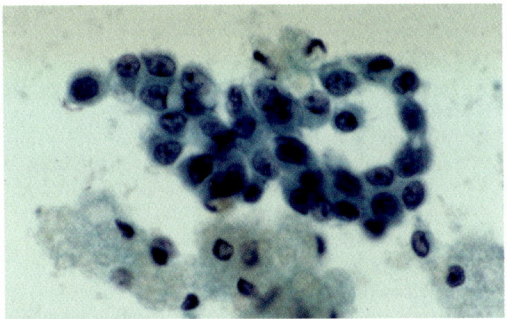

Fig. 4.50
FNAC ovary. Mucinous cystadenoma. The macroscopic appearance of the aspirated fluid is usually gelatinous. Cells are bland, epithelial and secrete mucin. Mucinous tumours are invariably excised

Liesegang rings are laminated ring-like structures that are occasionally found in benign cysts and abscesses. They have been confused with parasites (especially eggs), algae, calcifications and psammoma bodies. Liesegang rings are best seen with Pap, haematoxylin-eosin, Masson's trichrome, acid-fast bacilli (AFB) and Gram stains, which accentuate the concentrically laminated morphology. An amorphous electron-dense core and fibrillary lucent concentric rings can be seen with transmission electron microscopy. Liesegang rings are composed of organic substances most likely formed by periodic precipitation from a supersaturated solution within cystic fluid. Awareness of the Liesegang phenomenon within cystic lesions will decrease the possibility of erroneous misdiagnosis as another type of pathological process [120].

References

1. Dejmek A, Lindholm K. Fine needle aspiration biopsy of cystic lesions of the head and neck, excluding the thyroid. Acta Cytol 1990;34(3):443–8
2. Kadhim AL, Sheahan P, Colreavy MP, Timon CV. Pearls and pitfalls in the management of branchial cyst. J Laryngol Otol 2004;118(12):946–50
3. Bardales RH, Suhrland MJ, Korourian S, Schaefer RF, Hanna EY, Stanley MW. Cytologic findings in thyroglossal duct carcinoma. Am J Clin Pathol 1996;106(5):615–9
4. Gourin CG, Johnson JT. Incidence of unsuspected metastases in lateral cervical cysts. Laryngoscope 2000;110(10 Pt 1):1637–41
5. Zimmermann CE, von Domarus H, Moubayed P. Carcinoma in situ in a lateral cervical cyst. Head Neck 2002;24(10):965–9
6. Girvigian MR, Rechdouni AK, Zeger GD, Segall H, Rice DH, Petrovich Z. Squamous cell carcinoma arising in a second branchial cleft cyst. Am J Clin Oncol 2004;27(1):96–100
7. Briggs RD, Pou AM, Schnadig VJ. Cystic metastasis versus branchial cleft carcinoma: a diagnostic challenge. Laryngoscope 2002;112(6):1010–4
8. Bernstein A, Scardino PT, Tomaszewki MM, Cohen MH. Carcinoma arising in a branchial cleft cyst. Cancer 1976;37(5):2417–22
9. Khafif RA, Prichep R, Minkowitz S. Primary branchiogenic carcinoma. Head Neck 1989;11(2):153–63
10. Pisharodi LR. False-negative diagnosis in fine-needle aspirations of squamous-cell carcinoma of head and neck. Diagn Cytopathol 1997;17(1):70–3
11. Nasuti JF, Braccia MG, Roberts S, Baloch ZW. Utility of cytomorphologic criteria and p53 immunolocalization in distinguishing benign from malignant cystic squamous-lined lesions of the neck on fine-needle aspiration. Diagn Cytopathol 2002;27(1):10–4
12. Nordemar S, Tani E, Hogmo A, Jangard M, Auer G, Munck-Wikland E. Image cytometry DNA-analysis of fine needle aspiration cytology to aid cytomorphology in the distinction of branchial cleft cyst from cystic metastasis of squamous cell carcinoma: a prospective study. Laryngoscope 2004;114(11):1997–2000
13. Nordemar S, Hogmo A, Lindholm J, Tani E, Sjostrom B, Auer G, et al. The clinical value of image cytometry DNA analysis in distinguishing branchial cleft cysts from cystic metastases of head and neck cancer. Laryngoscope 2002;112(11):1983–7

14. Lopez-Rios F, Diaz-Bustamante T, Serrano-Egea A, Jimenez J, de Agustin P. Amylase crystalloids in salivary gland lesions: report of a case with a review of the literature. Diagn Cytopathol 2001;25(1):59–62
15. Vicandi B, Jimenez-Heffernan JA, Lopez-Ferrer P, Patron M, Gamallo C, Colmenero C, et al. HIV-1 (p24)-positive multinucleated giant cells in HIV-associated lymphoepithelial lesion of the parotid gland. A report of two cases. Acta Cytol 1999;43(2):247–51
16. Favia G, Capodiferro S, Scivetti M, Lacaita MG, Filosa A, Lo Muzio L. Multiple parotid lymphoepithelial cysts in patients with HIV-infection: report of two cases. Oral Dis 2004;10(3):151–4
17. Raymond MR, Yoo JH, Heathcote JG, McLachlin CM, Lampe HB. Accuracy of fine-needle aspiration biopsy for Warthin's tumours. J Otolaryngol 2002;31(5):263–70
18. Sheahan P, Fitzgibbon J, O'Leary G, Lee G. Efficacy and pitfalls of fine needle aspiration in the diagnosis of neck masses. Surgeon 2004;2(3):152–6
19. Postema RJ, van Velthuysen ML, van den Brekel MW, Balm AJ, Peterse JL. Accuracy of fine-needle aspiration cytology of salivary gland lesions in The Netherlands Cancer Institute. Head Neck 2004;26(5):418–24
20. Chae SW, Sohn JH, Shin HS, Choi JJ, Kim YB. Unilateral, multicentric Warthin's tumor mimicking a tumor metastatic to a lymph node. A case report. Acta Cytol 2004;48(2):229–33
21. Caglar M, Tuncel M, Usubutun A. Increased uptake on I-131 whole-body scintigraphy in Warthin tumor despite false-negative Tc-99m pertechnetate salivary gland scintigraphy. Clin Nucl Med 2003;28(11):945–6
22. Ali SZ. Acinic-cell carcinoma, papillary-cystic variant: a diagnostic dilemma in salivary gland aspiration. Diagn Cytopathol 2002;27(4):244–50
23. Takeshita T, Tanaka H, Harasawa A, Kaminaga T, Imamura T, Furui S. Benign pleomorphic adenoma with extensive cystic degeneration: unusual MR findings in two cases. Radiat Med 2004;22(5):357–61
24. Viguer JM, Vicandi B, Jimenez-Heffernan JA, Lopez-Ferrer P, Limeres MA. Fine needle aspiration cytology of pleomorphic adenoma. An analysis of 212 cases. Acta Cytol 1997;41(3):786–94
25. Pisharodi LR. Low grade papillary adenocarcinoma of minor salivary gland origin. Diagnosis by fine needle aspiration cytology. Acta Cytol 1997;41(5):1407–11
26. Baschinsky D, Hameed A, Keyhani-Rofagha S. Fine-needle aspiration cytological features of dermoid cyst of the parotid gland: a report of two cases. Diagn Cytopathol 1999;20(6):387–8
27. Jayaram G, Jayalakshmi P. Follicular adenoma with squamous metaplasia and cystic change: report of a case with fine needle aspiration cytological and histological features. Malays J Pathol 1999;21(2):101–4
28. Seven H, Gurkan A, Cinar U, Vural C, Turgut S. Incidence of occult thyroid carcinoma metastases in lateral cervical cysts. Am J Otolaryngol 2004;25(1):11–7
29. Lin JD, Huang BY. Comparison of the results of diagnosis and treatment between solid and cystic well-differentiated thyroid carcinomas. Thyroid 1998;8(8):661–6
30. Papotti M, Volante M, Saggiorato E, Deandreis D, Veltri A, Orlandi F. Role of galectin-3 immunodetection in the cytological diagnosis of thyroid cystic papillary carcinoma. Eur J Endocrinol 2002;147(4):515–21
31. Pathan SK, Francis IM, Das DK, Mallik MK, Sheikh ZA, Hira PR. Fine needle aspiration cytologic diagnosis of toxoplasma lymphadenitis. A case report with detection of a Toxoplasma bradycyst in a Papanicolaou-stained smear. Acta Cytol 2003;47(2):299–303
32. Absher KJ, Truong LD, Khurana KK, Ramzy I. Parathyroid cytology: avoiding diagnostic pitfalls. Head Neck 2002;24(2):157–64
33. Mevio E, Gorini E, Sbrocca M, Artesi L, Mullace M, Lecce S. Parathyroid cysts: description of two cases and review of the literature. Acta Otorhinolaryngol Ital 2004;24(3):161–4
34. Espinoza Colindres L, Molina Rodriguez MA, Gonzalez Casado I, Gracia Bouthelier R. [Parathyroid cyst in the differential diagnosis of neck masses. A case report]. An Pediatr (Barc) 2003;58(2):188–90
35. Alvi A, Myssiorek D, Wasserman P. Parathyroid cyst: current diagnostic and management principles. Head Neck 1996;18(4):370–3
36. Turner A, Lampe HB, Cramer H. Parathyroid cysts. J Otolaryngol 1989;18(6):311–3
37. Lin CC, Chen CH, Lin LM, Chen YK, Wright JM, Kessler HP, et al. Calcifying odontogenic cyst with ameloblastic fibroma: report of three cases. Oral Surg Oral Med Oral Pathol Oral Radiol Endod 2004;98(4):451–60
38. Goldenberg D, Sciubba J, Koch W, Tufano RP. Malignant odontogenic tumors: a 22-year experience. Laryngoscope 2004;114(10):1770–4
39. Chapelle KA, Stoelinga PJ, de Wilde PC, Brouns JJ, Voorsmit RA. Rational approach to diagnosis and treatment of ameloblastomas and odontogenic keratocysts. Br J Oral Maxillofac Surg 2004;42(5):381–90
40. Kerr JT, Steger J, Sorensen D. Midline maxillary odontogenic keratocyst. Ann Otol Rhinol Laryngol 2004;113(9):688–90
41. Amorim RF, Godoy GP, Galvao HC, Souza LB, Freitas RA. Immunohistochemical assessment of extracellular matrix components in syndrome and non-syndrome odontogenic keratocysts. Oral Dis 2004;10(5):265–70
42. Osny FJ, Azevedo LR, Sant'Ana E, Lara VS. Glandular odontogenic cyst: case report and review of the literature. Quintessence Int 2004;35(5):385–9

43. Babuccu O, Isiksacan Ozen O, Hosnuter M, Kargi E, Babuccu B. The place of fine-needle aspiration in the preoperative diagnosis of the congenital sublingual teratoid cyst. Diagn Cytopathol 2003;29(1):33–7
44. Wakoh M, Yonezu H, Otonari T, Sano T, Matsuzaka K, Inoue T, et al. Two cases of schwannoma with marked cystic changes. Dentomaxillofac Radiol 2005;34(1):44–50
45. Rios A, Rodriguez JM, Martinez E, Parrilla P. Cavernous hemangioma of the thyroid. Thyroid 2001;11(3):279–80
46. Hilborne LH, Glasgow BJ, Layfield LJ. Fine-needle aspiration cytology of juvenile hemangioma of the parotid gland: a case report. Diagn Cytopathol 1987;3(2):152–5
47. Bosch-Princep R, Castellano-Megias VM, Alvaro-Naranjo T, Martinez-Gonzalez S, Salvado-Usach MT. Fine needle aspiration cytology of a cervical lymph node lymphangioma in an adult. A case report. Acta Cytol 1999;43(3):442–6
48. Gutmann EJ. Lymphangioma presenting as a primary parotid neoplasm in an adult. Report of a case with the diagnosis suggested by fine needle aspiration biopsy. Acta Cytol 1994;38(5):747–50
49. Henke AC, Cooley ML, Hughes JH, Timmerman TG. Fine-needle aspiration cytology of lymphangioma of the parotid gland in an adult. Diagn Cytopathol 2001;24(2):126–8
50. Kosmahl M, Pauser U, Anlauf M, Sipos B, Peters K, Luttges J, et al. [Cystic pancreas tumors and their classification: features old and new.]. Pathologe 2005;26(1):22–30
51. Kosmahl M, Pauser U, Peters K, Sipos B, Luttges J, Kremer B, et al. Cystic neoplasms of the pancreas and tumor-like lesions with cystic features: a review of 418 cases and a classification proposal. Virchows Arch 2004;445(2):168–78.
52. Michael H, Gress F. Diagnosis of cystic neoplasms with endoscopic ultrasound. Gastrointest Endosc Clin N Am 2002;12(4):719–33
53. Frossard JL, Amouyal P, Amouyal G, Palazzo L, Amaris J, Soldan M, et al. Performance of endosonography-guided fine needle aspiration and biopsy in the diagnosis of pancreatic cystic lesions. Am J Gastroenterol 2003;98(7):1516–24
54. Hernandez LV, Mishra G, Forsmark C, Draganov PV, Petersen JM, Hochwald SN, et al. Role of endoscopic ultrasound (EUS) and EUS-guided fine needle aspiration in the diagnosis and treatment of cystic lesions of the pancreas. Pancreas 2002;25(3):222–8
55. Fritscher-Ravens A, Izbicki JR, Sriram PV, Krause C, Knoefel WT, Topalidis T, et al. Endosonography-guided, fine-needle aspiration cytology extending the indication for organ-preserving pancreatic surgery. Am J Gastroenterol 2000;95(9):2255–60
56. Salvia R, Festa L, Butturini G, Tonsi A, Sartori N, Biasutti C, et al. Pancreatic cystic tumors. Minerva Chir 2004;59(2):185–207
57. Ahrendt SA, Komorowski RA, Demeure MJ, Wilson SD, Pitt HA. Cystic pancreatic neuroendocrine tumors: is preoperative diagnosis possible? J Gastrointest Surg 2002;6(1):66–74
58. Kloppel G, Kosmahl M. Cystic lesions and neoplasms of the pancreas. The features are becoming clearer. Pancreatology 2001;1(6):648–55
59. Levy MJ, Clain JE. Evaluation and management of cystic pancreatic tumors: emphasis on the role of EUS FNA. Clin Gastroenterol Hepatol 2004;2(8):639–53
60. Brugge WR, Lewandrowski K, Lee-Lewandrowski E, Centeno BA, Szydlo T, Regan S, et al. Diagnosis of pancreatic cystic neoplasms: a report of the cooperative pancreatic cyst study. Gastroenterology 2004;126(5):1330–6
61. Lewandrowski KB, Southern JF, Pins MR, Compton CC, Warshaw AL. Cyst fluid analysis in the differential diagnosis of pancreatic cysts. A comparison of pseudocysts, serous cystadenomas, mucinous cystic neoplasms, and mucinous cystadenocarcinoma. Ann Surg 1993;217(1):41–7
62. Jayaram G, Chaturvedi KU, Jindal RK, Venugopal S, Kapoor R. Papillary cystic neoplasm of the pancreas. Report of a case diagnosed by fine needle aspiration cytology. Acta Cytol 1990;34(3):429–33
63. Kosmahl M, Wagner J, Peters K, Sipos B, Kloppel G. Serous cystic neoplasms of the pancreas: an immunohistochemical analysis revealing alpha-inhibin, neuron-specific enolase, and MUC6 as new markers. Am J Surg Pathol 2004;28(3):339–46
64. Fabiani A, Delia GJ, De Rosa R, Pombo MT, Molfino O, Ferraina P, et al. Pancreatic serous cystadenomas. Report of 8 cases with a mean follow up of 7 years. HPB Surg 1996;9(4):215–7
65. O'Toole D, Palazzo L, Hammel P, Ben Yaghlene L, Couvelard A, Felce-Dachez M, et al. Macrocystic pancreatic cystadenoma: The role of EUS and cyst fluid analysis in distinguishing mucinous and serous lesions. Gastrointest Endosc 2004;59(7):823–9
66. Kloppel G, Kosmahl M, Luttges J. [Intraductal neoplasms of the pancreas: cystic and common.]. Pathologe 2005;26(1):31–6
67. Recine M, Kaw M, Evans DB, Krishnamurthy S. Fine-needle aspiration cytology of mucinous tumors of the pancreas. Cancer 2004;102(2):92–9
68. Bardales RH, Centeno B, Mallery JS, Lai R, Pochapin M, Guiter G, et al. Endoscopic ultrasound-guided fine-needle aspiration cytology diagnosis of solid-pseudopapillary tumor of the pancreas: a rare neoplasm of elusive origin but characteristic cytomorphologic features. Am J Clin Pathol 2004;121(5):654–62
69. Master SS, Savides TJ. Diagnosis of solid-pseudopapillary neoplasm of the pancreas by EUS-guided FNA. Gastrointest Endosc 2003;57(7):965–8

70. Nadler EP, Novikov A, Landzberg BR, Pochapin MB, Centeno B, Fahey TJ, et al. The use of endoscopic ultrasound in the diagnosis of solid pseudopapillary tumors of the pancreas in children. J Pediatr Surg 2002;37(9):1370–3
71. Kosmahl M, Peters K, Anlauf M, Sipos B, Pauser U, Luttges J, et al. [Solid pseudopapillary neoplasms Weiblich orientiert und ratselhaft.]. Pathologe 2005;26(1):41–5
72. Brunner A, Ladurner R, Kosmahl M, Mikuz G, Tzankov A. Mucinous non-neoplastic cyst of the pancreas accompanied by non-parasitic asymptomatic liver cysts. Virchows Arch 2004;444(5):482–4.
73. Couvelard A, Terris B, Hammel P, Palazzo L, Belghiti J, Levy P, et al. [Acinar cystic transformation of the pancreas (or acinar cell cystadenoma), a rare and recently described entity]. Ann Pathol 2002;22(5):397–400
74. Chatelain D, Paye F, Mourra N, Scoazec JY, Baudrimont M, Parc R, et al. Unilocular acinar cell cystadenoma of the pancreas an unusual acinar cell tumor. Am J Clin Pathol 2002;118(2):211–4
75. Zamboni G, Terris B, Scarpa A, Kosmahl M, Capelli P, Klimstra DS, et al. Acinar cell cystadenoma of the pancreas: a new entity? Am J Surg Pathol 2002;26(6):698–704
76. Mandavilli SR, Port J, Ali SZ. Lymphoepithelial cyst (LEC) of the pancreas: cytomorphology and differential diagnosis on fine-needle aspiration (FNA). Diagn Cytopathol 1999;20(6):371–4
77. Liu J, Shin HJ, Rubenchik I, Lang E, Lahoti S, Staerkel GA. Cytologic features of lymphoepithelial cyst of the pancreas: two preoperatively diagnosed cases based on fine-needle aspiration. Diagn Cytopathol 1999;21(5):346–50
78. Bolis GB, Farabi R, Liberati F, Maccio T. Lymphoepithelial cyst of the pancreas. Report of a case diagnosed by fine needle aspiration biopsy. Acta Cytol 1998;42(2):384–6
79. Cappellari JO. Fine-needle aspiration cytology of a pancreatic lymphoepithelial cyst. Diagn Cytopathol 1993; 9(1):77–81
80. Capitanich P, Iovaldi ML, Medrano M, Malizia P, Herrera J, Celeste F, et al. Lymphoepithelial cysts of the pancreas: case report and review of the literature. J Gastrointest Surg 2004;8(3):342–5
81. Pauser U, Kosmahl M, Sipos B, Kloppel G. [Mesenchymal tumors of the pancreas Uberraschend, aber nicht ungewohnlich.]. Pathologe 2005;26(1):52–8
82. Pinto MM, Kaye AD. Fine needle aspiration of cystic liver lesions. Cytologic examination and carcinoembryonic antigen assay of cyst contents. Acta Cytol 1989;33(6):852–6
83. Pinto MM, Monteferrante M, Kaye AD. Carcinoembryonic antigen in fine-needle aspirate of liver: a diagnostic adjunct to cytology. Diagn Cytopathol 1991;7(1):23–6
84. Shariff S, Thomas JA, Kaliaperumal VG. An experience with ultrasonically guided liver aspirates from south India. Cytopathology 1993;4(5):291–8
85. Kuo FY, Chen WJ, Lu SN, Wang JH, Eng HL. Fine needle aspiration cytodiagnosis of liver tumors. Acta Cytol 2004;48(2):142–8
86. Hollerbach S, Willert J, Topalidis T, Reiser M, Schmiegel W. Endoscopic ultrasound-guided fine-needle aspiration biopsy of liver lesions: histological and cytological assessment. Endoscopy 2003;35(9):743–9
87. Das DK, Bhambhani S, Pant CS. Ultrasound guided fine-needle aspiration cytology: diagnosis of hydatid disease of the abdomen and thorax. Diagn Cytopathol 1995;12(2):173–6
88. Fava C, Patetta R, Cozzi L, Assi A. [Renal hydatid cyst: cytological diagnosis using fine needle biopsy (FNA)]. Pathologica 1999;91(2):115–8
89. Laforga JB, Bordallo A, Ara FI. Vascular adrenal pseudocyst: cytologic and immunohistochemical study. Diagn Cytopathol 2000;22(2):110–2
90. Jennings TA, Ng B, Boguniewicz A, Khan M, Rice D, Figge J. Adrenal pseudocysts: evidence of their posthemorrhagic nature. Endocr Pathol 1998;9(1):353–361
91. Todd TD, Dhurandhar B, Mody D, Ramzy I, Truong LD. Fine-needle aspiration of cystic lesions of the kidney. Morphologic spectrum and diagnostic problems in 41 cases. Am J Clin Pathol 1999;111(3):317–28
92. Brierly RD, Thomas PJ, Harrison NW, Fletcher MS, Nawrocki JD, Ashton-Key M. Evaluation of fine-needle aspiration cytology for renal masses. BJU Int 2000;85(1):14–8
93. Truong LD, Todd TD, Dhurandhar B, Ramzy I. Fine-needle aspiration of renal masses in adults: analysis of results and diagnostic problems in 108 cases. Diagn Cytopathol 1999;20(6):339–49
94. Wang S, Filipowicz EA, Schnadig VJ. Abundant intracytoplasmic hemosiderin in both histiocytes and neoplastic cells: A diagnostic pitfall in fine-needle aspiration of cystic papillary renal-cell carcinoma. Diagn Cytopathol 2001;24(2):82–5
95. Devaney K, Kragel PJ, Devaney EJ. Fine-needle aspiration cytology of multicystic mesothelioma. Diagn Cytopathol 1992;8(1):68–72
96. Moriwaki Y, Kobayashi S, Harada H, Kunizaki C, Imai S, Kido Y, et al. Cystic mesothelioma of the peritoneum. J Gastroenterol 1996;31(6):868–74
97. Staniscia G, Tidona V, Sardellone A, De Nicola E. [Benign peritoneal multicystic mesothelioma]. Ann Ital Chir 2003;74(5):579–82
98. Di Blasi A, Boscaino A, De Dominicis G, Marsilia GM, D'Antonio A, Nappi O. Multicystic mesothelioma of the liver with secondary involvement of peritoneum and inguinal region. Int J Surg Pathol 2004;12(1):87–91

99. Varma R, Wallace R. Multicystic benign mesothelioma of the peritoneum presenting as postmenopausal bleeding and a solitary pelvic cyst--a case report. Gynecol Oncol 2004;92(1):334–6
100. Sawh RN, Malpica A, Deavers MT, Liu J, Silva EG. Benign cystic mesothelioma of the peritoneum: a clinicopathologic study of 17 cases and immunohistochemical analysis of estrogen and progesterone receptor status. Hum Pathol 2003;34(4):369–74
101. Eloubeidi MA, Cohn M, Cerfolio RJ, Chhieng DC, Jhala N, Jhala D, et al. Endoscopic ultrasound-guided fine-needle aspiration in the diagnosis of foregut duplication cysts: the value of demonstrating detached ciliary tufts in cyst fluid. Cancer 2004;102(4):253–8
102. Wildi SM, Hoda RS, Fickling W, Schmulewitz N, Varadarajulu S, Roberts SS, et al. Diagnosis of benign cysts of the mediastinum: the role and risks of EUS and FNA. Gastrointest Endosc 2003;58(3):362–8
103. Kuroki S, Nasu K, Murakami K, Hayashi T, Sekiguchi R, Nishida H, et al. Thymic MALT lymphoma: MR imaging findings and their correlation with histopathological findings on four cases. Clin Imaging 2004;28(4):274–7
104. Silverman JF, Olson PR, Dabbs DJ, Landreneau R. Fine-needle aspiration cytology of a mediastinal seminoma associated with multilocular thymic cyst. Diagn Cytopathol 1999;20(4):224–8
105. Pinto MM, Dovgan D, Kaye AD, Chinniah A. Fine needle aspiration for diagnosing a thymoma producing CA-125. A case report. Acta Cytol 1993;37(6):929–32
106. Annema JT, Veselic M, Versteegh MI, Rabe KF. Mediastinitis caused by EUS-FNA of a bronchogenic cyst. Endoscopy 2003;35(9):791–3
107. Varadarajulu S, Eloubeidi MA Frequency and significance of acute intracystic hemorrhage during EUS-FNA of cystic lesions of the pancreas. Gastrointest Endosc 2004;60(4):631–5
108. Hindle WH, Arias RD, Florentine B, Whang J. Lack of utility in clinical practice of cytologic examination of nonbloody cyst fluid from palpable breast cysts. Am J Obstet Gynecol 2000;182(6):1300–5
109. Corkill ME, Sneige N, Fanning T, el-Naggar A. Fine-needle aspiration cytology and flow cytometry of intracystic papillary carcinoma of breast. Am J Clin Pathol 1990;94(6):673–80
110. Jeffrey PB, Ljung BM. Benign and malignant papillary lesions of the breast. A cytomorphologic study. Am J Clin Pathol 1994;101(4):500–7
111. Cheng L, Lee WY, Chang TW. Benign mucocelelike lesion of the breast: how to differentiate from mucinous carcinoma before surgery. Cytopathology 2004;15(2):104–8
112. Wong NL, Wan SK. Comparative cytology of mucocelelike lesion and mucinous carcinoma of the breast in fine needle aspiration. Acta Cytol 2000;44(5):765–70
113. Matthai SM, Kini U. Aspiration cytology of sarcomatoid carcinoma of the breast: Report of a case with cystic change. Diagn Cytopathol 2004;31(1):10–3
114. Papaevangelou A, Pougouras I, Liapi G, Pierrakakis S, Tibishrani M, Setakis N. Cystic adenomyoepithelioma of the breast. Breast 2004;13(4):356–8
115. Galindo LM, Shienbaum AJ, Dwyer-Joyce L, Garcia FU. Atypical hemangioma of the breast: a diagnostic pitfall in breast fine-needle aspiration. Diagn Cytopathol 2001;24(3):215–8
116. Perez-Guillermo M, Garcia-Solano J, Sanchez-Sanchez C, Montalban-Romero S, Acosta-Ortega J. Diagnostic limitations in testicular cytopathology: to what extent is fine-needle aspiration reliable for the diagnosis of epidermoid cyst of the testis? Diagn Cytopathol 2004;31(2):83–6
117. Parwani AV, Fatani IY, Burger PC, Erozan YS, Ali SZ. Colloid cyst of the third ventricle: cytomorphologic features on stereotactic fine-needle aspiration. Diagn Cytopathol 2002;27(1):27–31
118. Dodd LG, Layfield LJ. Fine-needle aspiration cytology of ganglion cysts. Diagn Cytopathol 1996;15(5):377–81
119. Mulvany NJ. Aspiration cytology of ovarian cysts and cystic neoplasms. A study of 235 aspirates. Acta Cytol 1996;40(5):911–20
120. Raso DS, Greene WB, Finley JL, Silverman JF. Morphology and pathogenesis of Liesegang rings in cyst aspirates: report of two cases with ancillary studies. Diagn Cytopathol 1998;19(2):116–9

Chapter 5

Diagnostic Dilemmas in FNAC Practice: Lymphoid Infiltrates

Contents

5.1.	**Granulomatous Infiltrates**	91
5.1.1	Tuberculous Lymphadenitis	91
5.1.2	Sarcoidosis	92
5.1.3	Kikuchi-Fujimoto Disease	92
5.1.4	Cat-Scratch Disease	94
5.1.5	Leishmania Lymphadenitis	94
5.1.6	Kimura's disease	95
5.1.7	Sinus Histiocytosis with Massive Lymphadenopathy	96
5.1.8	Foreign-Body Granulomatous Inflammatory Response	96
5.1.9	Malignant Lymphomas	97
5.2	**Lymphoid Infiltrates in Extranodal Sites**	99
5.2.1	Lymphoid Infiltrates in the Thyroid	99
5.2.2	Lymphoid Processes in the Salivary Gland	103
5.2.3	Lymphoid Infiltrates of the Orbit	105
5.2.4	Lymphoid Lesions in the Breast	107
5.3	**Neoplasms Containing Lymphocytes**	107
5.3.1	Dilemmas in the Cytological Diagnosis of Lymphomas	108
5.3.2	Solid Neoplasms Containing Lymphocytes	109
References		110

Diagnostic dilemmas associated with the presence of lymphoid cells in FNAC samples are usually considered to be associated with the diagnosis of lymphomas. However, whilst the majority of lymphomas can be diagnosed without difficulty, there are other aspects of lymphoid infiltrates in FNAC samples that may be either misleading or difficult. This chapter gives some examples of the conditions where observing the details of lymphoid infiltrates may be important in making the diagnosis.

5.1. Granulomatous Infiltrates

Granulomatous infiltrates refer to the lymphoid infiltrates in which aggregates of histiocytes/epithelioid cells and/or multinucleate giant histiocytes are present. The spectrum of conditions showing this change is wide and includes both benign and malignant processes. Granulomata represent either the main pathology or a secondary reaction to it. In both instances, their presence is highly relevant. Most commonly, granulomata point to additional features that may lead to a correct diagnosis. The following are examples of some of the granulomatous conditions encountered in FNAC cytology.

5.1.1 Tuberculous Lymphadenitis

This is probably the most commonly seen granulomatous lymphadenitis in FNAC practice. Although a relatively rare cause of lymphadenopathy in adults in the Western world, in HIV-positive African patients with superficial lymphadenopathy, it is more common than is generally appreciated [1]. Regardless of the geographic distribution, in the absence of pulmonary tuberculosis, tuberculous lymphadenitis is sometimes difficult to differentiate clinically from other diseases. Although the classical FNAC features of epithelioid cells, multinucleate giant cells and caseous necrosis are present in most cases, the early lesions may not be so apparent (Fig. 5.1). FNAC predicts the correct diagnosis in 62% of cases and has a high false-negative rate (38%) due to the absence of granulomata/necrosis in smears from cases of early tuberculosis [2]. Detection of AFB is positive in less than half of cases [3]. In addition, antiretroviral therapy has introduced new morphological patterns of mycobacterial infection as part of the seroconversion that occurs following treatment [4, 5]. Presently, as well as the detection of AFB, PCR of mycobacteria is used as the gold standard for diagnosis. The best results are achieved when FNAC and PCR are used in combination [1, 3, 6–13].

sarcoidosis is not capable of differentiating the lesions from TB on the basis of imaging alone. It may be diagnosed from EUS-FNAC of lymph nodes by demonstrating non-caseating granulomata without necrosis. Annema et al. report an accuracy rate of 82% when using FNAC for the final diagnosis of sarcoidosis [14]. Aspirated material can be sent for mycobacterial culture [15, 16]. Sarcoidosis may affect multiple other sites that can potentially be subjected to FNAC, including the salivary glands (Fig. 5.2). Caution is needed, however, since granulomatous transformation of the lymphoid stroma resembling sarcoidosis may be seen in the lymphoid component of Warthin's tumour of the salivary gland. It is rare, may be associated with previous FNAC and should be considered within the spectrum of secondary changes in adenolymphoma [17].

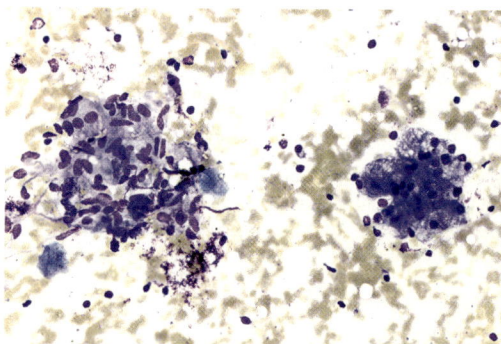

Fig. 5.2
FNAC parotid. Sarcoidosis. Sarcoidosis may affect multiple sites that are potentially subjected to FNAC, including the salivary glands

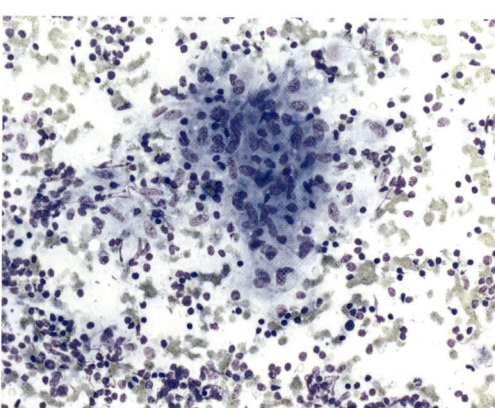

Fig. 5.1
FNAC lymph node. Granulomatous lymphadenitis. Aggregates of epithelioid cells in large aggregates in a case of tuberculous lymphadenitis

5.1.3 Kikuchi-Fujimoto Disease

Also known as histiocytic necrotising lymphadenitis, this is a benign disorder that is characterised histologically by necrotic foci surrounded by histiocytic aggregates, and with the absence of neutrophils. The disease most commonly affects young women. It has a worldwide distribution, but with a higher prevalence among Asiatic people. Its cause is unknown and its exact pathogenesis has not yet been clarified. Many investigators have postulated a viral aetiology, connecting

5.1.2 Sarcoidosis

This is a chronic multisystem granulomatous disease that is often diagnosed after a finding of hilar and mediastinal lymphadenopathy on a chest X-ray. EUS of mediastinal lymph nodes in it with Epstein-Barr virus, human herpes simplex virus 6 Parvo B 19 and with toxoplasmic infection. Kikuchi-Fujimoto disease is usually manifested by acute tender, cervical lymphadenopathy, predominantly in the posterior cervical region, a low-grade fever and is associated with lymphopaenia, splenomegaly and hepatomegaly with abnormal liver function tests, arthralgia and weight loss [18]. The disease has the tendency toward spontaneous remission, with a mean duration of 3 months. Single recurrent episodes of Kikuchi's disease have been reported with gaps of many years between episodes. Kikuchi's disease has been reported to precede, coexist with or follow the diagnosis of systemic lupus erythematosus (SLE) [18, 19]. Final diagnosis is usually established on the basis of lymph node biopsy. As Kikuchi's disease does not have any classical clinical features or laboratory characteristics, it may lead to diagnostic confusion and erroneous treatment. FNAC smears contain a random polymorphous lymphoid population: plasmacytoid monocytes, immunoblasts, small and large lymphocytes, abundant karyorrhectic debris and prominent histiocytes, many of which are small and eccentrically placed, have crescent nuclei and are thought to be characteristic of Kikuchi's [20] (Fig. 5.3). The overall accuracy of FNAC diagnosis in a series by Tong et al. was 56.25%. They found that morphological overlap between Kikuchi's and tuberculous lymphadenitis could have been the reason for the false-negative diagnoses [21]. Some of the cases do not show typical cytological findings and are indistinguishable from other non-specific reactive lymphadenopathies. However, when typical cytological findings are present in an adequate clinical context (cervical nodes in young patients), a precise diagnosis is possible, avoiding unnecessary biopsy procedures [22]. Histological findings include paracortical areas of coagulative necrosis with abundant karyorrhectic debris. Karyorrhectic foci consist of various types of both histiocytes and lymphocytes, as described above. There is an abundance of T cells with predominance of CD8+ over CD4+ T cells. Lymphadenopathy in a patient with fever of unknown origin could be clinically mistaken for a lymphoma, lymphadenitis associated with SLE, tuberculosis, metastatic carcinoma, toxoplasmosis and infectious mononucleosis, or even a submandibular tumour [23, 24]. Kikuchi's lymphadenitis is an uncommon, self-limited and perhaps underdiagnosed process with an excellent prognosis. Accurate clinicopathological recognition is crucial, particularly because it can be mistaken for malignant lymphoma [18–32].

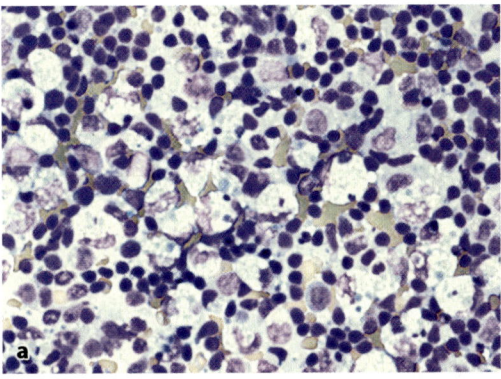

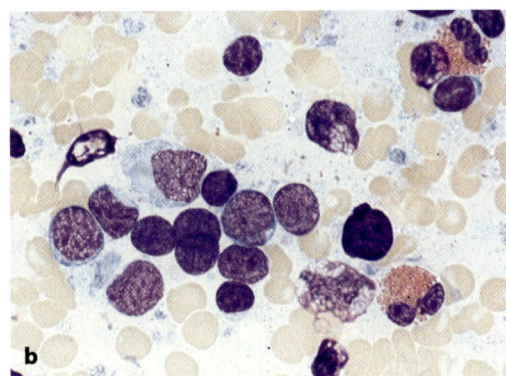

Fig. 5.3
FNA lymph node. Kikuchi's lymphadenitis. **a** FNAC smears contain abundant karyorrhectic debris and prominent histiocytes, many of which are small and eccentrically placed, crescent-shaped nuclei and are thought to be characteristic of Kikuchi's. **b** A polymorphous lymphoid population consists of plasmacytoid monocytes, immunoblasts, and small and large lymphocytes

When SLE patients develop lymphadenopathy, FNAC helps differentiate lupus adenopathy from infectious conditions such as tuberculous adenitis, and from Kikuchi's lymphadenitis although, as mentioned earlier, the latter may be associated with or mimic SLE changes [19, 29, 30]. FNAC in these cases shows predominantly typical and atypical immunoblasts, plasma cells, occasional Reed-Sternberg-like cells and dispersed haematoxylin bodies. Smears are negative for AFB. A similarity between lupus adenopathy to the multicentric Castleman's disease has been described [33–35].

5.1.4 Cat-Scratch Disease

Cat-scratch disease was initially described in 1931, but the aetiologic agent (Bartonella henselae) was not elucidated until decades later. This disease is the most common cause of chronic lymphadenopathy among children and adolescents, characteristically manifesting as subacute regional lymphadenitis with an associated inoculation site due to a cat scratch or bite, often accompanied by fever. The hallmark histological lesion is granulomatous inflammation with a central stellate microabscess. FNAC of nodes in the axilla, parotid, epitrochlear, neck and submental and intraclavicular areas have all been described. Due to the sometimes dramatic clinical presentation of a sizeable swelling, neoplasia may initially be suspected clinically in 38% of the cases [36]. Most patients give a history of cat exposure on subsequent interview. Typical FNAC features of cat-scratch fever include confluent epithelioid cells with the associated and central scattering of neutrophils against a background of polymorphic inflammatory cells (Fig. 5.4). A varying number of medium-sized to large lymphoid cells with an appearance suggestive of monocytoid B lymphocytes may be associated with the epithelioid cells. FNAC is an effective method for diagnosis, despite its heterogeneous appearance and, when combined with clinical information and silver staining, it may be possible to avoid excision. Cytological differential diagnosis includes bacterial abscess and lymphoproliferative disorders. Granulomata or suppurative inflammation are not seen in all cases of cat-scratch fever. The most frequently seen features include granulomata (77%), neutrophils (62%), dispersed epithelioid histiocytes (46%) and suppurative granulomata (38%). A modified silver stain (Warthin-Starry) shows silver-positive organisms in 69% of cases and is not limited to those preparations with suppurative granulomata [36]. Numerous atypical manifestations of the disease have been described, and these often lack the characteristic superficial lymphadenopathy and inoculation site papule. These atypical forms may be misdiagnosed initially as other infectious processes or neoplasms [37–40].

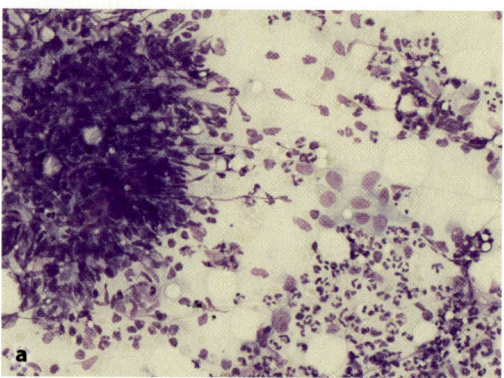

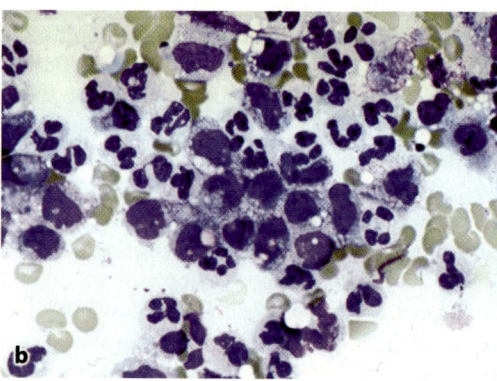

Fig. 5.4
FNAC lymph node. Cat-scratch fever. **a** Typical FNAC features of cat-scratch fever include confluent epithelioid cells with the associated and central scattering of neutrophils against a background of polymorphic inflammatory cells. **b** High-power view showing a varying number of medium-sized to large lymphoid cells with an appearance suggestive of monocytoid B lymphocytes, associated with the epithelioid cells

5.1.5 Leishmania Lymphadenitis

Leishmaniasis is an uncommon cause of cervical lymphadenitis, but should be considered in the differential diagnosis of unexplained lymphadenopathy in endemic countries. FNAC smears reveal a polymorphic population of cells composed of lymphocytes, histiocytes, giant cells, abnormal plasma cells and tingible body macrophages. Leishman Donovan bodies can be identified in all cases, but their number may differ from case to case. Granulomata, dendritic cells, mast cells and lymphoglandular bodies may be identified. Depending upon the presence of characteristic cytological findings, the cases may be divided into five major groups: acute inflammation with giant cells, histiocytic granulomata, epithelioid cell granulomata, plasma cell type and mixed histioplasmacytic type. Demonstration of Leishman Donovan bodies is necessary for the diagnosis of this self-limited condition, for which no treatment is required [41, 42].

5.1.6 Kimura's disease

This is a rare chronic inflammatory disorder with a benign course affecting lymphoid tissue and is seen primarily in young Asian males [43]. Patients usually present with painless subcutaneous swellings in the head and neck region or in the salivary glands (parotid, submandibular and/or lymph node masses), peripheral eosinophilia and markedly elevated serum immunoglobulin E levels [43, 44]. FNAC is characterised by Warthin-Finkeldey-type giant cells against a background of a mixed population of lymphocytes and a significant number of eosinophils [45–47] (Fig. 5.5). Multiple epithelioid granulomata with central eosinophilic abscesses and necrosis have also been described [48]. Excision biopsy is important in order to exclude malignant lymphoma, Langerhans cell histiocytosis, angiolymphoid hyperplasia with eosinophilia and other reactive lymphadenopathies [47, 49, 50]. FNAC may be valuable in the diagnosis of recurrent lesions of Kimura's disease and may spare the patient from repeated biopsy procedures (Fig. 5.6).

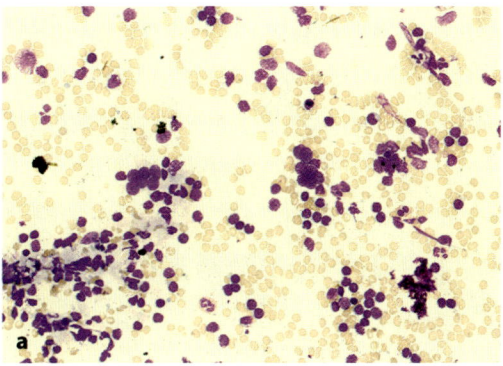
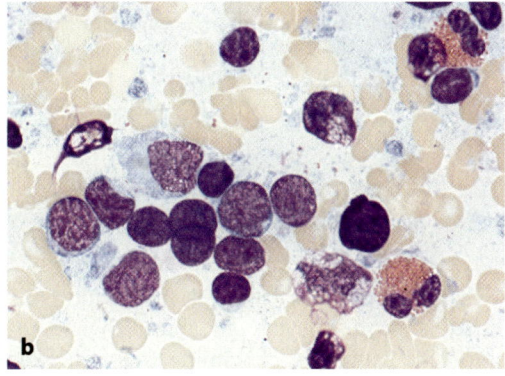

Fig. 5.5
FNAC lymph node. Kimura's disease. FNAC is characterised by the Warthin-Finkeldey-type giant cells against a background of a mixed population of lymphocytes and a significant number of eosinophils. Multiple epithelioid granulomata with central eosinophilic abscesses and necrosis have also been described

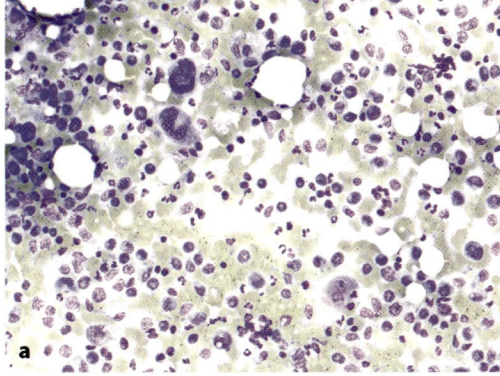

Fig. 5.6
Langerhans cell histiocytosis. **a** low power.

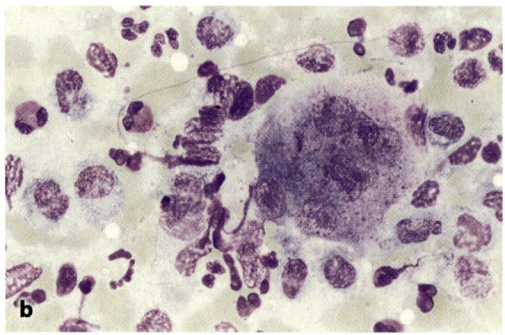

Fig. 5.6
FNAC lymph node. Langerhans cell histiocytosis. **b** Numerous multinucleate giant cells, epithelioid histiocytes and eosinophils. The lesion should be distinguished from Kimura's disease.

5.1.7 Sinus Histiocytosis with Massive Lymphadenopathy

This is also known as Rosai-Dorfman syndrome. FNAC shows histiocytes with abundant pale, eosinophilic cytoplasm containing well-preserved lymphocytes (lymphophagocytosis, emperipolesis), reactive lymphocytes, occasional plasma cells and granulocytes [51, 52]. Immunophenotypic analysis of the histiocytes shows reactivity for S-100 protein and alpha-1-antichymotrypsin and negativity for lysozyme. These features, which are characteristic of sinus histiocytosis with massive lymphadenopathy, demonstrate the reliability of FNAC in making the diagnosis of this disorder [53].

5.1.8 Foreign-Body Granulomatous Inflammatory Response

Foreign-body granulomatous inflammatory response as a result of regionally disseminated foreign-body material (e.g. silicone particles from an orthopaedic prosthesis or from breast silicone implants) may result in lymphadenopathy and be mistaken for a different pathology (Figs. 5.7–5.9). An artificial joint implant may fail due to mechanical mishap, and migration of wear particles can create granulomatous inflammation and node enlargement. This may contain pigment that may be mistaken for a metastatic melanoma [54, 55].

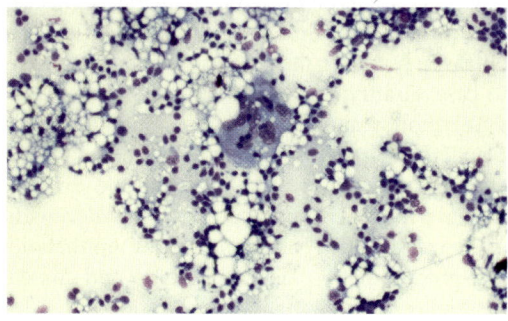

Fig. 5.7
FNAC breast nodule. Patient had a history of silicone implant several years earlier. Now presenting with several firm nodules in the breast. FNAC shows island of fatty cells associated with multinucleate giant cells and histiocytes, presumably as a reaction to the silicone

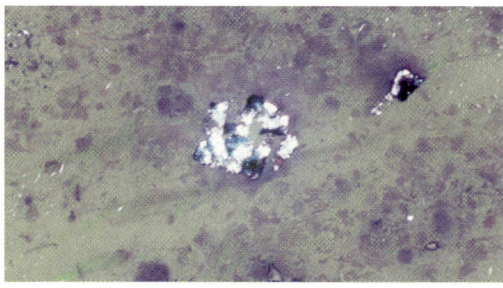

Fig. 5.8
FNAC nodule in the scar. Under polarised light, refractile foreign-body material is seen in the multinucleate giant cells confirming the iatrogenic cause of this process, in this instance, starch granules

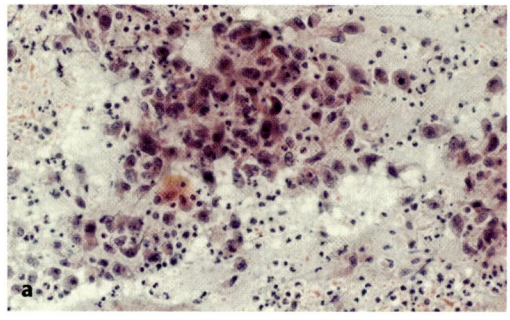

Fig. 5.9
FNAC operation site. (see next page)

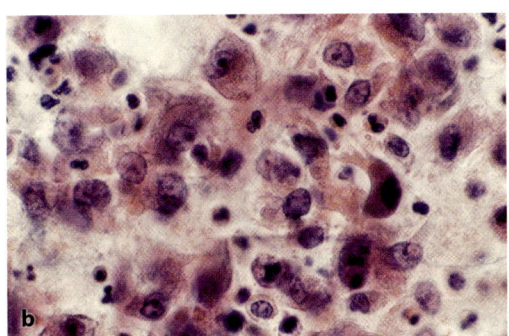

Fig. 5.9
FNAC operation site. **a** (previous page) Smears show a florid granulation tissue response with numerous fibroblasts, histiocytes, endothelial and inflammatory cells. **b** If not expected, the granulations cells seen in this high-power view may be alarming

5.1.9 Malignant Lymphomas

Malignant lymphomas and solid tumours that mimic or are associated with epithelioid granulomas are important in the cytological differential diagnosis of granulomatous infiltrates [56]. Metastatic SqCC with an extensive granulomatous response, Hodgkin's disease (HD) with exuberant granulomatous response, diffuse large cell lymphoma, anaplastic carcinoma of the thyroid, lymphoepithelial carcinoma, marginal zone lymphoma [57] and others may all be associated with granulomata and contain tumour cells mimicking epithelioid histiocytes, making the diagnosis difficult on FNAC [53–60] (Figs. 5.10–5.13). Cytological differential diagnosis of a granulomatous process should include malignant neoplasms [56] (Case history 5.1).

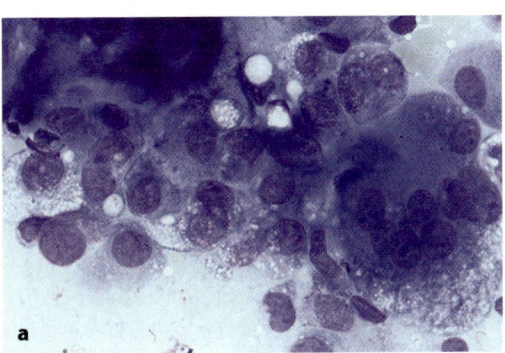

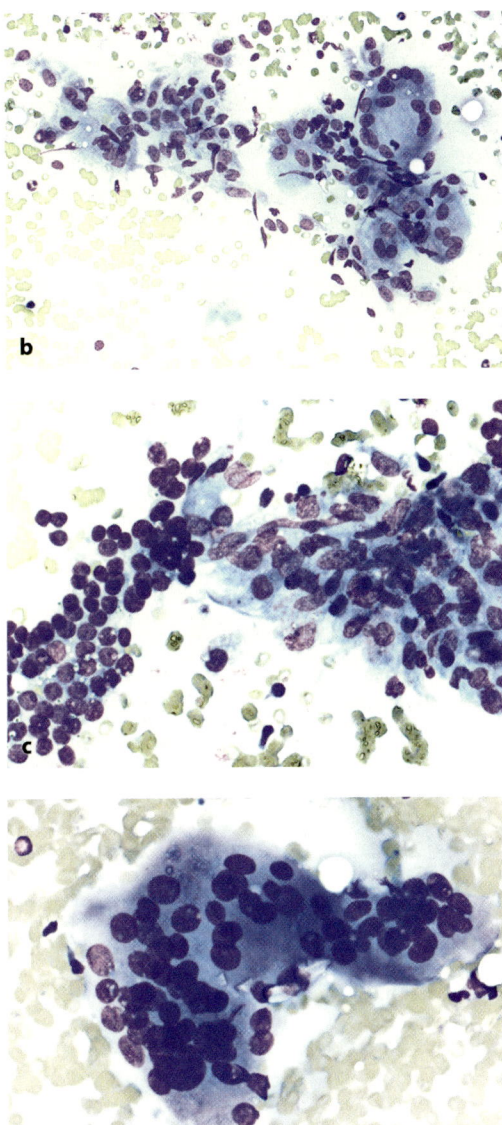

Fig. 5.10
FNAC thyroid. **a** Papillary carcinomas often contain multinucleate giant cells, which may mislead the observer into thinking that the lesion is an inflammatory, granulomatous process. **b** Subacute thyroiditis contains numerous multinucleate giant cells and epithelioid cells. **c** High-power view of epithelioid cells and thyroid epithelium. **d** Multinucleate giant cells are commonly found in Hashimoto's thyroiditis

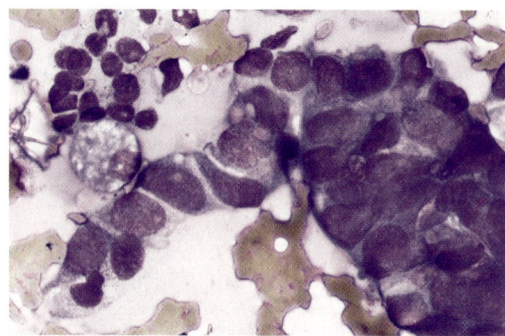

Fig. 5.11
FNAC thyroid. Anaplastic carcinoma of the thyroid may contain multinucleate giant cells

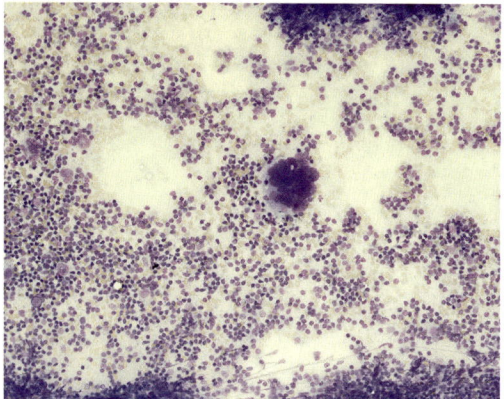

Fig. 5.12
FNAC lymph node. Hodgkin lymphoma may contain giant cells of the Reed-Sternberg type but may also contain epithelioid cells and histiocyte-type giant cells as part of the tumour

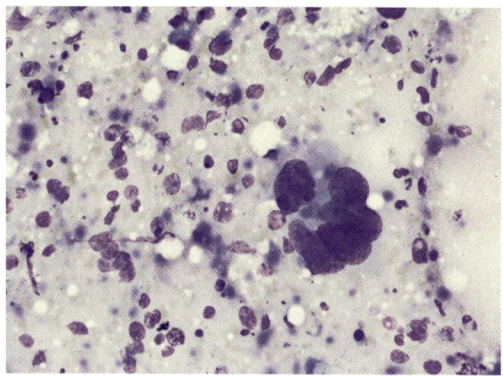

Fig. 5.13
FNAC mediastinum. Tumour giant cells in a case of mediastinal germ cell tumour (seminoma)

Case history 5.1: A 64-year-old patient with a history of a recent resection of an SqCC of the left tonsil presented with a swelling in the ipsilateral supraclavicular fossa. FNAC yielded thick keratinous material. Microscopy revealed an inflammatory background with anucleate squamous cells, multinucleate giant cells and very occasional viable squamous cells, some showing cytological atypia. A diagnosis of metastatic SqCC was given. At a multidisciplinary meeting, it was revealed that patient had had an epider moid cyst at this site prior to the operation and that the area had been subsequently irradiated. The cytologist issued a correction to the original report stating that the features would be consistent with a ruptured epidermoid cyst. Histology confirmed the lesion as benign (Fig. 5.14)

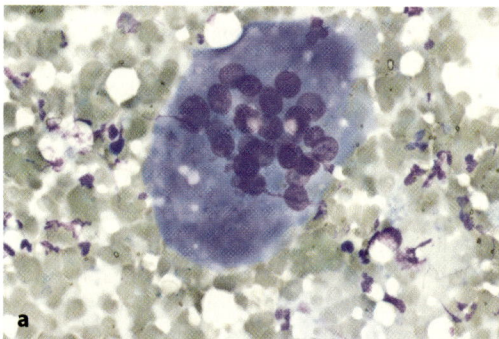

a

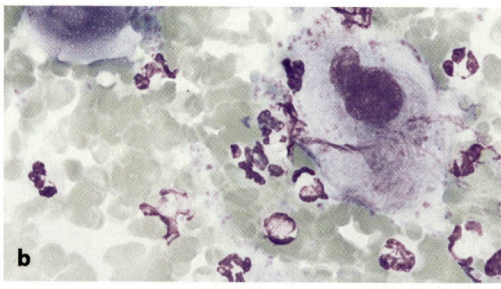

b

Fig. 5.14
FNAC supraclavicular mass. **a** Inflammatory background with anucleate squamous cells, multinucleate giant cells and **b** very occasional viable squamous cells, some showing cytological atypia. A diagnosis of metastatic SqCC was given. The lesion was in fact a raptured epidermoid cyst within the a radiation field for treatment of SqCC

Granulomatous processes elsewhere in the body can be diagnosed by means of FNAC. Some examples include Wegener's granuloma and fat necrosis (Figs. 5.15 and 5.16).

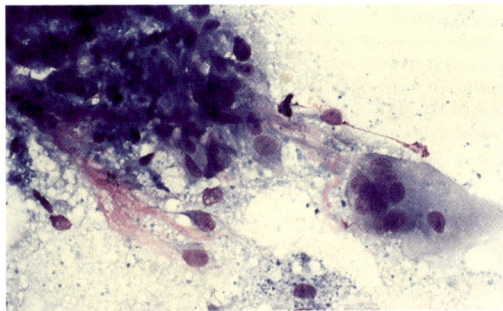

Fig. 5.15
FNAC breast. Fat necrosis. Multinucleate giant cells, macrophages, debris and fragments of fat are typical of this condition. Microcalcifications may cause diagnostic dilemma on imaging and lesion may be clinically suspicious of malignancy

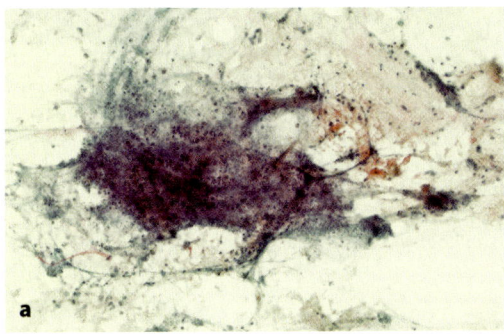

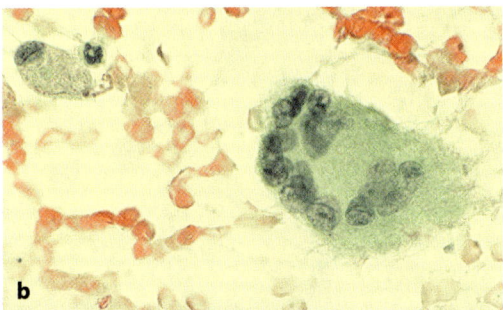

Fig. 5.16
FNAC lung. Wegener's granuloma. **a** FNAC material often contains much necrosis and polymorphs. **b** Occasional multinucleate giant cells are noted. A diagnosis of granulomatous condition can me made. Differential diagnosis includes tuberculosis and malignancy. Staining for acid-fast bacilli is negative

5.2 Lymphoid Infiltrates in Extranodal Sites

The finding of lymphoid cells in FNAC samples from extranodal sites is always noteworthy. In these cases, lymphoid cells may define the underlying pathology and contribute to an accurate diagnosis. Most frequently, lymphocytes form part of an inflammatory exudate, are reactive and may explain some of the cytological changes and processes. The ratio between neutrophils and lymphocytes usually indicates the stage of the inflammatory process. The presence of non-circulating lymphoid cells indicates the presence of lymphoid follicles and may be significant for diagnosis. The following are some examples of lymphoid cells in extranodal sites, including differential diagnoses and pitfalls.

5.2.1 Lymphoid Infiltrates in the Thyroid

Lymphocytic (Hashimoto's) thyroiditis is a condition that is exemplified by the association between lymphoid and epithelial cells. It is the second most common thyroid lesion diagnosed on FNAC, after endemic goitre, in iodine-deficient areas [61]. Patients usually present either with diffuse and rubbery thyroid enlargement or, less frequently, with one or two prominent nodules [62]. FNAC is highly sensitive in diagnosing Hashimoto's thyroiditis, with a diagnostic accuracy rate of 92% [62]. FNAC preparations characteristically show a dual population of follicular epithelium (some or most of which may undergo oncocytic - Hurthle cell - change) and lymphoid cell infiltrate composed of lymphoid follicle cells including mature lymphocytes, centroblasts, plasma cells and follicular dendritic cells (Fig. 5.17). Hurthle cells may show a variable degree of cytological atypia, namely anisonucleosis and macronucleosis (Fig. 5.18). Lymphoid cells may also exhibit variable forms including that of atypical immunoblasts (Fig. 5.19). Diagnosis of Hashimoto's thyroiditis may be not be apparent in FNAC preparations, which reveal cytological evidence of hyperplasia or abundant colloid with sparse lymphoid cells. On the other hand, the diagnosis of lymphocytic thyroiditis should not be made when only a few lymphocytes are present. Pleomorphic Hurthle cells may be present in aspirates from Hurthle cell neoplasms and may be misdiagnosed as Hashimoto's thyroiditis, especially when they are associated with a few lymphocytes [63] (Fig. 5.20). The differential diagnosis between a hyperplastic nodule and a follicular neoplasm and between a Hurthle cell nodule and a Hurthle cell tumour is impossible in some cases and may result in a false-positive interpretation. In equivocal cases, multiple aspirates and immunological investigations are helpful. In antibody-negative cases, a repeat FNAC at follow-up is useful. Marked lymphocytic infiltration and Hurthle cell change may indicate a hypothyroid state, but hormonal levels are required for clinical management [61].

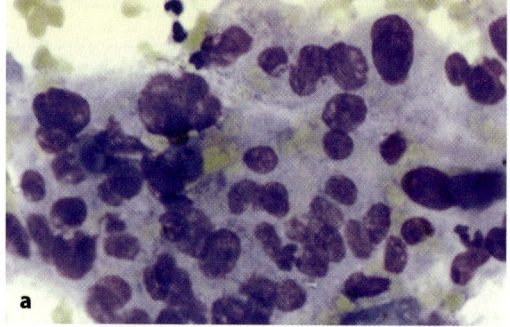

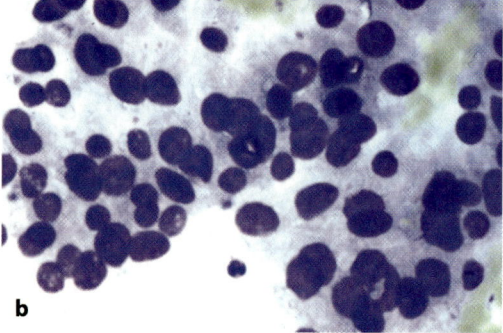

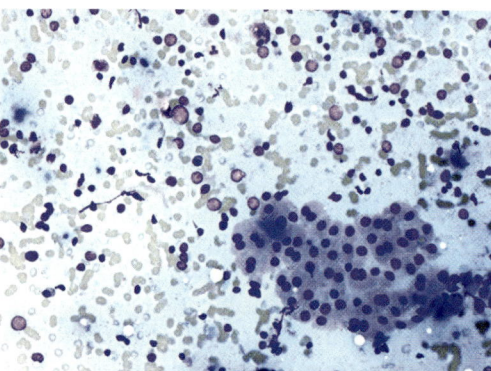

Fig. 5.18
FNAC thyroid. **a** Hashimoto's thyroiditis. Hurthle cells may show a variable degree of cytological atypia, namely anisonucleosis and macronucleosis. **b** Follicular carcinoma of the thyroid may show similar nuclear features. A careful examination of the whole sample and search for lymphoid cell usually clarifies the diagnosis

Fig. 5.17
FNAC thyroid. Hashimoto's thyroiditis. Preparations characteristically show a dual population of follicular epithelium, some or most of which may undergo oncocytic (Hurthle cell) changes, and lymphoid cell infiltrate composed of lymphoid follicle cells including mature lymphocytes, centroblasts, plasma cells and follicular dendritic cells

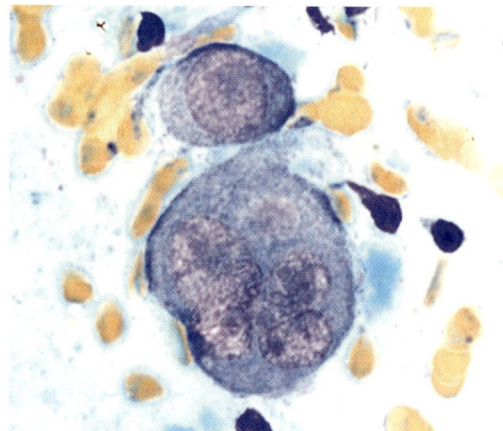

Fig. 5.19
FNAC thyroid. Lymphoid cells may also show variable forms including atypical immunoblasts

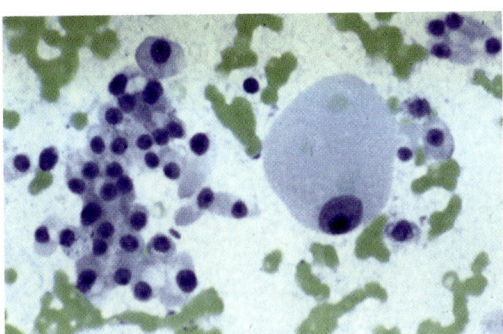

Fig. 5.20
FNAC thyroid. Oncocytic tumour. Pleomorphic Hurthle cells may be present in aspirates from oncocytic cell neoplasms and misdiagnosed as Hashimoto's thyroiditis, especially when they are associated with a few lymphocytes

Some investigators have found an increased incidence of PTC in patients with Hashimoto's thyroiditis, which raises the possibility that there may be more than an incidental association between these two diseases (Fig. 5.21). The frequency of carcinoma in Hashimoto's thyroiditis varies between 0.5 and 23.7%, depending on the stringency of diagnostic criteria applied [64–66]. Similarly, the prevalence of Hashimoto's thyroiditis is significantly higher in patients with PTC [67]. In addition to epidemiological data, there is an overlap in the morphological features, immunohistochemical staining pattern and molecular profile between the two conditions (Fig. 5.21). Although considered a benign condition, Hashimoto's thyroiditis almost always harbours a genetic rearrangement that is strongly associated with and is highly specific for PTC [68]. Focal PTC-like immunophenotypic changes in Hashimoto's thyroiditis suggest the possibility of early, focal pre-malignant transformation in some cases [69]. In addition, p53 is commonly expressed in both PTC and Hashimoto's thyroiditis, suggesting another potential biological link between the two disorders [70]. Patients with PTC associated with Hashimoto's thyroiditis typically have a dominant nodule, 44% of which are discovered incidentally upon routine examination [67]. FNAC has a sensitivity of 91% for the identification of PTC and is unaffected by the presence of co-existent Hashimoto's thyroiditis [67]. However, Hashimoto-associated PTCs may frequently display prominent stromal desmoplasia and a pseudovascular pattern, both of which may present diagnostic difficulties in the cytological diagnosis because of the marked obliteration of the tumour by fibrosis [71]. All palpable nodules in the same gland should be investigated by FNAC in order to improve diagnostic sensitivity and identify occult neoplasms [72]. Focal thyroiditis may be confused with Hashimoto's thyroiditis, especially when adjacent to a neoplasm. Surgical exploration should be performed in cases of severe lymphocytic thyroiditis diagnosed by FNAC, which has a repeatedly negative antibody titres, in order to exclude neoplasm [73]. The survival of patients who have PTC may be superior in the presence of the coexistent Hashimoto's thyroiditis [74].

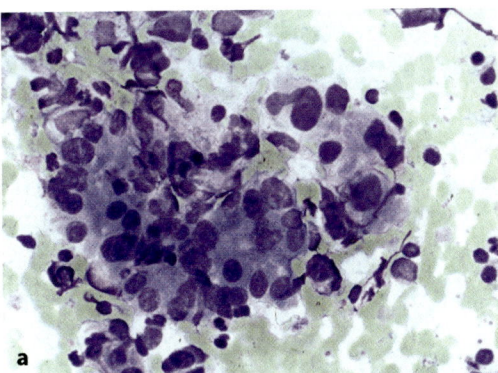

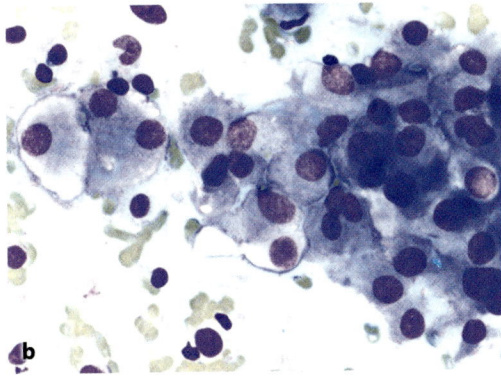

Fig. 5.21
FNAC thyroid. (see next page)

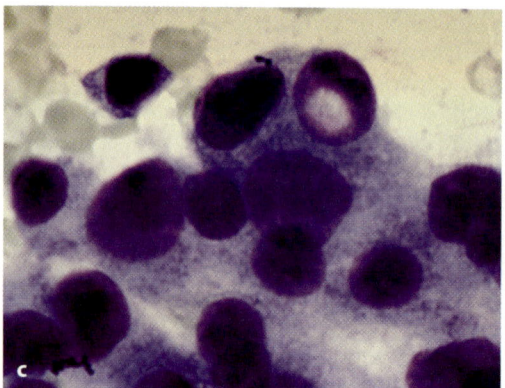

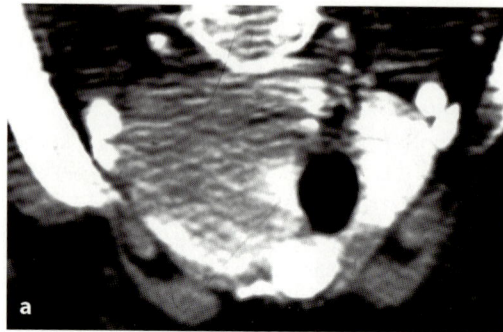

Fig. 5.21
FNAC thyroid. There is an overlap in the morphological features, immunohistochemical staining pattern and molecular profile between the papillary carcinoma and Hashimoto's thyroiditis. **a** Papillary carcinoma cell clusters with well-defined scalloped cytoplasm and a surrounding lymphoid infiltrate. **b** Hashimoto's thyroiditis showing oncocytic type cells and lymphoid infiltrate. **c** Some nuclei may have intranuclear inclusions (see Fig. 5.18)

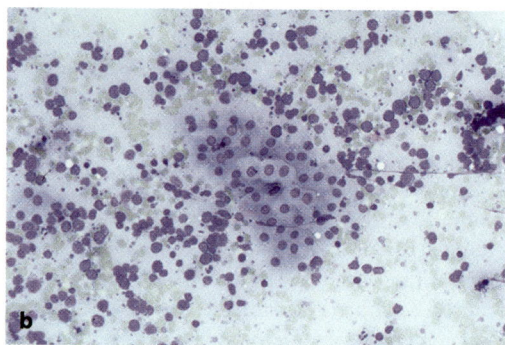

Hashimoto's thyroiditis is a risk factor for thyroid lymphoma. This is usually a DLBL, but can also be a low-grade B-cell MALT lymphoma. Up to 40% of all DLBLs appear to have undergone transformation from a MALT lymphoma, but they behave in a similar fashion to DLBLs. DLBLs can be correctly diagnosed by FNAC (Fig. 5.22). MALT may be diagnosed as lymphoma, suspicious of lymphoma or be mistaken for Hashimoto's thyroiditis [75]. False-negative results are usually caused by sampling error because of the frequent coexistence of Hashimoto's thyroiditis and lymphoma [76, 77]. Clonality analysis of FNAC material or tissue samples by PCR currently holds the promise of a diagnosis in difficult cases, but is not always conclusive [78–80]. MALT lymphomas of the thyroid are indolent, comprising approximately 6–27% of thyroid lymphomas and, when localised to the thyroid, respond well to total thyroidectomy or radiation, with a complete response rate of more than 90%. The overall 5-year survival for the DLBL aggressive group is less then 50%. Surgery is rarely beneficial [81].

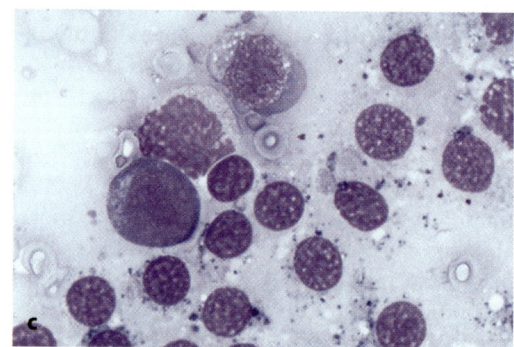

Fig. 5.22
FNAC thyroid. **a** CT scan of a patient with a thyroid mass shows deviation of the trachea. **b** DLBL can be correctly diagnosed by FNAC. Large atypical blasts are found in close proximity to thyroid epithelium.
c High-power view of the neoplastic lymphoid cell blasts showing scant basophilic cytoplasm

5.2.2 Lymphoid Processes in the Salivary Gland

Lymphoid proliferations of the salivary glands can be either reactive or neoplastic. Reactive lesions include lymphoepithelial cyst and the lymphoepithelial sialadenitis of Sjogren's syndrome (so-called benign lymphoepithelial lesion or myoepithelial sialadenitis -MESA). This lymphoid proliferation involves the infiltration of ductal epithelium by lymphocytes of the marginal zone or monocytoid B-cell type, forming lymphoepithelial lesions (epimyoepithelial islands) (Fig. 5.23). Patients with lymphoepithelial sialadenitis have a 44-fold increased risk of developing salivary gland or extrasalivary lymphoma, of which 80% are the marginal zone/MALT type. Broad strands of marginal zone or monocytoid B cells around lymphoepithelial lesions and monotypic immunoglobulin detection by immunohistochemistry are considered diagnostic of MALT lymphoma (Fig. 5.24). B-cell clones are detected in over 50% of cases of MESA by molecular genetic methods, but this does not correlate with lymphoma. Nodal-type B-cell lymphomas of the salivary glands are either follicular lymphoma (35%), which may arise in intra-salivary gland lymph nodes and behave similarly to follicular lymphoma in other sites, or DLBL (30%), which may arise de novo or secondary to either MALT or follicular lymphomas [82].

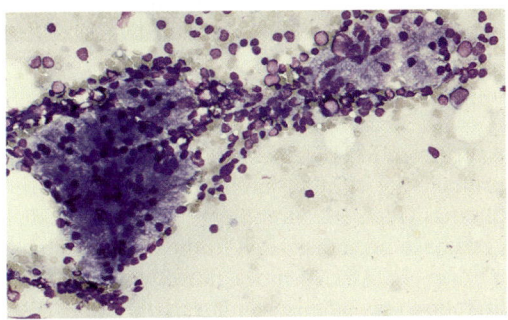

Fig. 5.23
FNAC salivary gland. Myoepithelial sialadenitis (MESA). This lymphoid proliferation involves infiltration of ductal epithelium by lymphocytes of marginal zone or monocytoid B-cell type, forming lymphoepithelial lesions (epimyoepithelial islands)

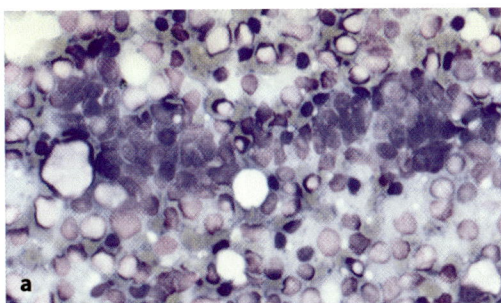

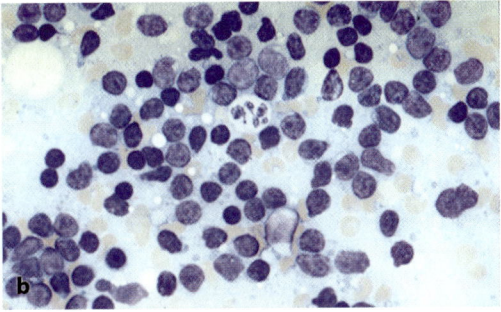

Fig. 5.24
FNAC salivary gland. MALT lymphoma. **a** Low-power features are almost indistinguishable from MESA. Broad strands of marginal zone or monocytoid B cells around lymphoepithelial lesions and monotypic immunoglobulin detection by immunohistochemistry are considered diagnostic of MALT lymphoma. **b** The diagnosis of MESA versus marginal zone B-cell lymphoma of the MALT type still relies largely on the evaluation of morphological features. Bland centrocyte-like cells dominate the aspirate

The diagnosis of MESA versus marginal zone B-cell lymphoma of the MALT type still relies largely on the evaluation of morphological features. It seems that molecular genetic analysis has little or no practical role in the clinical diagnosis of salivary gland lymphoma in the setting of MESA and Sjogren's syndrome [83]. Clinically, reactive intraparotid lymph nodes, myoepithelial sialadenitis and lymphomas all present as parotid enlargements that are indistinguishable from pleomorphic adenomas and are therefore part of a differential diagnosis of mass lesions in the parotid. Warthin's tumour of the parotid (see Chap. 4), although typically containing a lymphoid infiltrate, may present as a diagnostic pitfall if there is prominence of squamous metaplasia/atypia, mucoid/mucinous background, spindle-shaped cells, and cystic/inflammatory debris [84]. Warthin's tumour may mimic chronic sialadenitis/MESA in some cases (Fig. 5.25).

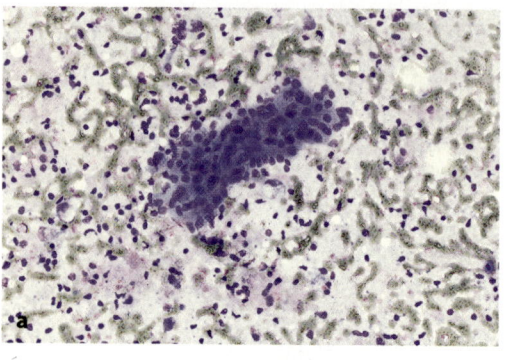

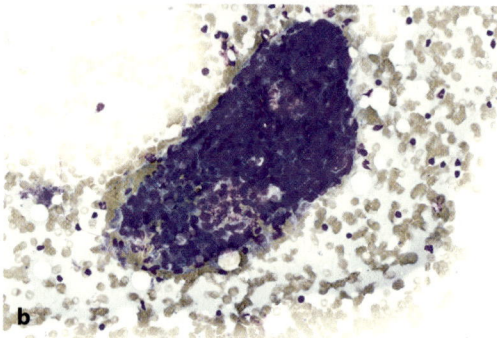

Fig. 5.25
FNAC salivary gland. **a** Warthin's tumour, although typically containing a lymphoid infiltrate, may present as a diagnostic pitfall if there is a prominence of squamous metaplasia/atypia, mucoid/mucinous background, spindle-shaped cells, and cystic/inflammatory debris [84]. It may mimic chronic sialadenitis/MESA in some cases. **b** Chronic sialadenitis often contains only ductal epithelium against a background of inflammatory cells and can mimic Warthin's tumour

In a review of over 6,000 cases of salivary FNAC, Hughes et al. found that intraparotid lymph node (36%) and granulomatous sialadenitis (10%) are amongst the most common false-positive diagnoses in FNAC salivary gland [85], salivary gland lymphoma being the most common false-negative FNAC diagnosis (57%) followed by ACC (49%), low-grade mucoepidermoid carcinoma (43%), and adenoid cystic carcinoma (33%). Flow cytometric cell-surface-marker analysis may be helpful to determine the clonality of the B-cell proliferations [86].

Case history 2: A 53-year-old female patient presented with a mass at the left angle of mandible following a parotidectomy for MALT lymphoma on the contralateral side 10 years previously. FNAC Smears showed a monotonous lymphoid cell population with a residual follicular pattern. PCR revealed monoclonal bands identical to those in the other parotid. A diagnosis of MALT lymphoma was made. The patient underwent left parotidectomy. Three years later, a new mass appeared in the proximity of the resection site. This time, MALT cells had transformed into a high-grade lymphoma (DLBL). Immunocytochemistry showed strong proliferative activity in the marginal zone cells. PCR showed the same IgH monoclonal bands as observed in the previous tumours (Figs. 5.26 and 5.27).

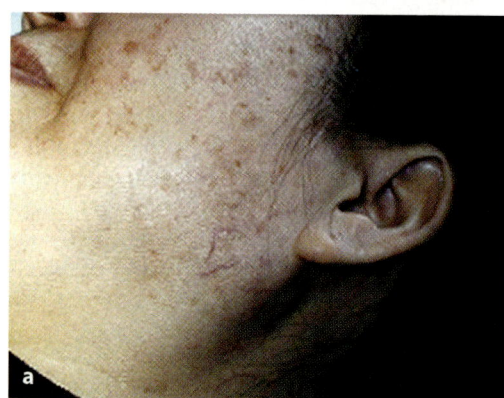

Fig. 5.26 a
Patien with a left parotid tumour

Apart from MALT, the salivary gland can be the primary site of other low- and high-grade lymphomas (Figs. 5.28 and 5.29). Lymphoepithelial cysts have been discussed in the previous chapter (see Fig. 4.6). At times, florid lymphoid proliferation may be mistaken for a lymphoma (Fig. 5.30).

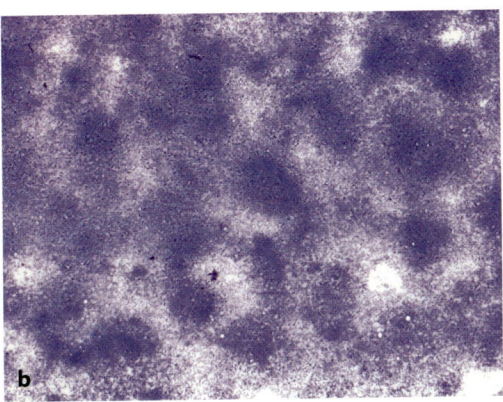

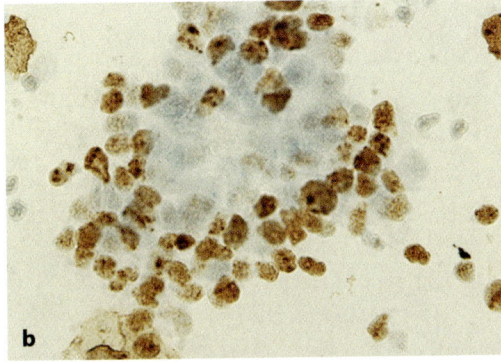

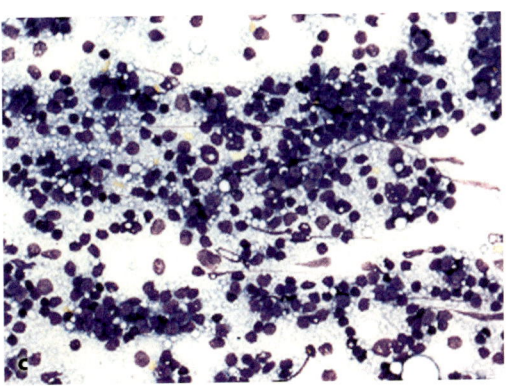

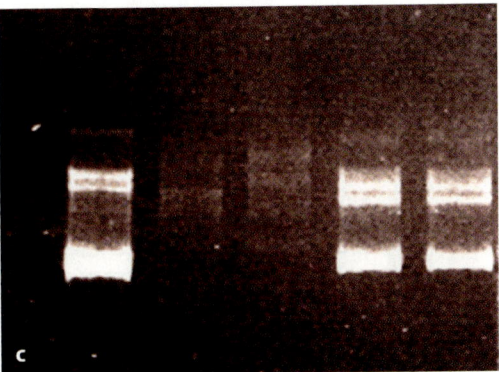

Fig. 5.26
Salivary gland tumour. **b** Low power view shows residual "follicular pattern" in a very cellular lymphoid aspirate. population, **c** High power view shows monotonous centrocyte like cells in close proximity to salivary gland epithelium.

Fig. 5.27
Same patient as in Fig. 5.26, FNAC cheek lump, several years later: **a** In addition to small, there are transformed lymphocytes consistent with DLBL. **b** MIB 1 proliferation marker shows strong positivity in the cells from a marginal zone. PCR of FNAC salivary gland. **c** IgH shows monoclonal bands, identical to those from the previous tumour, confirming the diagnosis

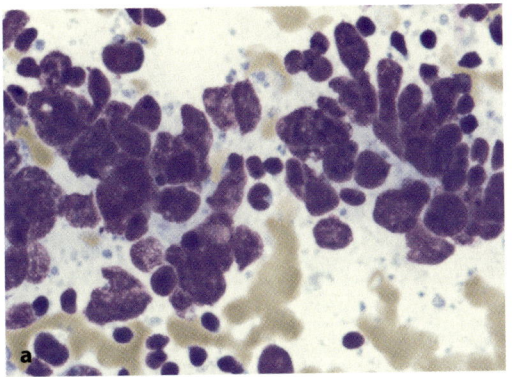

5.2.3 Lymphoid Infiltrates of the Orbit

In a review of the diagnoses for 79 FNAC samples from the orbit, Nassar et al. found that lymphoproliferative diagnoses accounted for 54%, including cases diagnosed as lymphoma/atypical lymphocytic infiltrate, inflammation or abscess, plasmacytoma and Langerhans' cell histiocytosis [87]. Lymphoid infiltrate can manifest as a solitary mass that can simulate an iris melanoma [88]. Vitreous cytology in conjunction with ancillary studies may be a sensitive procedure in the diagnosis of intraocular lymphoma [89].

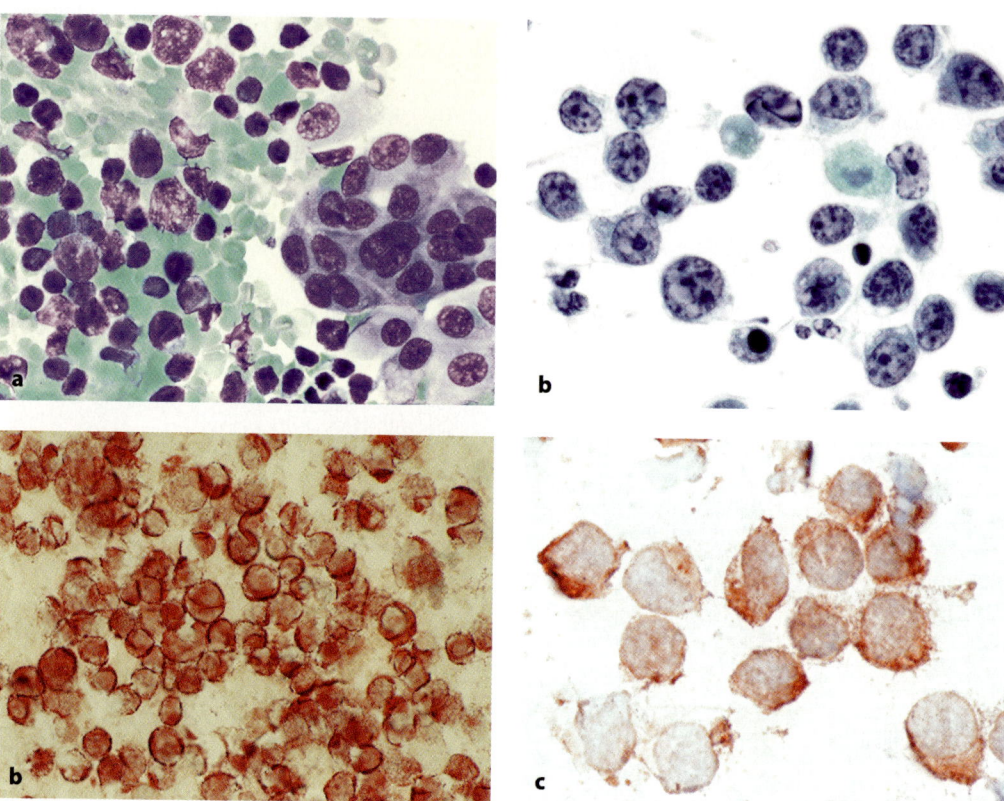

Fig. 5.28
FNAC salivary gland. Low-grade T-cell lymphoma.
a Salivary duct epithelium seen in the proximity of medium-sized lymphoid cells showing little cellular pleomorphism. **b** CD3 immunocytochemistry confirms the cells to be of T-cell origin and outlines the convoluted nuclear contours (alkaline phosphatase anti-alkaline phosphatase staining)

Fig. 5.29
FNAC parotid. DLBL. **a** MGG-stained high-power view of lymphoid blast cells. **b** Pap staining reveals details of the nuclear chromatin. **c** CD79a (a B-cell marker) confirms the B-cell phenotype of this lymphoma

Fig. 5.30
FNAC breast. Lymphocytic mastitis. Sparse lymphoid follicle centre cells are found in breast aspirates of patients with diabetes

5.2.4 Lymphoid Lesions in the Breast

FNAC is an inexpensive but highly useful diagnostic tool with which to distinguish between primary lymphoma and carcinoma of the breast. This helps with clinical management in avoiding unnecessary surgical procedures [74, 90]. Breast lumps resulting from lymphocytic mastopathy may present a clinical pitfall in diabetic patients and patients with a history of breast carcinoma. These cases can be resolved by FNAC sampling of the lumps, which show mature lymphocytes and follicle centre cells [91, 92] (Fig. 5.31). Lymphoepithelioma-like carcinoma is a rare tumour composed of sheets of epithelioid cells arranged as single cells or in cords that are partially obscured by a dense lymphocytic infiltrate. The epithelioid cells extensively express cytokeratin stain, but do not express E-cadherin. It has a good prognosis and should be considered as a possible diagnosis in breast tumours with an intense lymphocytic infiltrate [93]. Medullary carcinoma is a tumour with a lymphoid infiltrate, a favourable prognosis and a low frequency of metastases (Fig. 5.31). Lymphoid infiltrate of medullary carcinomas is related to beta-actin fragments exposed by apoptotic cells. Myofibroblastic tumour of the breast is a rare and unusual inflammatory lesion with occasional aggregates of cellular connective tissue fragments, sheets of uniform ductal epithelial cells with myoepithelial cells, spindle cells, lymphocytes and histiocyte-like cells. Clinically and on imaging, it resembles a carcinoma [94].

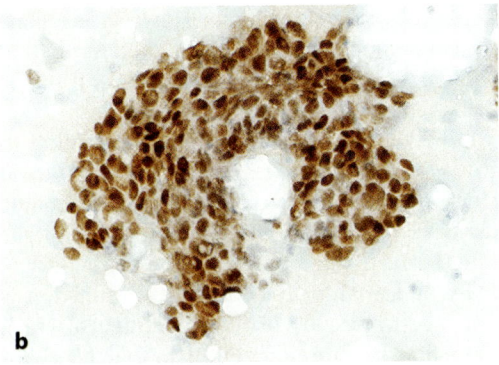

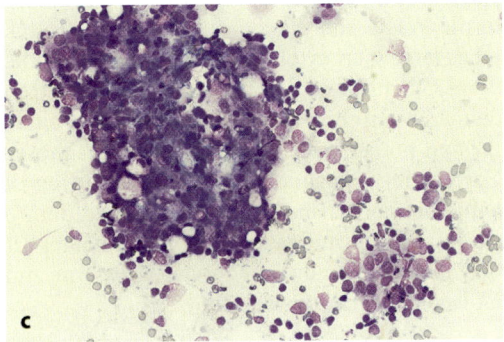

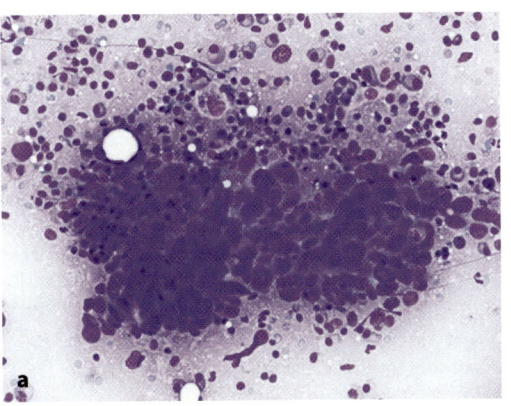

Fig. 5.31
FNAC breast. Medullary carcinoma. **a** Lymphoid infiltrate, a hallmark of this tumour conveys a favourable prognosis and low frequency of metastasis. It is related to beta-actin fragments exposed by apoptotic cells. **b** Oestrogen receptor positivity in epithelial cells from a medullary carcinoma

FNAC may be a very useful triaging procedure in the diagnosis of lymphoid infiltrates in other extranodal sites including the pancreas, bone, thyroid, kidney, abdomen, mediastinum, pancreas and soft tissues [76, 95–104].

5.3 Neoplasms Containing Lymphocytes

Neoplasms containing lymphoid cells may be either primary lymphoid neoplasms (i.e. lymphomas) or other non-haemopoietic neoplasms that typically contain lymphocytes as part of their morphological appearance. Lymphomas will be described in general terms with emphasis on the diagnostic pitfalls. However, neoplasms containing lymphocytes will be described in some detail, in keeping with the general theme of this chapter.

NHLs are currently diagnosed according to the World Health Organisation (WHO) classification [105]. This classification still broadly divides lymphomas according to the phenotype into B- and T-cell types. Since the availability of FNAC material for phenotyping is limited, it is note worthy that 90% of NHLs are B cell, of which more than half are either DLBL or follicular lymphomas (31% and 22%, respectively). According to the WHO, morphological diagnosis of NHL relies largely on cytological detail, although the development of new technologies has helped to define several clinical entities. Morphology alone is often not sufficient for a definitive diagnosis. Current recommendations for the reporting of lymphoid neoplasms suggest that in addition to clinical features and morphology, the final report may include: immunophenotype, karyotype and molecular characteristics [106].

5.3.1 Dilemmas in the Cytological Diagnosis of Lymphomas

Cytological assessment of the sample taken with FNAC is often the first-line morphological investigation of lymphoma [107, 108]. Some lymphomas have characteristic cytological appearances, and it is generally possible to diagnose most, at least in general terms, on the basis of the initial morphology [109]. With an overall accuracy rate of 96–99% and a typing accuracy rate of 96.5%, FNAC yields a high rate of conclusive cytological diagnoses in the assessment of metastatic malignancies, high-grade NHL (79–90%) and HD (with the exception of the lymphocytic predominance variant of HD), but has significant limitations in the assessment of low-grade NHL and precise Revised European American Lymphoma classification (REAL) typing [110–113]. Some centres successfully use a combination of cytology and flow cytometry as an initial approach [114–116]. The combination of FNAC and core biopsy in the diagnosis of lymphoma can further reduce the rate of inadequate samples and improve the typing of lymphomas [117]. The techniques are best used to complement rather than compete with one another. Examples of morphological difficulties include distinguishing between the following: (1) low-grade lymphoma from reactive lymph node hyperplasia; (2) variants of small lymphocytic lymphomas and lymphoma from metastases, particularly of small round-cell tumours (SRCT), such as peripheral neuroectodermal tumour, rhabdomyosarcoma (RMS), and small cell carcinoma (SCC); (3) HD from ALCL; (4) ALCL from non-lymphoid tumours. Although most of these can be resolved with the help of immunocytochemistry, there are sometimes problems with immunophenotyping on cytological preparations, partly as a result of the small amount of material available [118]. Grading follicular lymphomas on FNAC specimens cannot clearly distinguish between grades 2 and 3 [119]. Despite the best efforts of morphology and immunophenotyping, some lymphomas are impossible to diagnose on FNAC [120]. Future algorithms for the diagnosis of lymphoma should include FNAC as a preferred method of initial lymphoma diagnostic triage, RNA or protein extraction, followed by high throughput genomic or proteomic analysis and tissue biopsy, where necessary [121] (Fig. 5.32; reproduced with permission from J Clin Pathol).

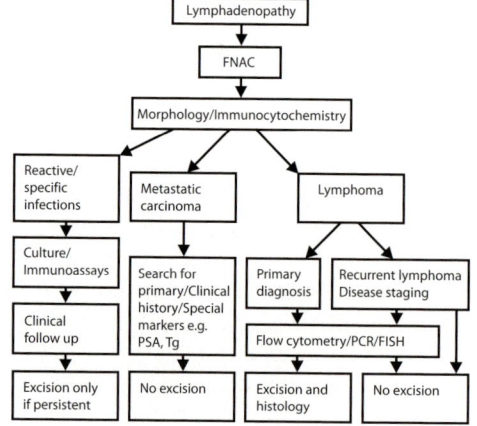

Fig. 5.32
Algorithm for FNAC lymph nodes (FISH, fluorescence in situ hybridisation; PSA, prostate-specific antigen) [121]

The cytological diagnosis of HD can be challenging when classical Reed-Sternberg cells are absent. Contributing factors for a false-negative diagnosis include obscuring reactive inflammatory cells, fibrosis of the involved lymph nodes, partial involvement of the lymph node by HD, sampling error and misinterpretation. The lymphocyte-depleted type of HD may be particularly difficult to diagnose in FNAC samples [122, 123].

5.3.2 Solid Neoplasms Containing Lymphocytes

A pronounced lymphocytic reaction is a hallmark in 10% of ACCs. Both the variety of tumour cell differentiation and the pronounced lymphocytic reaction observed in FNAC may result in confusion with other salivary gland lesions. The differential diagnosis of ACC encompasses adenocarcinoma, mucoepidermoid carcinoma, pleomorphic adenoma, Warthin's tumour, sebaceous lymphadenoma, benign lymphoepithelial lesion, sialoadenosis, sialadenitis caused by radiotherapy and lymphadenitis [124]. Paediatric follicular carcinomas of the thyroid have an associated lymphocytic infiltrate in the tumour and/or adjacent thyroid, however, this is more commonly the case in papillary carcinomas [125] (Fig. 5.21). Lymphoepithelioma-like carcinoma is an undifferentiated carcinoma with a dense lymphoid stroma. It has been mentioned earlier as occurring in the breast, but it has also been reported in diverse organs and shows variable association with Epstein-Barr virus, which can be demonstrated in the tumour cells [126–134]. Nasopharyngeal carcinoma typically contains mature lymphocytes intermingled with clusters of cohesive tumour cells, most of which are undifferentiated with medium-sized, oval, vesicular nuclei and prominent nucleoli. The cytoplasm is generally pale with ill-defined boundaries. Mitoses are present in 75% of cases [135] (Fig. 5.33). Testicular seminoma has characteristically a variable numbers of lymphocytes and plasma cells admixed with the dispersed cell population of large cells with scant to moderately abundant cytoplasm, round nuclei (which may be slightly irregular), finely granular chromatin and either one central prominent nucleolus or two to three smaller nucleoli (Fig. 5.34). Epithelioid histiocytes or the characteristic tigroid background may be seen [136]. The majority subset of the lymphoid infiltrate is composed of cytotoxic T-lymphocytes infiltrating seminoma tumour nests [137]. Sebaceous lymphadenoma is a rare, benign neoplasm that is characterised histologically by proliferating islands of epithelium with sebaceous glandular differentiation in a dense, lymphocytic background. The parotid gland is the most common site, and the patient usually presents with a well-circumscribed, enlarging and painless mass. Primary sebaceous lesions of the salivary glands are very rare entities and must be differentiated from the more common, potentially malignant tumours [138].

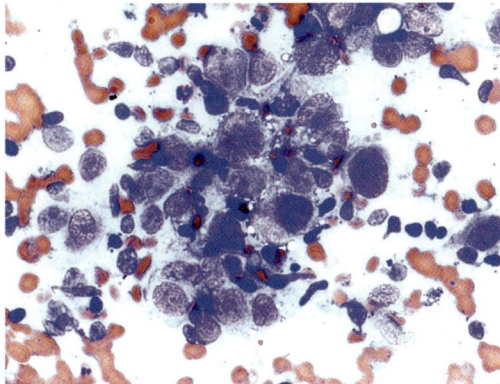

Fig. 5.33
FNAC neck mass. Nasopharyngeal carcinoma is an undifferentiated carcinoma with a dense lymphoid stroma. It has been reported in diverse organs and shows variable association with Epstein-Barr virus that can be demonstrated in the tumour cells

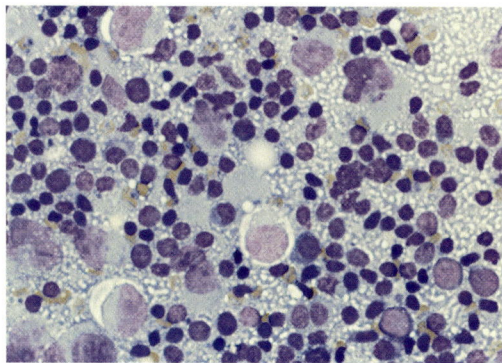

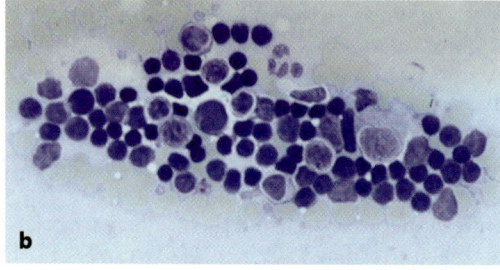

Fig. 5.35
FNAC mediastinum. **a** Thymoma is characterised by a biphasic epithelial and lymphoid population and irregular cohesive tissue fragments of varying proportions of lymphoid and epithelial cells. **b** Lymphocytes tend to be of the small type. Epithelium may be atypical

Fig. 5.34
FNAC lymph node. Seminoma has characteristically a variable number of lymphocytes and plasma cells admixed with the dispersed cell population of large cells, with scant to moderately abundant cytoplasm, round nuclei (which may be slightly irregular), finely granular chromatin and either one central prominent nucleolus or two to three smaller nucleoli

Lymphocytic infiltrates in medullary carcinoma of the breast and Warthin's tumour of the salivary gland have been described earlier in this chapter. Thymomas are characterised by a biphasic epithelial and lymphoid population and irregular cohesive tissue fragments of varying proportions of lymphoid and epithelial cells (Fig. 5.35). The presence of cytological atypia of epithelial cells may be helpful in predicting aggressiveness. However, the absence of atypia and necrosis may not imply a benign course. Correlation with clinical and radiographic findings should be sought [139, 140].

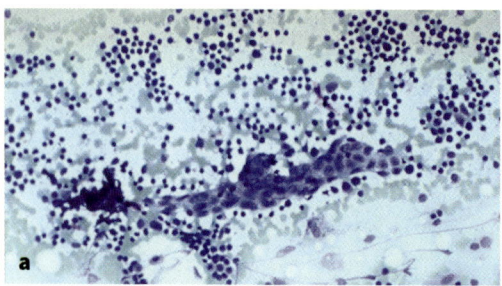

References

1. Bem C. Human immunodeficiency virus-positive tuberculous lymphadenitis in Central Africa: clinical presentation of 157 cases. Int J Tuberc Lung Dis 1997;1(3):215–9
2. Aljafari AS, Khalil EA, Elsiddig KE, El Hag IA, Ibrahim ME, Elsafi ME, et al. Diagnosis of tuberculous lymphadenitis by FNAC, microbiological methods and PCR: a comparative study. Cytopathology 2004;15(1):44–8
3. Handa U, Palta A, Mohan H, Punia RP. Fine needle aspiration diagnosis of tuberculous lymphadenitis. Trop Doct 2002;32(3):147–9
4. Kocjan G, Miller R. The cytology of HIV-induced immunosuppression. Changing pattern of disease in the era of highly active antiretroviral therapy. Cytopathology 2001;12(5):281–96
5. Whitely W, Tariq A, Peters B, Kocjan G, Miller RF. Pyrexia of undetermined origin in the era of HAART. Sex Transm Infect 2000;76(6):484–8
6. Baek CH, Kim SI, Ko YH, Chu KC. Polymerase chain reaction detection of Mycobacterium tuberculosis from fine-needle aspirate for the diagnosis of cervical tuberculous lymphadenitis. Laryngoscope 2000;110(1):30–4
7. Ersoz C, Polat A, Serin MS, Soylu L, Demircan O. Fine needle aspiration (FNA) cytology in tuberculous lymphadenitis. Cytopathology 1998;9(3):201–7
8. Lau SK, Wei WI, Hsu C, Engzell UC. Efficacy of fine needle aspiration cytology in the diagnosis of tuberculous cervical lymphadenopathy. J Laryngol Otol 1990;104(1):24–7
9. Manitchotpisit B, Kunachak S, Kulapraditharom B, Sura T. Combined use of fine needle aspiration cytology and polymerase chain reaction in the diagnosis of cervical tuberculous lymphadenitis. J Med Assoc Thai 1999;82(4):363–8

10. Oberborsch K, Maurer HM, Hess T, Kroner T. [Rational diagnostic strategy for tuberculous lymphadenitis]. Schweiz Med Wochenschr 2000;130(44):1702–5
11. Ueda T, Murayama T, Hasegawa Y, Bando K. [Tuberculous lymphadenitis: a clinical study of 23 cases]. Kekkaku 2004;79(5):349–54
12. Shariff S, Thomas JA. Fine needle aspiration cytodiagnosis of clinically suspected tuberculosis in tissue enlargements. Acta Cytol 1991;35(3):333–6
13. Perenboom RM, Richter C, Swai AB, Kitinya J, Mtoni I, Chande H, et al. Diagnosis of tuberculous lymphadenitis in an area of HIV infection and limited diagnostic facilities. Trop Geogr Med 1994;46(5):288–92
14. Annema JT, Veselic M, Rabe KF. Endoscopic ultrasound-guided fine-needle aspiration for the diagnosis of sarcoidosis. Eur Respir J 2005;25(3):405–9
15. Fritscher-Ravens A, Sriram PV, Topalidis T, Hauber HP, Meyer A, Soehendra N, et al. Diagnosing sarcoidosis using endosonography-guided fine-needle aspiration. Chest 2000;118(4):928–35
16. Mishra G, Sahai AV, Penman ID, Williams DB, Judson MA, Lewin DN, et al. Endoscopic ultrasonography with fine-needle aspiration: an accurate and simple diagnostic modality for sarcoidosis. Endoscopy 1999;31(5):377–82
17. Ryska A, Seifert G. Adenolymphoma (Warthin's tumor) with multiple sarcoid-like granulomas. Pathol Res Pract 1999;195(12):835–9
18. Toll A, Gilaberte M, Matias-Guiu X, Camacho L, Alomar A, Gonzalez-Gay MA, et al. Kikuchi's disease (necrotizing lymphadenitis) with cutaneous involvement associated with subacute cutaneous lupus erythematosus. Clin Exp Dermatol 2004;29(3):240–3
19. Santana A, Lessa B, Galrao L, Lima I, Santiago M. Kikuchi-Fujimoto's disease associated with systemic lupus erythematosus: case report and review of the literature. Clin Rheumatol 2005;24(1):60–3. Epub 2004 Oct 27
20. Kung IT, Ng WF, Yuen RW, Chan JK. Kikuchi's histiocytic necrotizing lymphadenitis. Diagnosis by fine needle aspiration. Acta Cytol 1990;34(3):323–8
21. Tong TR, Chan OW, Lee KC. Diagnosing Kikuchi disease on fine needle aspiration biopsy: a retrospective study of 44 cases diagnosed by cytology and 8 by histopathology. Acta Cytol 2001;45(6):953–7
22. Viguer JM, Jimenez-Heffernan JA, Perez P, Lopez-Ferrer P, Gonzalez-Peramato P, Vicandi B. Fine-needle aspiration cytology of Kikuchi's lymphadenitis: a report of ten cases. Diagn Cytopathol 2001;25(4):220–4
23. Bosch X, Guilabert A, Miquel R, Campo E. Enigmatic Kikuchi-Fujimoto disease: a comprehensive review. Am J Clin Pathol 2004;122(1):141–52
24. Chiang YC, Chen RM, Chao PZ, Yang TH, Lee FP. Pediatric Kikuchi-Fujimoto disease masquerading as a submandibular gland tumor. Int J Pediatr Otorhinolaryngol 2004;68(7):971–4
25. Dokic M, Begovic V, Bojic I, Tasic O, Stamatovic D. [Kikuchi-Fujimoto disease]. Vojnosanit Pregl 2003;60(5):625–30
26. Hsueh EJ, Ko WS, Hwang WS, Yam LT. Fine-needle aspiration of histiocytic necrotizing lymphadenitis (Kikuchi's disease). Diagn Cytopathol 1993;9(4):448–52
27. Loo CK, Greenberg ML. Role of fine-needle biopsy in an atypical case of lupus lymphadenopathy. Diagn Cytopathol 1994;10(2):162–4
28. Mannara GM, Boccato P, Rinaldo A, La Rosa F, Ferlito A. Histiocytic necrotizing lymphadenitis (Kikuchi-Fujimoto disease) diagnosed by fine needle aspiration biopsy. ORL J Otorhinolaryngol Relat Spec 1999;61(6):367–71
29. Pai MR, Adhikari P, Coimbatore RV, Ahmed S. Fine needle aspiration cytology in systemic lupus erythematosus lymphadenopathy. A case report. Acta Cytol 2000;44(1):67–9
30. Pai SA. Kikuchi-like lymphadenitis may be an early manifestation of SLE. J Indian Med Assoc 2004;102(6):330
31. Sathiyasekaran M, Varadharajan R, Shivbalan S. Kikuchi's disease. Indian Pediatr 2004;41(2):192–4
32. Tsang WY, Chan JK. Fine-needle aspiration cytologic diagnosis of Kikuchi's lymphadenitis. A report of 27 cases. Am J Clin Pathol 1994;102(4):454–8
33. Van de Voorde K, De Raeve H, De Block CE, Van Regenmortel N, Van Offel JF, De Clerck LS, et al. Atypical systemic lupus erythematosus or Castleman's disease. Acta Clin Belg 2004;59(3):161–4
34. Taylor GB, Smeeton IW. Cytologic demonstration of „dysplastic" follicular dendritic cells in a case of hyaline-vascular Castleman's disease. Diagn Cytopathol 2000;22(4):230–4
35. Meyer L, Gibbons D, Ashfaq R, Vuitch F, Saboorian MH. Fine-needle aspiration findings in Castleman's disease. Diagn Cytopathol 1999;21(1):57–60
36. Donnelly A, Hendricks G, Martens S, Strovers C, Wiemerslage S, Thomas PA. Cytologic diagnosis of cat scratch disease (CSD) by fine-needle aspiration. Diagn Cytopathol 1995;13(2):103–6
37. Lamps LW, Scott MA. Cat-scratch disease: historic, clinical, and pathologic perspectives. Am J Clin Pathol 2004;121(Suppl):S71–80
38. Godet C, Roblot F, Le Moal G, Roblot P, Frat JP, Becq-Giraudon B. Cat-scratch disease presenting as a breast mass. Scand J Infect Dis 2004;36(6–7):494–5
39. Povoski SP, Spigos DG, Marsh WL. An unusual case of cat-scratch disease from Bartonella quintana mimicking inflammatory breast cancer in a 50-year-old woman. Breast J 2003;9(6):497–500

40. Sakellaris G, Kampitakis E, Karamitopoulou E, Scoulica E, Psaroulaki A, Mihailidou E, et al. Cat scratch disease simulating a malignant process of the chest wall with coexistent osteomyelitis. Scand J Infect Dis 2003;35:6–7
41. Kumar PV, Moosavi A, Karimi M, Safaei A, Noorani H, Abdollahi B, et al. Subclassification of localized Leishmania lymphadenitis in fine needle aspiration smears. Acta Cytol 2001;45(4):547–54
42. Tallada N, Raventos A, Martinez S, Compano C, Almirante B. Leishmania lymphadenitis diagnosed by fine-needle aspiration biopsy. Diagn Cytopathol 1993;9(6):673–6
43. Shetty AK, Beaty MW, McGuirt WF, Jr., Woods CR, Givner LB. Kimura's disease: a diagnostic challenge. Pediatrics 2002;110(3):e39
44. Boccato P, Mannara GM, Rinaldo A, La Rosa F, Ferlito A. Kimura's disease of the intraparotid lymph nodes: fine needle aspiration biopsy findings. ORL J Otorhinolaryngol Relat Spec 1999;61(4):227–31
45. Kini U, Shariff S. Cytodiagnosis of Kimura's disease. Indian J Pathol Microbiol 1998;41(4):473–7
46. Jayaram G, Peh KB. Fine-needle aspiration cytology in Kimura's disease. Diagn Cytopathol 1995;13(4):295–9
47. Chow LT, Yuen RW, Tsui WM, Ma TK, Chow WH, Chan SK. Cytologic features of Kimura's disease in fine-needle aspirates. A study of eight cases. Am J Clin Pathol 1994;102(3):316–21
48. Hosaka N, Minato T, Yoshida S, Toki J, Yang G, Hisha H, et al. Kimura's disease with unusual eosinophilic epithelioid granulomatous reaction: a finding possibly related to eosinophil apoptosis. Hum Pathol 2002;33(5):561–4
49. Deshpande AH, Nayak S, Munshi MM, Bobhate SK. Kimura's disease. Diagnosis by aspiration cytology. Acta Cytol 2002;46(2):357–63
50. Nyrop M. Kimura's disease: case report and brief review of the literature. J Laryngol Otol 1994;108(11):1005–7
51. Deshpande V, Verma K. Fine needle aspiration (FNA) cytology of Rosai Dorfman disease. Cytopathology 1998;9(5):329–35
52. Schmitt FC. Sinus histiocytosis with massive lymphadenopathy (Rosai-Dorfman disease): cytomorphologic analysis on fine-needle aspirates. Diagn Cytopathol 1992;8:596–9
53. Pettinato G, Manivel JC, d'Amore ES, Petrella G. Fine needle aspiration cytology and immunocytochemical characterization of the histiocytes in sinus histiocytosis with massive lymphadenopathy (Rosai-Dorfman syndrome). Acta Cytol 1990;34(6):771–7
54. Peoc'h M, Duprez D, Grice G, Fabre-Bocquentin B, Gressin R, Pasquier B. Silicone lymphadenopathy mimicking a lymphoma in a patient with a metatarsophalangeal joint prosthesis. J Clin Pathol 2000;53(7):549–51
55. Xin W, Davenport RD, Chang AE, Michael CW. Exaggerated pigmented granulomatous reaction to the artificial joint implant mimics metastatic melanoma. Diagn Cytopathol 2004;30(3):198–200
56. Khurana KK, Stanley MW, Powers CN, Pitman MB. Aspiration cytology of malignant neoplasms associated with granulomas and granuloma-like features: diagnostic dilemmas. Cancer 1998;84(2):84–91
57. Vaillo A, Gutierrez-Martin A, Ballestin C, Ruiz-Liso JM. Marginal zone B-cell lymphoma of the parotid gland associated with epithelioid granulomas. Report of a case with fine needle aspiration. Acta Cytol 2004;48(3):420–4
58. Lui PC, Chow LT, Tsang RK, Chan AB, Tse GM. Fine needle aspiration cytology of lymph node with metastatic undifferentiated carcinoma and granulomatous (sarcoid-like) reaction. Pathology 2004;36(3):273–4
59. Komatsu M, Itoh N, Yazawa M, Kobayashi S, Inoue K, Kuroda T. Sarcoid reaction in thyroid diseases: report of a case of thyroid carcinoma demonstrating sarcoid reaction in regional lymph nodes. Endocr J 1997;44(5):697–700
60. Iyengar KR, Mutha S. Discrete epithelioid cells: useful clue to Hodgkin's disease cytodiagnosis. Diagn Cytopathol 2002;26(3):142–4
61. Kumar N, Ray C, Jain S. Aspiration cytology of Hashimoto's thyroiditis in an endemic area. Cytopathology 2002;13(1):31–9
62. Nguyen GK, Ginsberg J, Crockford PM, Villanueva RR. Hashimoto's thyroiditis: cytodiagnostic accuracy and pitfalls. Diagn Cytopathol 1997;16(6):531–6
63. MacDonald L, Yazdi HM. Fine needle aspiration biopsy of Hashimoto's thyroiditis. Sources of diagnostic error. Acta Cytol 1999;43(3):400–6
64. Pisanu A, Piu S, Cois A, Uccheddu A. Coexisting Hashimoto's thyroiditis with differentiated thyroid cancer and benign thyroid diseases: indications for thyroidectomy. Chir Ital 2003;55(3):365–72
65. Carson HJ, Castelli MJ, Gattuso P. Incidence of neoplasia in Hashimoto's thyroiditis: a fine-needle aspiration study. Diagn Cytopathol 1996;14(1):38–42
66. Kollur SM, El Sayed S, El Hag IA. Follicular thyroid lesions coexisting with Hashimoto's thyroiditis: incidence and possible sources of diagnostic errors. Diagn Cytopathol 2003;28(1):35–8
67. Singh B, Shaha AR, Trivedi H, Carew JF, Poluri A, Shah JP. Coexistent Hashimoto's thyroiditis with papillary thyroid carcinoma: impact on presentation, management, and outcome. Surgery 1999;126(6):1070–6; discussion 1076–7
68. Arif S, Blanes A, Diaz-Cano SJ. Hashimoto's thyroiditis shares features with early papillary thyroid carcinoma. Histopathology 2002;41(4):357–62
69. Prasad ML, Huang Y, Pellegata NS, de la Chapelle A, Kloos RT. Hashimoto's thyroiditis with papillary thyroid carcinoma (PTC)-like nuclear alterations express molecular markers of PTC. Histopathology 2004;45(1):39–46

70. Unger P, Ewart M, Wang BY, Gan L, Kohtz DS, Burstein DE. Expression of p63 in papillary thyroid carcinoma and in Hashimoto's thyroiditis: a pathobiologic link? Hum Pathol 2003;34(8):764–9
71. Di Pasquale M, Rothstein JL, Palazzo JP. Pathologic features of Hashimoto's-associated papillary thyroid carcinomas. Hum Pathol 2001;32(1):24–30
72. Zeppa P, Benincasa G, Lucariello A, Palombini L. Association of different pathologic processes of the thyroid gland in fine needle aspiration samples. Acta Cytol 2001;45(3):347–52
73. Tseleni-Balafouta S, Kyroudi-Voulgari A, Paizi-Biza P, Papacharalampous NX. Lymphocytic thyroiditis in fine-needle aspirates: differential diagnostic aspects. Diagn Cytopathol 1989;5:362–5
74. Singh NG, Kapila K, Dawar R, Verma K. Fine needle aspiration cytology diagnosis of lymphoproliferative disease of the breast. Acta Cytol 2003;47(5):739–43
75. Al-Marzooq YM, Chopra R, Younis M, Al-Mulhim AS, Al-Mommatten MI, Al-Omran SH. Thyroid low-grade B-cell lymphoma (MALT type) with extreme plasmacytic differentiation: report of a case diagnosed by fine-needle aspiration and flow cytometric study. Diagn Cytopathol 2004;31(1):52–6
76. Sangalli G, Serio G, Zampatti C, Lomuscio G, Colombo L. Fine needle aspiration cytology of primary lymphoma of the thyroid: a report of 17 cases. Cytopathology 2001;12(4):257–63
77. Jayaram G, Rani S, Raina V, Singh CH, Chandra M, Marwaha RK. B cell lymphoma of the thyroid in Hashimoto's thyroiditis monitored by fine-needle aspiration cytology. Diagn Cytopathol 1990;6:130–3
78. Saxena A, Alport EC, Moshynska O, Kanthan R, Boctor MA. Clonal B cell populations in a minority of patients with Hashimoto's thyroiditis. J Clin Pathol 2004;57(12):1258–63
79. Hsi ED, Singleton TP, Svoboda SM, Schnitzer B, Ross CW. Characterization of the lymphoid infiltrate in Hashimoto thyroiditis by immunohistochemistry and polymerase chain reaction for immunoglobulin heavy chain gene rearrangement. Am J Clin Pathol 1998;110(3):327–33
80. Yamauchi A, Tomita Y, Takakuwa T, Hoshida Y, Nakatsuka S, Sakamoto H, et al. Polymerase chain reaction-based clonality analysis in thyroid lymphoma. Int J Mol Med 2002;10(1):113–7
81. Widder S, Pasieka JL. Primary thyroid lymphomas. Curr Treat Options Oncol 2004;5(4):307–13
82. Harris NL. Lymphoid proliferations of the salivary glands. Am J Clin Pathol 1999;111(1 Suppl 1):S94–103
83. Carbone A, Gloghini A, Ferlito A. Pathological features of lymphoid proliferations of the salivary glands: lymphoepithelial sialadenitis versus low-grade B-cell lymphoma of the malt type. Ann Otol Rhinol Laryngol 2000;109(12 Pt 1):1170–5
84. Parwani AV, Ali SZ. Diagnostic accuracy and pitfalls in fine-needle aspiration interpretation of Warthin tumor. Cancer 2003;99(3):166–71
85. Hughes JH, Volk EE, Wilbur DC. Pitfalls in salivary gland fine-needle aspiration cytology: lessons from the College of American Pathologists Interlaboratory Comparison Program in Nongynecologic Cytology. Arch Pathol Lab Med 2005;129(1):26–31
86. MacCallum PL, Lampe HB, Cramer H, Matthews TW. Fine-needle aspiration cytology of lymphoid lesions of the salivary gland: a review of 35 cases. J Otolaryngol 1996;25(5):300–4
87. Nassar DL, Raab SS, Silverman JF, Kennerdell JS, Sturgis CD. Fine-needle aspiration for the diagnosis of orbital hematolymphoid lesions. Diagn Cytopathol 2000;23(5):314–7
88. Sharma MC, Shields CL, Shields JA, Eagle RC, Jr., Demirci H, Wiley L. Benign lymphoid infiltrate of the iris simulating a malignant melanoma. Cornea 2002;21(4):424–5
89. Karikehalli S, Nazeer T, Lee CY. Intraocular large B-cell lymphoma. A case report. Acta Cytol 2004;48(2):207–10
90. Levine PH, Zamuco R, Yee HT. Role of fine-needle aspiration cytology in breast lymphoma. Diagn Cytopathol 2004;30(5):332–40
91. Salto-Tellez M, Kocjan G. Lymphocytic mastopathy in a patient with previous breast cancer diagnosed by fine-needle aspirate. Diagn Cytopathol 2000;23(2):141–2
92. Valdez R, Thorson J, Finn WG, Schnitzer B, Kleer CG. Lymphocytic mastitis and diabetic mastopathy: a molecular, immunophenotypic, and clinicopathologic evaluation of 11 cases. Mod Pathol 2003;16(3):223–8
93. Sanati S, Ayala AG, Middleton LP. Lymphoepithelioma-like carcinoma of the breast: report of a case mimicking lymphoma. Ann Diagn Pathol 2004;8(5):309–15
94. Zardawi IM, Clark D, Williamsz G. Inflammatory myofibroblastic tumor of the breast. A case report. Acta Cytol 2003;47(6):1077–81
95. Nayer H, Weir EG, Sheth S, Ali SZ. Primary pancreatic lymphomas: a cytopathologic analysis of a rare malignancy. Cancer 2004;102(5):315–21
96. Lin F, Staerkel G, Fanning TV. Cytodiagnosis of primary lymphoma of bone on fine-needle aspiration cytology specimens: review of 25 cases. Diagn Cytopathol 2003;28(4):205–11
97. Mayall F, Darlington A, Harrison B. Fine needle aspiration cytology in the diagnosis of uncommon types of lymphoma. J Clin Pathol 2003;56(11):821–5
98. Truong LD, Caraway N, Ngo T, Laucirica R, Katz R, Ramzy I. Renal lymphoma. The diagnostic and therapeutic roles of fine-needle aspiration. Am J Clin Pathol 2001;115(1):18–31

99. Liu K, Mann KP, Vitellas KM, Paulson EK, Nelson RC, Gockerman JP, et al. Fine-needle aspiration with flow cytometric immunophenotyping for primary diagnosis of intra-abdominal lymphomas. Diagn Cytopathol 1999;21(2):98–104
100. Yu GH, Salhany KE, Gokaslan ST, Cajulis RS, De Frias DV. Thymic epithelial cells as a diagnostic pitfall in the fine-needle aspiration diagnosis of primary mediastinal lymphoma. Diagn Cytopathol 1997;16(5):460–5
101. Das DK, Gupta SK, Francis IM, Ahmed MS. Fine-needle aspiration cytology diagnosis of non-Hodgkin lymphoma of thyroid: a report of four cases. Diagn Cytopathol 1993;9(6):639–45
102. Zeppa P, Picardi M, Marino G, Troncone G, Fulciniti F, Vetrani A, et al. Fine-needle aspiration biopsy and flow cytometry immunophenotyping of lymphoid and myeloproliferative disorders of the spleen. Cancer 2003;99(2):118–27
103. Boni L, Benevento A, Dionigi G, Cabrini L, Dionigi R. Primary pancreatic lymphoma. Surg Endosc 2002;16(7):1107–8. Epub 2002 May 3
104. Soderlund V, Tani E, Skoog L, Bauer HC, Kreicbergs A. Diagnosis of skeletal lymphoma and myeloma by radiology and fine needle aspiration cytology. Cytopathology 2001;12(3):157–67
105. Harris NL, Jaffe ES, Diebold J, Flandrin G, Muller-Hermelink HK, Vardiman J, et al. The World Health Organization classification of neoplasms of the hematopoietic and lymphoid tissues: report of the Clinical Advisory Committee meeting--Airlie House, Virginia, November, 1997. Hematol J 2000;1(1):53–66
106. Jaffe ES, Banks PM, Nathwani B, Said J, Swerdlow SH. Recommendations for the reporting of lymphoid neoplasms: A report from the Association of Directors of Anatomic and Surgical Pathology. Mod Pathol 2004;17(1):131–5
107. Daskalopoulou D, Harhalakis N, Maouni N, Markidou SG. Fine needle aspiration cytology of non-Hodgkin's lymphomas. A morphologic and immunophenotypic study. Acta Cytol 1995;39(2):180–6
108. Liu K, Stern RC, Rogers RT, Dodd LG, Mann KP. Diagnosis of hematopoietic processes by fine-needle aspiration in conjunction with flow cytometry: A review of 127 cases. Diagn Cytopathol 2001;24(1):1–10
109. Hehn ST, Grogan TM, Miller TP. Utility of fine-needle aspiration as a diagnostic technique in lymphoma. J Clin Oncol 2004;22(15):3046–52
110. Lioe TF EH, Allen DC, Spence RA. . The role of fine needle aspiration cytology (FNAC) in the investigation of superficial lymphadenopathy; uses and limitations of the technique. Cytopathology 1999;10(5):291–7
111. Kocjan G. The role of FNAC in diagnosis of lymph node enlargements. Cytopathology 1997;8(Suppl)::2–3
112. Dong HY, Harris NL, Preffer FI, Pitman MB. Fine-needle aspiration biopsy in the diagnosis and classification of primary and recurrent lymphoma: a retrospective analysis of the utility of cytomorphology and flow cytometry. Mod Pathol 2001;14(5):472–81
113. Young NA, Al-Saleem T. Diagnosis of lymphoma by fine-needle aspiration cytology using the revised European-American classification of lymphoid neoplasms. Cancer 1999;87(6):325–45
114. Young NA, Al-Saleem TI, Ehya H, Smith MR. Utilization of fine-needle aspiration cytology and flow cytometry in the diagnosis and subclassification of primary and recurrent lymphoma. Cancer 1998;84(4):252–61
115. Henrique RM, Sousa ME, Godinho MI, Costa I, Barbosa IL, Lopes CA. Immunophenotyping by flow cytometry of fine needle aspirates in the diagnosis of lymphoproliferative disorders: A retrospective study. J Clin Lab Anal 1999;13(5):224–8
116. Meda BA, Buss DH, Woodruff RD, Cappellari JO, Rainer RO, Powell BL, et al. Diagnosis and subclassification of primary and recurrent lymphoma. The usefulness and limitations of combined fine-needle aspiration cytomorphology and flow cytometry. Am J Clin Pathol 2000;113(5):688–99
117. Mourad WA, Tulbah A, Shoukri M, Al Dayel F, Akhtar M, Ali MA, et al. Primary diagnosis and REAL/WHO classification of non-Hodgkin's lymphoma by fine-needle aspiration: cytomorphologic and immunophenotypic approach. Diagn Cytopathol 2003;28(4):191–5
118. Mourad WA, al Nazer M, Tulbah A. Cytomorphologic differentiation of Hodgkin's lymphoma and Ki-1+ anaplastic large cell lymphoma in fine needle aspirates. Acta Cytol 2003;47(5):744–8
119. Hans CP, Weisenburger DD, Vose JM, Hock LM, Lynch JC, Aoun P, et al. A significant diffuse component predicts for inferior survival in grade 3 follicular lymphoma, but cytologic subtypes do not predict survival. Blood 2003;101(6):2363–7
120. Medeiros LJ, Carr J. Overview of the role of molecular methods in the diagnosis of malignant lymphomas. Arch Pathol Lab Med 1999;123(12):1189–207
121. Kocjan G. Cytological and molecular diagnosis of lymphoma. J Clin Pathol 2005;58:561–567
122. Chhieng DC, Cangiarella JF, Symmans WF, Cohen JM. Fine-needle aspiration cytology of Hodgkin disease: a study of 89 cases with emphasis on false-negative cases. Cancer 2001;93(1):52–9
123. Grosso LE, Collins BT, Dunphy CH, Ramos RR. Lymphocyte-depleted Hodgkin's disease: diagnostic challenges by fine-needle aspiration. Diagn Cytopathol 1998;19(1):66–9
124. Nagel H, Laskawi R, Buter JJ, Schroder M, Chilla R, Droese M. Cytologic diagnosis of acinic-cell carcinoma of salivary glands. Diagn Cytopathol 1997;16(5):402–12

125. Van Savell H, Jr., Hughes SM, Bower C, Parham DM. Lymphocytic infiltration in pediatric thyroid carcinomas. Pediatr Dev Pathol 2004;7(5):487–92. Epub 2004 Jul 30
126. Si MW, Thorson JA, Lauwers GY, DalCin P, Furman J. Hepatocellular lymphoepithelioma-like carcinoma associated with Epstein Barr virus: a hitherto unrecognized entity. Diagn Mol Pathol 2004;13(3):183–9
127. Thompson MB, Nestok BR, Gluckman JL. Fine needle aspiration cytology of lymphoepithelioma-like carcinoma of the parotid gland. A case report. Acta Cytol 1994;38(5):782–6
128. Huang Y, Tsung JS, Lin CW, Cheng TY. Intrahepatic cholangiocarcinoma with lymphoepithelioma-like carcinoma component. Ann Clin Lab Sci 2004;34(4):476–80
129. Ilvan S, Celik V, Ulker Akyildiz E, Senel Bese N, Ramazanoglu R, Calay Z. Lymphoepithelioma-like carcinoma of the breast: is it a distinct entity? Clinicopathological evaluation of two cases and review of the literature. Breast 2004;13(6):522–6
130. Abe T, Tanabe Y, Watanabe S, Fujita N, Matsumoto N, Moriyama H, et al. [A case of recurrent pulmonary lymphoepithelioma-like carcinoma responding to treatment with CBDCA/paclitaxel combined chemotherapy]. Gan To Kagaku Ryoho 2004;31(8):1215–7
131. Hernandez Vazquez J, de Miguel Diez J, Llorente Inigo D, Pedraza Serrano F, Serrano Saiz JL, Alvarez Fernandez E. [Large cell lymphoepithelioma-like carcinoma of the lung]. Arch Bronconeumol 2004;40(8):381–3
132. Mrad K, Ben Brahim E, Driss M, Abbes I, Marakchi M, Ben Romdhane K. Lymphoepithelioma-like carcinoma of the submandibular salivary gland associated with Epstein-Barr virus in a North African woman. Virchows Arch 2004;445(4):419–20. Epub 2004 Jul 17
133. Izquierdo-Garcia FM, Garcia-Diez F, Fernandez I, Perez-Rosado A, Saez A, Suarez-Vilela D, et al. Lymphoepithelioma-like carcinoma of the bladder: three cases with clinicopathological and p53 protein expression study. Virchows Arch 2004;444(5):420–5. Epub 2004 Apr 6
134. El Hossini Soua A, Trabelsi A, Laarif M, Mutijima E, Sriha B, Mokni M, et al. [Lymphoepithelioma-like carcinoma of the uterine cervix: case report]. J Gynecol Obstet Biol Reprod (Paris) 2004;33(1 Pt 1):47–50
135. Chan MK, McGuire LJ, Lee JC. Fine needle aspiration cytodiagnosis of nasopharyngeal carcinoma in cervical lymph nodes. A study of 40 cases. Acta Cytol 1989;33(3):344–50
136. Caraway NP, Fanning CV, Amato RJ, Sneige N. Fine-needle aspiration cytology of seminoma: a review of 16 cases. Diagn Cytopathol 1995;12(4):327–33
137. Yakirevich E, Lefel O, Sova Y, Stein A, Cohen O, Izhak OB, et al. Activated status of tumour-infiltrating lymphocytes and apoptosis in testicular seminoma. J Pathol 2002;196(1):67–75
138. Boyle JL, Meschter SC. Fine needle aspiration cytology of a sebaceous lymphadenoma: a case report. Acta Cytol 2004;48(4):551–4
139. Chhieng DC, Rose D, Ludwig ME, Zakowski MF. Cytology of thymomas: emphasis on morphology and correlation with histologic subtypes. Cancer 2000;90(1):24–32
140. Ali SZ, Erozan YS. Thymoma. Cytopathologic features and differential diagnosis on fine needle aspiration. Acta Cytol 1998;42(4):845–54

Chapter 6

Diagnostic Dilemmas in FNAC Practice: Metastatic Tumours

Contents

6.1	Metastatic Carcinomas	118
6.1.1	Establishing the Diagnosis of Malignancy	118
6.1.2	Determining the Nature of the Tumour	120
6.1.3	Finding the Primary Tumour	124
6.1.4	The Role of Imaging in the FNAC of Metastases	129
6.2	Metastases of Non-Epithelial Tumours	129
	References	130

The diagnosis of metastatic tumours represents one of the main uses of FNAC. They represent the majority of findings in the FNAC of lymph nodes [1]. Establishing the stage of the tumour has major management implications. With the advancement of different treatment options, requirements for a more refined diagnosis are becoming greater. This chapter discusses some general principles and dilemmas associated with the FNAC diagnosis of metastatic tumours, regardless of the site and type.

As has been mentioned in the preceding chapters, metastatic tumours and their diagnosis require a close collaboration between the clinician and the pathologist. A full knowledge of the patient's clinical history is a prerequisite for a meaningful answer. A clear request to the pathologist will ensure an appropriate role of FNAC in patient management. Knowledge of the patient's history, previous diagnosis and, where appropriate, clinical staging, is essential in order for FNAC to be meaningful and clinically relevant. A review of previous diagnoses should be possible and management implications clarified. Any additional investigations that may be required should be discussed in advance. Only if these questions can be answered appropriately will the FNAC diagnosis of metastatic tumour be meaningful. Absence of clinical information may result in errors and is unacceptable. On their part, pathologists are expected to seek any clinical information that may be relevant to the diagnosis.

The Association of Directors of Anatomic and Surgical Pathology has published a set of recommendations including those for FNAC of lymph nodes intended specifically for those nodes being studied for metastatic neoplasms [2].

6.1 Metastatic Carcinomas

Metastatic carcinomas seen in FNAC practice are usually present in the material obtained from lymph nodes and rarely that from extranodal sites. A finding of malignant epithelial cells within the lymph has to be seen in the clinical context (i.e. with the knowledge of patient's clinical history and with the understanding of the management implications of the cytology report). There are several practical steps that may be useful to cytopathologists in order to avoid some of the pitfalls associated with FNAC diagnosis of metastatic tumours.

6.1.1 Establishing the Diagnosis of Malignancy

The pitfalls in the diagnosis of metastatic carcinoma are usually caused by several factors that may be summarised under the general heading of "absence of clinical correlation". Examples include benign disease that may mimic metastases (e.g. epithelial inclusions in the lymph nodes). These are either primary (Case history 6.1) or secondary, the latter as a result of FNAC sampling of adjacent tissues (e.g. epithelium of the skin adnexa in the FNAC; Figs. 6.1 and 6.2).

> **Case history 6.1:** A 37-year-old woman presented with an axillary mass that had recently grown since she became pregnant. There was no obvious palpable abnormality in the breasts; ultrasound showed no focal abnormality, but this finding was equivocal in view of the pregnancy. FNAC revealed clusters of benign breast epithelium, myoepithelium and stromal cells, in keeping with ectopic breast tissue. The patient was advised that the lesion was benign and was referred to the surgeon after the cessation of breast feeding (Fig. 6.2).

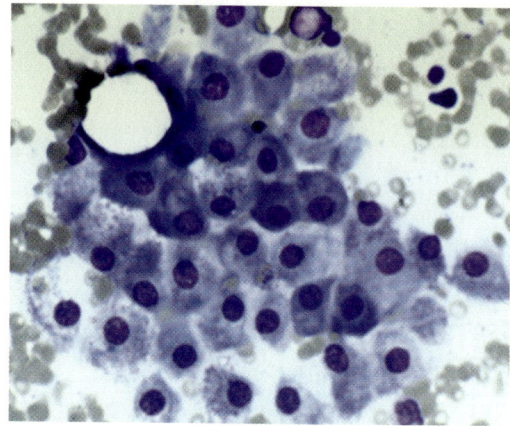

Fig. 6.1
FNAC axilla. Epithelium of the skin adnexa is present in the FNAC of an axillary lymph node. This may lead to a diagnostic pitfall in cases where axillary metastases are suspected

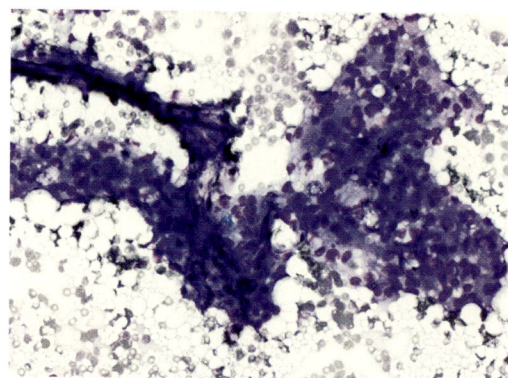

Fig. 6.2
FNAC axillary mass. FNAC revealed clusters of benign breast epithelium, myoepithelium and stromal cells in keeping with ectopic breast tissue

Secondary changes (e.g. squamous metaplasia in chronic sialadenitis) may mimic malignancy and pose as SqCC, particularly if a patient has a history of head and neck carcinoma followed by the neck radiation (Fig. 6.3). A false-positive diagnoses may result in radical neck dissection of the ipsilateral lymph nodes.

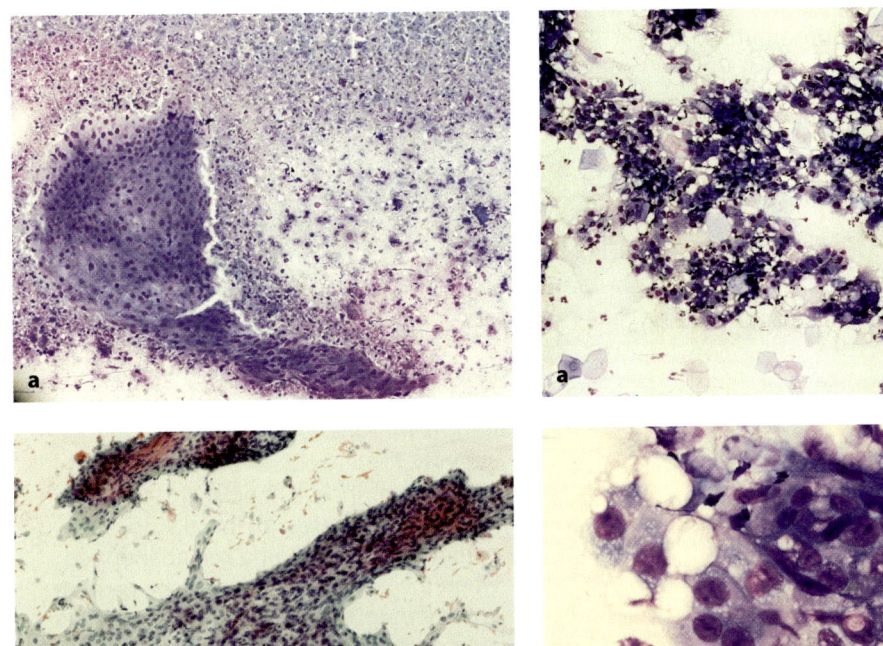

Fig. 6.3
FNAC salivary gland. Squamous metaplasia in a case of chronic sialadenitis following neck radiation for SqCC of the oral cavity. **a** MGG-stained preparations show a sheet of benign epithelium amidst the inflammatory exudates and debris. Features may be mistaken for metastatic SqCC. **b** Another case with similar features. Patients with history of neck radiation following the resection of oral cancer may present with chronic sialadenitis, which is clinically indistinguishable from a neck lymph node

Suture granuloma, radiation changes and other post-treatment changes may pose a difficult morphological problem in a patient where metastases need to be excluded (Fig. 6.4). Some other benign tumours (e.g. Warthin's tumour or paraganglioma) can pose a diagnostic challenge and be interpreted as carcinoma since they may present with a wide variety of morphological patterns [3] (Case history 6.2; Fig. 6.5).

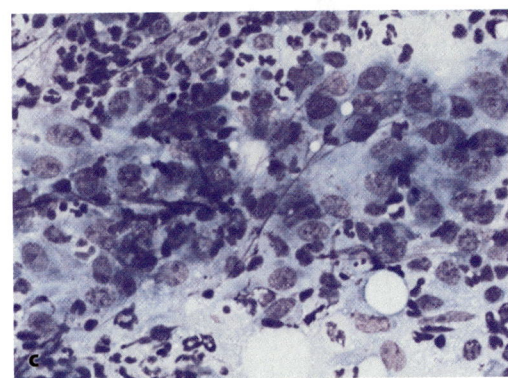

Fig. 6.4
FNAC nodule near the operation scar. Granulomatous inflammation. No evidence of malignancy. **a** Low-power view showing a mixed inflammatory background in which numerous medium- and large-sized cells are noted, apparently in a loosely cohesive aggregate.
b High-power view revealing a sheet of histiocytes mimicking epithelial cells. **c** The inflammatory exudate in another case may appear even more worrying due to the air drying, which makes aggregates of histiocytes and granulation cells appear larger

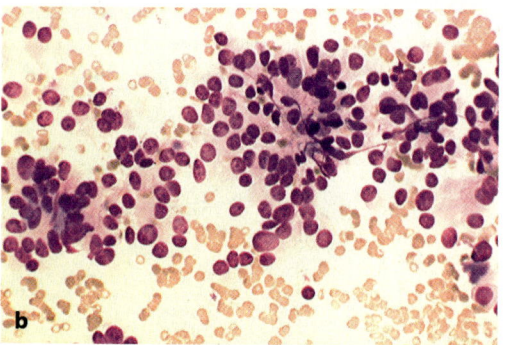
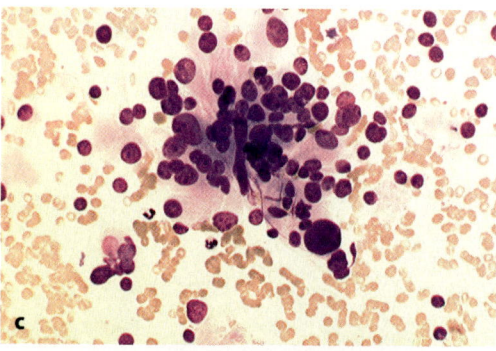
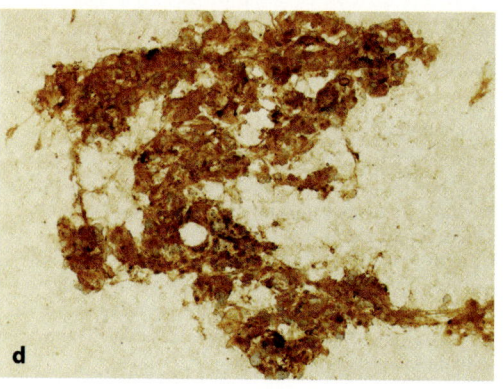
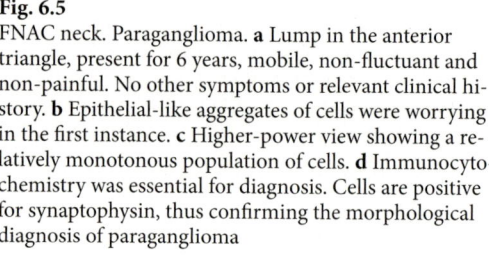

Fig. 6.5
FNAC neck. Paraganglioma. **a** Lump in the anterior triangle, present for 6 years, mobile, non-fluctuant and non-painful. No other symptoms or relevant clinical history. **b** Epithelial-like aggregates of cells were worrying in the first instance. **c** Higher-power view showing a relatively monotonous population of cells. **d** Immunocytochemistry was essential for diagnosis. Cells are positive for synaptophysin, thus confirming the morphological diagnosis of paraganglioma

Case history 6.2: A 45-year-old woman presented with a lump in the neck, present for the past 6 years. The lump was mobile, non-painful and had not changed in size recently. FNAC yielded cellular material (Fig. 6.5) composed of epithelial-like cells in loose aggregates. An initial suspicion of metastatic carcinoma was abandoned when the cells were proved to be positive for synaptophysin and negative for cytokeratin markers.

6.1.2 Determining the Nature of the Tumour

By definition, a metastasis is a secondary tumour deposit, the primary tumour arising elsewhere. Decisive factors in defining a metastasis are based on anatomical (i.e. the site of the lump, for example the axillary nodes in breast carcinoma) and morphological criteria (i.e. the cells are alien to the site). In the case of lymph nodes, this can be easily established, particularly if there is a residual lymphoid population present. However, as mentioned earlier, some tumours contain a significant lymphoid cell population (e.g. medullary carcinoma of the breast or seminoma; see Chap. 5, Figs. 5.13 and 5.31). Thus, the presence of a dissociated or mixed architectural pattern of large anaplastic cells and naked nuclei accompanied by an abundant lymphoid component, highly suggestive of undifferentiated nasopharyngeal carcinoma, may be mistaken for a metastasis or a lymphoma [4] (Fig. 6.6; Case history 6.3). Anatomically, if the mass subjected to FNAC contains only malignant cells, the diagnosis of

Case history 6.3: A 24-year-old man presented with a mass in the neck that was hard, immobile and had doubled in size within the past 2 months, preventing normal movement. Clinically, a lymphoma was suspected. However, FNAC yielded material that appeared at first glance to be from a carcinoma because of the presence of cell aggregates. Diagnosis was withheld until the results of immunocytochemistry, which proved the lesion to be a lymphoma (Fig. 6.6).

metastatic tumour has to be qualified; for example, a submandibular gland swelling containing cells from a keratinising SqCC could represent both a primary salivary gland tumour or a metastasis from an unknown oropharyngeal primary (Fig. 6.7). Malignant cells within the breast tissue may represent a metastasis from other tumours: melanoma, myeloma, rhabdomyosarcoma (RMS) or small cell carcinoma (SCC) of the lung, leukaemic deposit, lymphoma, choriocarcinoma and soft-tissue sarcomas have all been described to metastasise into the breast [5] (Figs. 6.8–6.10). Breast tumours can metastasise almost anywhere (Fig. 6.11). The pancreas may be the site of metastases from renal-cell carcinoma, melanoma, SCC, breast carcinoma, prostatic carcinoma, colon adenocarcinoma, SqCC and gastrointestinal stromal tumours [6] (Fig. 6.12). The cytomorphological features of meningioma metastatic to the neck overlap with those of more commonly aspirated head and neck tumours, such as ACC arising primarily in a salivary gland, metastatic papillary thyroid caricoma (PTC) and paraganglioma [7] (Fig. 6.13).

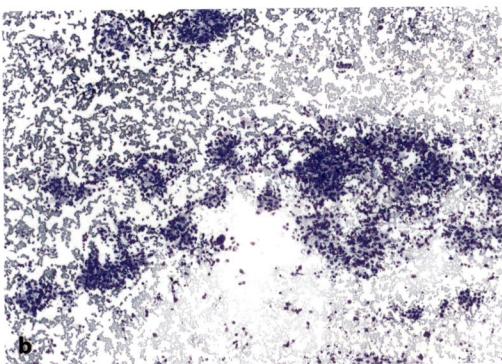

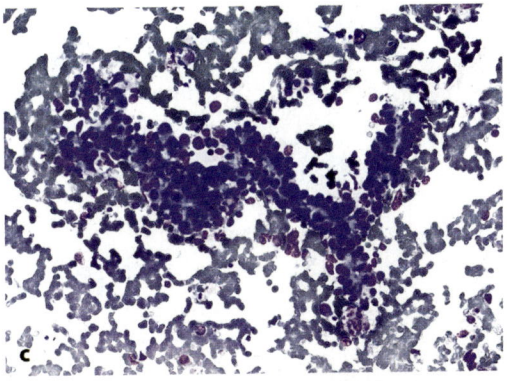

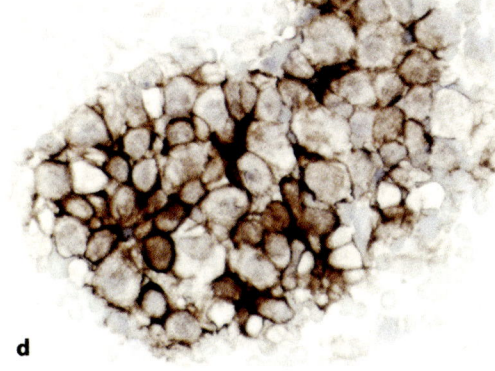

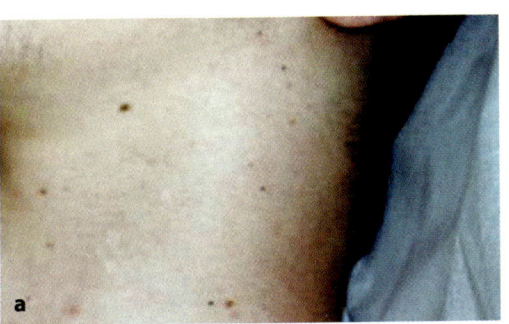

Fig. 6.6
Case history 3. **a** Neck mass (Case history 6.3) **b** FNAC shows apparent aggregates of cells mimicking an epithelial tumour. **c** High-power view showing pseudopapillary structures composed of medium-sized cells. **d** Immunocytochemistry shows positivity for CD79a, confirming that the cells are B-type. The lesion was a DLBL

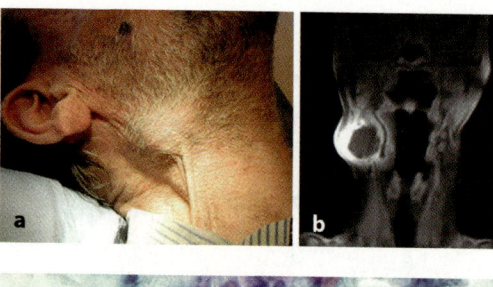
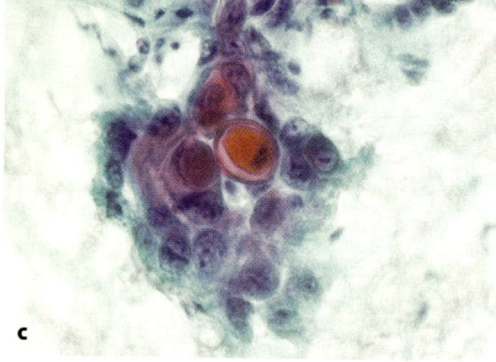

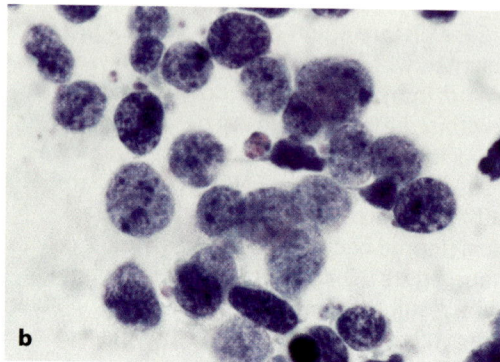

Fig. 6.8
FNAC breast. SCC. **a** Pap staining reveals almost bare nuclei with a characteristic granular chromatin pattern, nuclear moulding and absence of nucleoli. **b** MGG staining shows similar features with less crisp nuclear detail. The lung is the most likely primary site, although SCCs with neuroendocrine differentiation may be found in other sites, including the breast

Fig. 6.7
FNAC submandibular swelling. **a** This elderly male patient presented with a fixed hard mass in the region of the right parotid. **b** Magnetic resonance imaging showed a large cystic lesion with central necrosis in the lateral neck. **c** FNAC showed cells indicative of SqCC. It was not possible to establish the primary site of the tumour. In the absence of lymphoid cells or any normal structures, it is sometimes not possible to establish if the tumour is primary or secondary

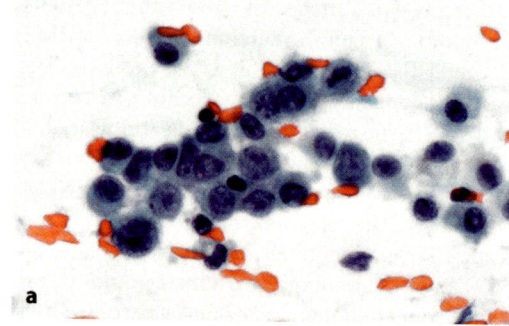

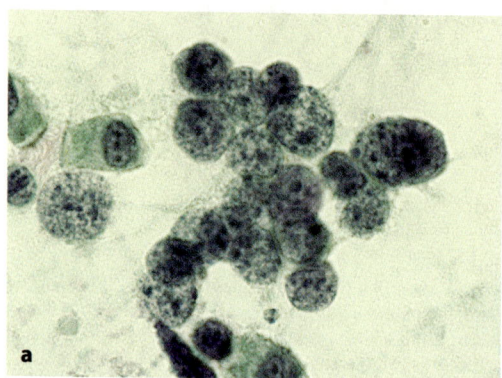

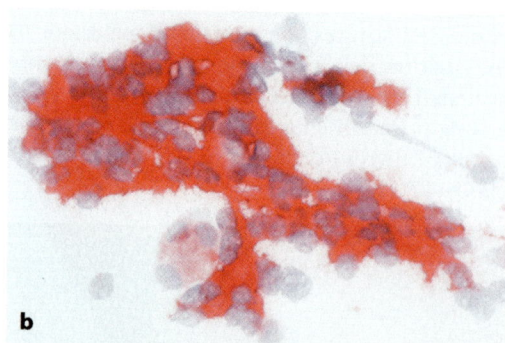

Fig. 6.9
FNAC breast. Carcinoid. **a** Pap-stained FNAC containing a relatively monotonous population of medium-sized cells with moderate amount of cytoplasm and prominent nucleoli. **b** CD56 staining is positive, indicating that the cells are of neuroendocrine origin. This is a primary carcinoid of the breast

Metastatic Tumours Chapter 6

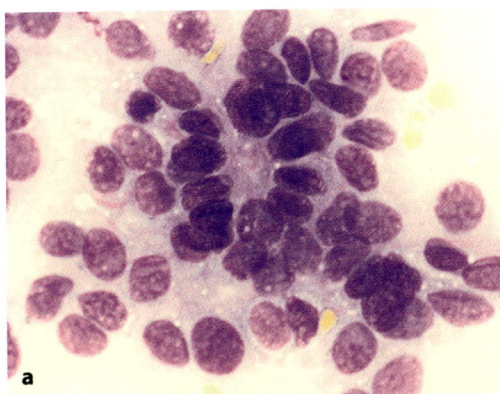

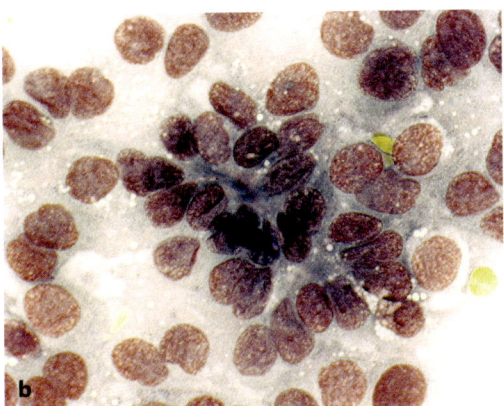

Fig. 6.10
FNAC breast. **a** Melanoma cells forming pseudoacini and mimicking a primary breast adenocarcinoma. **b** HMB 45 staining is positive in melanoma cells, confirming the diagnosis of metastatic tumour

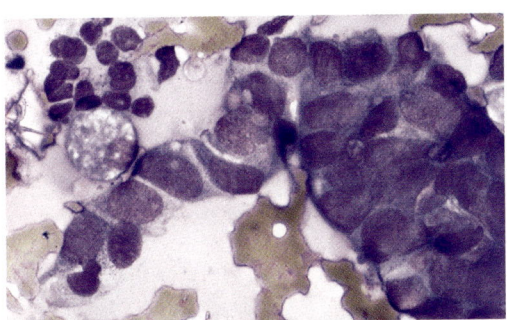

Fig. 6.11
FNAC thyroid. In addition to the normal follicular epithelium in one corner, there are large, pleomorphic cells forming an Indian-file-like pattern. In a patient with an appropriate clinical history, the features are consistent with metastatic carcinoma of the breast

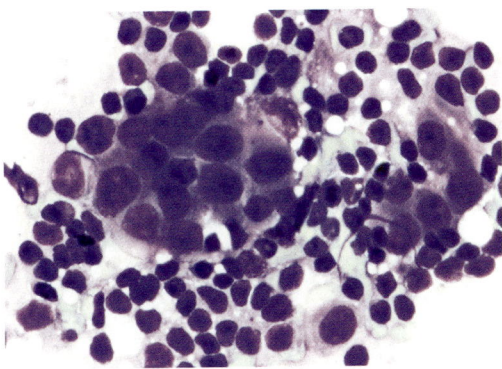

Fig. 6.12
FNAC lymph node. Malignant cells from an unknown primary. The patient had a history of carcinoma of the breast

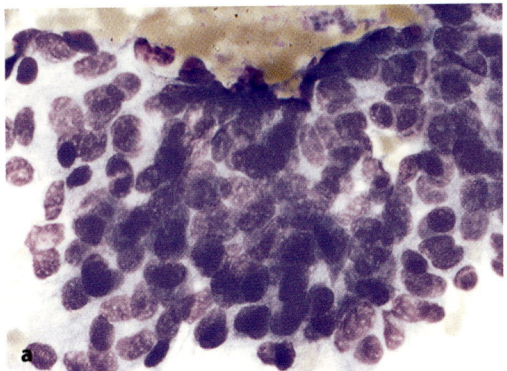

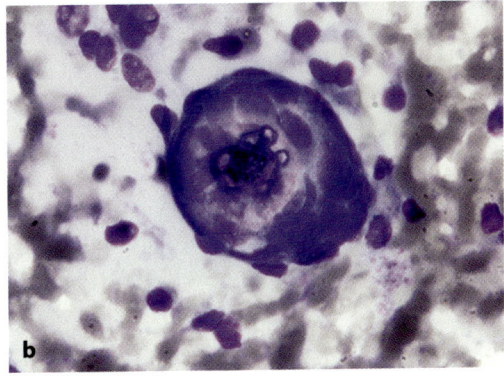

Fig. 6.13
FNAC neck. Meningioma. (see next page)

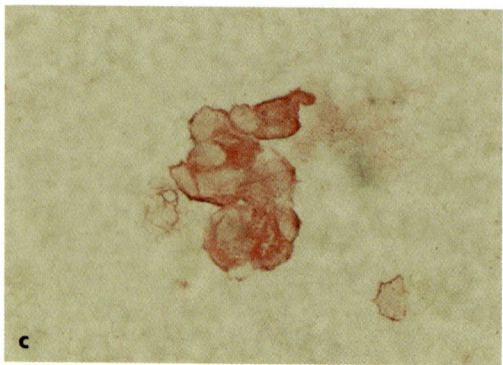

Fig. 6.13
Continued from previous page. **a** Cytomorphological features of meningioma metastatic to the neck overlap with those of more commonly aspirated head and neck tumours, such as ACC arising primarily in a salivary gland, metastatic PTC and paraganglioma. **b** Psammoma bodies may be seen within the papillary projections. **c** Tumour cells are vimentin positive. **d** Negative for epithelial membrane antigen (EMA) staining

6.1.3 Finding the Primary Tumour

Once the diagnosis of malignancy is established as a metastasis, the question of the primary tumour arises. In most cases, the primary tumour is clinically known and FNAC is merely a vehicle in the staging procedure. In cases where the primary tumour is unknown, FNAC should be used to attempt to narrow the search for the primary site. Some carcinomas can be identified by their morphological differentiation, for example adenocarcinomas by the acinar arrangement and mucin secretion, SqCCs by the keratinisation of the cytoplasm (Fig 6.14) and SCCs by their typical chromatin pattern (Fig 6.15). However, there are many instances where features of different tumours overlap and where the precise primary diagnosis remains obscure (Fig. 6.15). In these cases, it is important to be in consultation with clinicians and to clarify the importance of refining the diagnosis (Fig. 6.16). Often, morphology alone may be helpful (e.g. metastatic non-small-cell-carcinoma (NSCC) in the case of a lung primary may be the diagnosis that is sufficient for management). In most cases, however, immunocytochemistry is necessary in order to make a diagnosis with a major management implication (e.g. in the differentiation between carcinoma and lymphoma; Fig. 6.17). Awareness of rare subtypes of the more common tumours is also important (e.g. prostate adenocarcinoma is known to metastasise widely to bone, lung and the lymph nodes; Fig. 6.18). A rare, although distinctive neuroendocrine cytomorphology of metastatic prostatic adenocarcinoma on FNAC can mimic SCC [8].

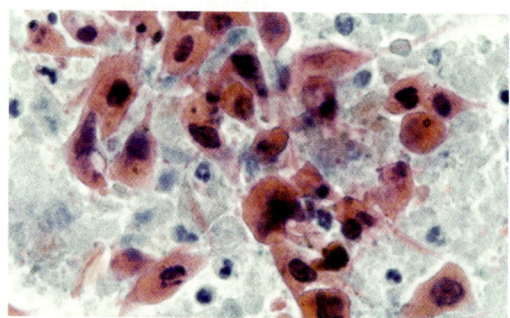

Fig. 6.14
FNAC lung. SqCC showing cytoplasmic keratinisation. Lung is the most probably primary site

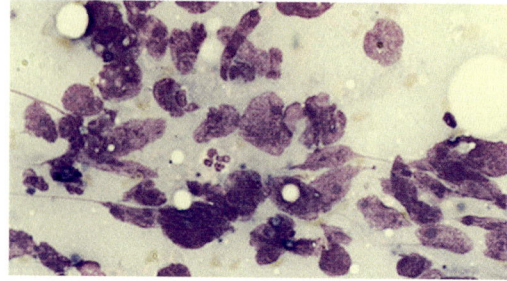

Fig. 6.15
FNAC neck. Nasopharyngeal carcinoma. Undifferentiated features of this tumour may cause difficulties in distinguishing it from a lymphoma

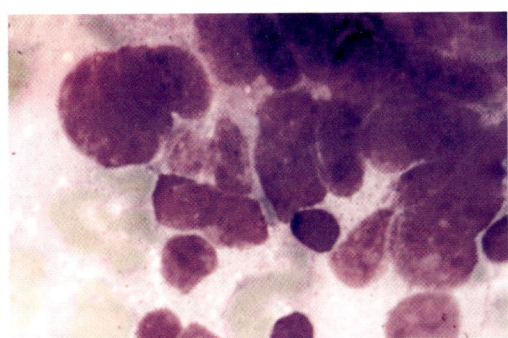

Fig. 6.16
FNAC mediastinum. Malignant thymoma. Undifferentiated malignant cells that are positive for epithelial markers. Clinical history of an enlarging mediastinal mass was important in reaching a diagnosis

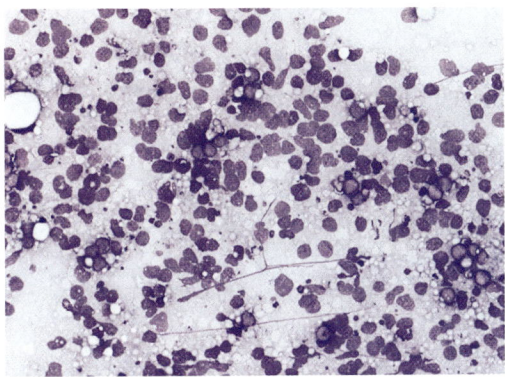

Fig. 6.17
FNAC neck mass. Undifferentiated malignant cells showed positivity with CD45 marker confirming their haemopoietic origin. The lesion was a high-grade NHL

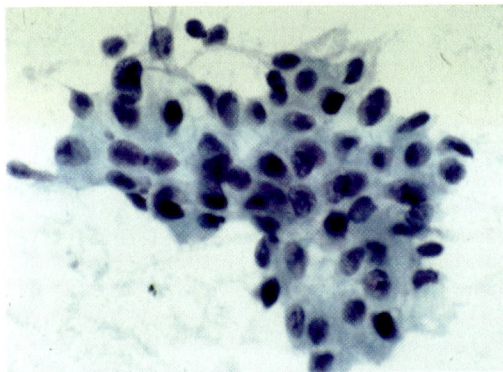

Fig. 6.18
FNAC lung. Metastatic adenocarcinoma. Malignant cells were PSA positive

Clear-cell tumours occur as primary neoplasms in several anatomical sites. Due to their overlapping morphological features, these tumours can be challenging for the cytopathologist, particularly when they present as metastatic lesions. Primary anatomical sites for clear-cell carcinoma may include kidney, ovary, salivary gland, cervix, lung, endometrium and germ-cell tumour. On light microscopy, these tumours have a similar appearance and are often indistinguishable. A history of prior malignancy and/or the presence of the concurrent tumour mass may be helpful (Fig. 6.19). Cytological examination, ancillary studies and clinical information can establish the anatomical site of origin in the majority (95%) of cases of clear-cell carcinoma [9].

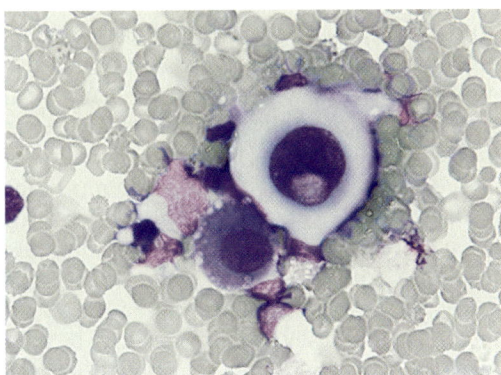

Fig. 6.19
Ascitic fluid. Clear-cell tumours occur as primary neoplasms in several anatomical sites. Due to their overlapping morphologic features, these tumours can be challenging for the cytologist, particularly when they present as metastatic lesions. On light microscopy, these tumours have a similar appearance and are often indistinguishable. In this case, the clear cell next to the mesothelial cells is from an ovarian clear-cell carcinoma

Immunocytochemistry has brought a major breakthrough in the typing of some tumours and in identifying some antigens common to certain groups of tumours. Immunocytochemistry markers specific for a single type of epithelium are rare (e.g. the prostate and thyroid both have specific markers), and melanoma and some germ-cell tumours may be identified accurately (Figs. 6.20 and 6.21). In others, immunocytochemistry helps to narrow down the possibilities [10–12] (Fig. 6.22). It has been shown that antibodies to thyroid transcription factor (TTF1) and the anti-lung-surfactant apoprotein monoclonal antibody PE-10 are fairly specific markers for primary lung tumours in histological specimens [13]. An accurate diagnosis of adrenal cortical neoplasm in FNAC specimens can often be difficult due to overlapping cytomorphological features with renal-cell carcinoma. CD10 immunostaining is helpful in separating metastatic renal-cell carcinoma from a primary adrenal cortical neoplasia and can be reliably performed on a cytological sample [14]. The cytopathological distinction between hepatocellular carcinoma and metastatic carcinoma in the liver can be problematic, especially in patients with poorly differentiated hepatocellular carcinoma, in whom a trabecular pattern, bile production and Mallory bodies may not be apparent on FNAC samples (e.g. metastatic hepatic adrenocortical carcinoma may mimic the features of hepatocellular carcinoma) [15]. HepPar1 antibody appears to be useful in making this distinction [16]. Uroplakin seems to be specific for transitional-cell carcinoma of the bladder in 66% of cases [17]. A careful scrutiny of the morphology for diagnostic clues, together with a careful clinical history remain the most valuable tools in the search for the primary tumour (Fig. 6.23). FNAC diagnosis may be used for establishing the tumour markers that may potentially be useful in treatment (e.g. HER-2/neu and hormonal receptors in the case of breast carcinoma) [18–29] (Fig. 6.24).

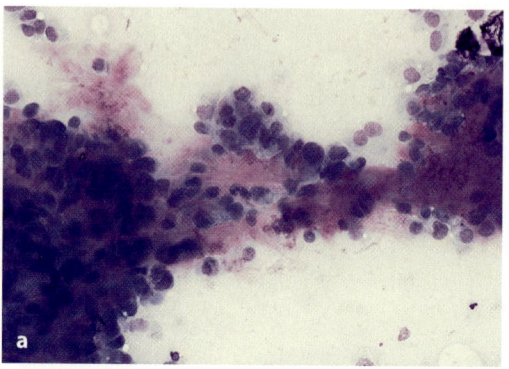

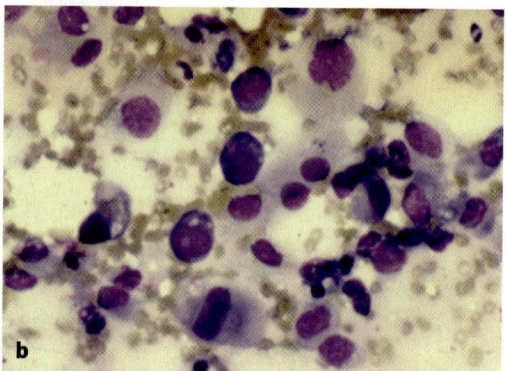

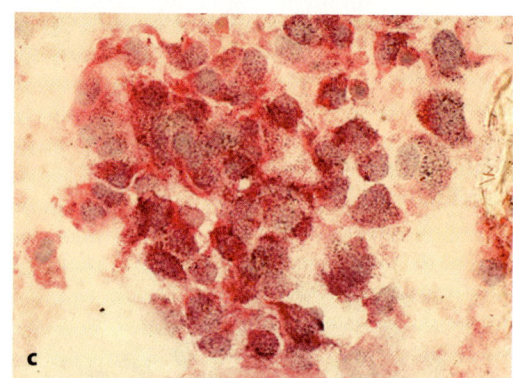

Fig. 6.20
FNAC neck node. Melanoma. **a** Tumour shows marked desmoplastic reaction. Morphologically, it could be mistaken for a soft-tissue tumour. **b** Different case of melanoma mimicking a lymphoma. **c** S100-positive tumour cells

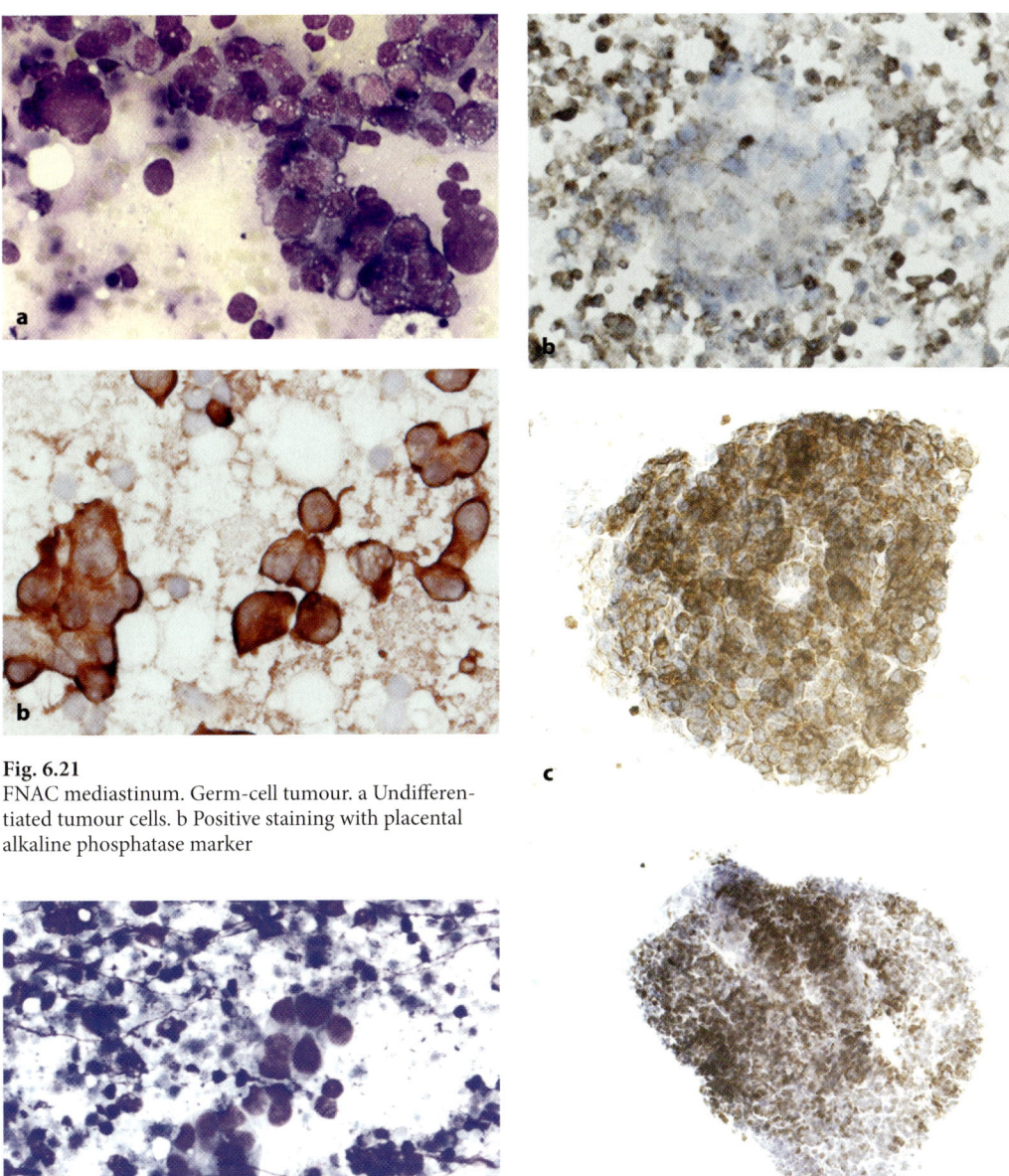

Fig. 6.21
FNAC mediastinum. Germ-cell tumour. a Undifferentiated tumour cells. b Positive staining with placental alkaline phosphatase marker

Fig. 6.22
Ascitic fluid. a Metastatic carcinoma cells. b CA 125-negative tumour cells. c Cells are positive for CK7. d Cells are positive for oestrogen receptors (ER). This panel of markers allows treatment of the patient for metastatic breast as opposed to ovarian carcinoma

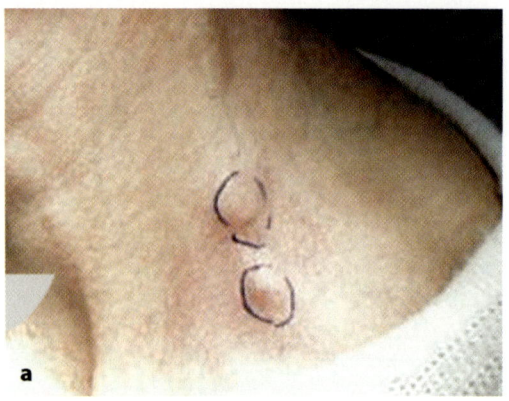
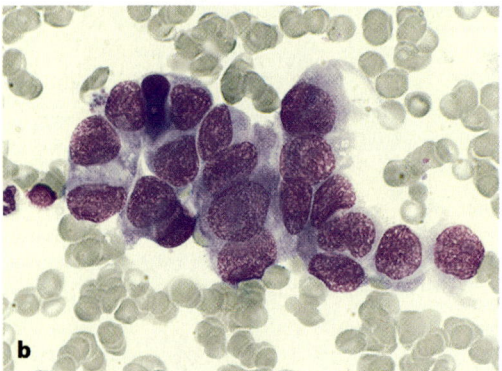
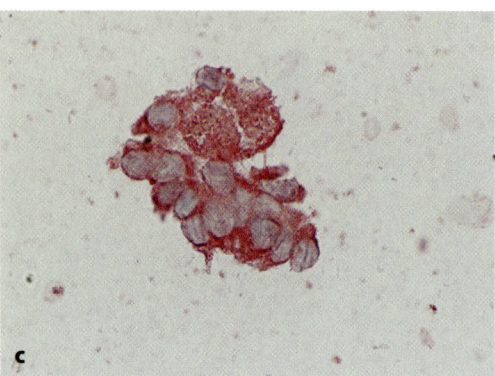

Fig. 6.23
FNAC neck nodes. Angiosarcoma. **a** Patient with a history of angiosarcoma treated with radiation. **b** Malignant cells in the neck nodes that may mimic metastatic carcinoma. **c** CD34 endothelial marker positivity in tumour cells

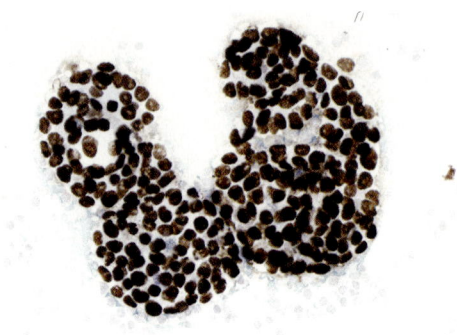

Fig. 6.24
FNAC breast. ER-positive cells from breast carcinoma

Although metastatic processes appear random, there are features in the behaviour of certain carcinomas that may help in diagnosis. A knowledge of areas of lymphatic drainage is helpful in excluding the tumours in the proximity of the metastases (e.g. cholangiocarcinoma, in the case of liver metastases, neck, in the case of PTC; Fig. 6.25). In the case of distant metastases, there are certain patterns that are more common in disease spread than others (e.g. Virchow's gland, in the case of abdominal and pelvic primary carcinomas, which tend to metastasise into the left supraclavicular fossa and constitute 88% of all metastatic tumours there) [1]. Bone is a site of metastases favoured by certain tumours (lung, breast, kidney, thyroid, prostate). FNAC is usually successful in sampling osteolytic bone metastases [30]. Melanoma can be found anywhere and can mimic any tumour type. Differentiation between the primary and metastatic tumour is important for both staging and treatment (e.g. a solitary lung and bone metastasis of a renal tumour may be mistaken for a stage IV lung carcinoma) [31].

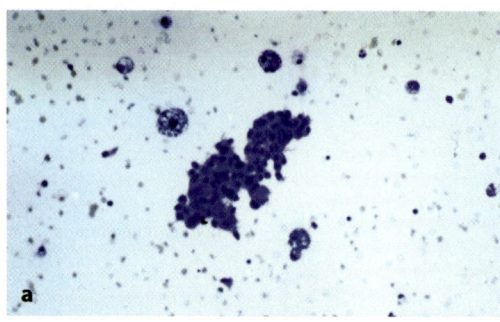

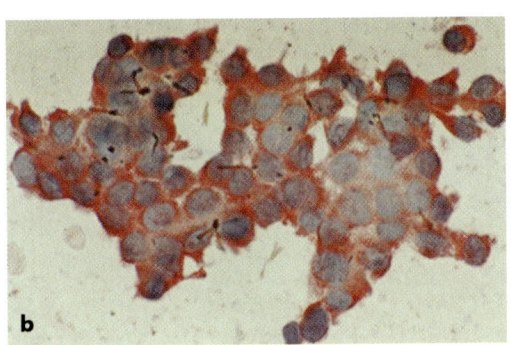

Fig. 6.25
FNAC neck node. **a** Epithelial cells within a cystic fluid of the neck node. **b** Papillary carcinoma cells confirmed by thyroglobulin stain

The importance of diagnosing metastases in staging malignancy has been shown to be paramount in giving the appropriate treatment (e.g. mediastinal lymph node metastases in patients with NSCC are a critical determinant of operability). Mediastinoscopy is invasive, requires general anaesthesia and carries appreciable morbidity. The development of minimally invasive techniques for the pathological staging of lung cancer is important [32]. Immediate cytological evaluation of EUS-FNAC specimens allows a diagnosis in all cases and contributes to the utility of EUS-FNAC as a diagnostic procedure for mediastinal adenopathy [33]. It is more accurate than CT for nodal staging of oesophageal carcinoma and impacts on therapy for these patients [34]. In the case of the adrenal gland, apart from diagnosing metastases, FNAC has been used to confirm that 29% of enlarged adrenal glands are actually benign [35].

6.1.4 The Role of Imaging in the FNAC of Metastases

Imaging techniques have an ever increasing ability to distinguish between reactive and malignant lymph nodes. Ultrasound is more sensitive than physical examination alone in determining axillary lymph-node involvement during the preliminary staging of breast carcinoma. Due to the occasional overlap of sonographic features of benign and indeterminate lymph nodes, FNAC of sonographically indeterminate/suspicious lymph nodes can provide a more definitive diagnosis than ultrasound alone. When used in the initial staging of breast carcinoma, EUS-FNAC of non-palpable lymph nodes had an overall sensitivity of 86.4%, a specificity of 100%, a diagnostic accuracy of 79.0%, a positive predictive value of 100% and a negative predictive value of 67% [36].

6.2 Metastases of Non-Epithelial Tumours

Non-epithelial tumours, which includes the majority of small round-cell tumours (see Chap. 7), sarcomas, melanomas, lymphoma/leukaemia and other miscellaneous tumours, can also be diagnosed by FNAC from their metastases (Figs. 6.5, 6.10, 6.13, 6.17, 6.20 and 6.23). These usually present as soft-tissue deposits or lung metastases. The diagnostic principles that apply for carcinomas are even more important for the non-epithelial tumours because of their less predictable metastatic spread. The knowledge of clinical history and written evidence of previous histology (preferably with the slides available) is essential when making a diagnosis of a metastatic non-epithelial tumour. Since these tumours are rarer than carcinomas, the original diagnosis may frequently have been made outside the referral institution. Since the effect of the errors involved may be grave, it is always important to compare the original histology with the present findings and repeat the markers if necessary. Distinction between lymphoma and carcinoma (e.g. nasopharyngeal carcinoma and DLBL) or sarcoma and lymphoma may be one of those fundamental decisions that has to be made based on the findings of a metastatic deposit and thus confirm or correct the initial diagnosis. Nowadays, it is common practice that such cases are discussed at multidisciplinary meetings where pathologists, radiologists and clinicians may exchange views about the different aspects of an individual case and reach a mutual decision about the management of that patient.

References

1. Nasuti JF, Mehrotra R, Gupta PK. Diagnostic value of fine-needle aspiration in supraclavicular lymphadenopathy: a study of 106 patients and review of literature. Diagn Cytopathol 2001;25(6):351–5
2. Lawrence WD. ADASP recommendations for processing and reporting of lymph node specimens submitted for evaluation of metastatic disease. Virchows Arch 2001;439(5):601–3
3. Gong Y, DeFrias DV, Nayar R. Pitfalls in fine needle aspiration cytology of extraadrenal paraganglioma. A report of 2 cases. Acta Cytol 2003;47(6):1082–6
4. Viguer JM, Jimenez-Heffernan JA, Lopez-Ferrer P, Banaclocha M, Vicandi B. Fine-needle aspiration cytology of metastatic nasopharyngeal carcinoma. Diagn Cytopathol 2005;32(4):233–237
5. Shukla R, Pooja B, Radhika S, Nijhawan R, Rajwanshi A. Fine-needle aspiration cytology of extramammary neoplasms metastatic to the breast. Diagn Cytopathol 2005;32(4):193–197
6. Volmar KE, Jones CK, Xie HB. Metastases in the pancreas from nonhematologic neoplasms: report of 20 cases evaluated by fine-needle aspiration. Diagn Cytopathol 2004;31(4):216–20
7. Tan LH. Meningioma presenting as a parapharyngeal tumor: report of a case with fine needle aspiration cytology. Acta Cytol 2001;45(6):1053–9
8. Parwani AV, Ali SZ. Prostatic adenocarcinoma metastases mimicking small cell carcinoma on fine-needle aspiration. Diagn Cytopathol 2002;27(2):75–9
9. Hughes JH, Jensen CS, Donnelly AD, Cohen MB, Silverman JF, Geisinger KR, et al. The role of fine-needle aspiration cytology in the evaluation of metastatic clear cell tumors. Cancer 1999;87(6):380–9
10. Simsir A, Wei XJ, Yee H, Moreira A, Cangiarella J. Differential expression of cytokeratins 7 and 20 and thyroid transcription factor-1 in bronchioloalveolar carcinoma: an immunohistochemical study in fine-needle aspiration biopsy specimens. Am J Clin Pathol 2004;121(3):350–7
11. Tot T, Samii S. The clinical relevance of cytokeratin phenotyping in needle biopsy of liver metastasis. APMIS 2003;111(12):1075–82
12. Hecht JL, Pinkus JL, Weinstein LJ, Pinkus GS. The value of thyroid transcription factor-1 in cytologic preparations as a marker for metastatic adenocarcinoma of lung origin. Am J Clin Pathol 2001;116(4):483–8. Write to the Help Desk NCBI | NLM | NIH Department of Health & Human Services Privacy Statement | Freedom of Information Act | Disclaimer
13. Chhieng DC, Cangiarella JF, Zakowski MF, Goswami S, Cohen JM, Yee HT. Use of thyroid transcription factor 1, PE-10, and cytokeratins 7 and 20 in discriminating between primary lung carcinomas and metastatic lesions in fine-needle aspiration biopsy specimens. Cancer 2001;93(5):330–6
14. Yang B, Ali SZ, Rosenthal DL. CD10 facilitates the diagnosis of metastatic renal cell carcinoma from primary adrenal cortical neoplasm in adrenal fine-needle aspiration. Diagn Cytopathol 2002;27(3):149–52
15. Serrano R, Rodriguez-Peralto JL, Santos-Briz A, de Agustin P. Fine needle aspiration cytology of metastatic hepatic adrenocortical carcinoma mimicking hepatocellular carcinoma: a case report. Acta Cytol 2001;45(5):768–70
16. Siddiqui MT, Saboorian MH, Gokaslan ST, Ashfaq R. Diagnostic utility of the HepPar1 antibody to differentiate hepatocellular carcinoma from metastatic carcinoma in fine-needle aspiration samples. Cancer 2002;96(1):49–52
17. Xu X, Sun TT, Gupta PK, Zhang P, Nasuti JF. Uroplakin as a marker for typing metastatic transitional cell carcinoma on fine-needle aspiration specimens. Cancer 2001;93(3):216–21
18. Beatty BG, Bryant R, Wang W, Ashikaga T, Gibson PC, Leiman G, et al. HER-2/neu detection in fine-needle aspirates of breast cancer: fluorescence in situ hybridization and immunocytochemical analysis. Am J Clin Pathol 2004;122(2):246–55
19. Bofin AM, Ytterhus B, Martin C, O'Leary JJ, Hagmar BM. Detection and quantitation of HER-2 gene amplification and protein expression in breast carcinoma. Am J Clin Pathol 2004;122(1):110–9
20. Sneige N. Utility of cytologic specimens in the evaluation of prognostic and predictive factors of breast cancer: current issues and future directions. Diagn Cytopathol 2004;30(3):158–65
21. Dagrada GP, Mezzelani A, Alasio L, Ruggeri M, Romano R, Pierotti MA, et al. HER-2/neu assessment in primary chemotherapy treated breast carcinoma: no evidence of gene profile changing. Breast Cancer Res Treat 2003;80(2):207–14
22. Bofin AM, Ytterhus B, Hagmar BM. TOP2A and HER-2 gene amplification in fine needle aspirates from breast carcinomas. Cytopathology 2003;14(6):314–9
23. Bofin AM, Ytterhus B, Fjosne HE, Hagmar BM. Abnormal chromosome 8 copy number in cytological smears from breast carcinomas detected by means of fluorescence in situ hybridization (FISH). Cytopathology 2003;14(1):5–11
24. Vesoulis Z, Rajappannair L, Define L, Beach J, Schnell B, Myers S. Quantitative image analysis of estrogen receptors in breast fine needle aspiration biopsies. Anal Quant Cytol Histol 2004;26(6):323–30

25. Krishnamurthy S, Dimashkieh H, Patel S, Sneige N. Immunocytochemical evaluation of estrogen receptor on archival Papanicolaou-stained fine-needle aspirate smears. Diagn Cytopathol 2003;29(6):309–14
26. Cano G, Milanezi F, Leitao D, Ricardo S, Brito MJ, Schmitt FC. Estimation of hormone receptor status in fine-needle aspirates and paraffin-embedded sections from breast cancer using the novel rabbit monoclonal antibodies SP1 and SP2. Diagn Cytopathol 2003;29(4):207–11
27. Pusztai L, Ayers M, Stec J, Clark E, Hess K, Stivers D, et al. Gene expression profiles obtained from fine-needle aspirations of breast cancer reliably identify routine prognostic markers and reveal large-scale molecular differences between estrogen-negative and estrogen-positive tumors. Clin Cancer Res 2003;9(7):2406–15
28. Lofgren L, Skoog L, von Schoultz E, Tani E, Isaksson E, Fernstad R, et al. Hormone receptor status in breast cancer--a comparison between surgical specimens and fine needle aspiration biopsies. Cytopathology 2003;14(3):136–42
29. Kuenen-Boumeester V, Timmermans AM, De Bruijn EM, Henzen-Logmans SC. Immunocytochemical detection of prognostic markers in breast cancer; technical considerations. Cytopathology 1999;10(5):308–16
30. Suterwala S, Volk EE, Danforth RD. Aspiration biopsy of osseous metastasis of occult hepatocellular carcinoma: Case report, literature review, and differential diagnosis. Diagn Cytopathol 2001;25(1):63–7
31. Griniatsos J, Michail PO, Menenakos C, Hatzianastasiou D, Koufos C, Bastounis E. Metastatic renal clear cell carcinoma mimicking stage IV lung cancer. Int Urol Nephrol 2003;35:15–7
32. Rintoul RC, Skwarski KM, Murchison JT, Hill A, Walker WS, Penman ID. Endoscopic and endobronchial ultrasound real-time fine-needle aspiration for staging of the mediastinum in lung cancer. Chest 2004;126(6):2020–2
33. Emery SC, Savides TJ, Behling CA. Utility of immediate evaluation of endoscopic ultrasound-guided transesophageal fine needle aspiration of mediastinal lymph nodes. Acta Cytol 2004;48(5):630–4
34. Vazquez-Sequeiros E, Wiersema MJ, Clain JE, Norton ID, Levy MJ, Romero Y, et al. Impact of lymph node staging on therapy of esophageal carcinoma. Gastroenterology 2003;125(6):1626–35
35. Jhala NC, Jhala D, Eloubeidi MA, Chhieng DC, Crowe DR, Roberson J, et al. Endoscopic ultrasound-guided fine-needle aspiration biopsy of the adrenal glands: analysis of 24 patients. Cancer 2004;102(5):308–14
36. Krishnamurthy S, Sneige N, Bedi DG, Edieken BS, Fornage BD, Kuerer HM, et al. Role of ultrasound-guided fine-needle aspiration of indeterminate and suspicious axillary lymph nodes in the initial staging of breast carcinoma. Cancer 2002;95(5):982–8

Chapter 7

Diagnostic Dilemmas in FNAC Cytology: Small Round Cell Tumours

Contents

7.1	**Small Round Cell Tumours of Childhood**	133
7.1.1	Ewing's Sarcoma/Primitive Neuroectodermal Tumour	134
7.1.2	Neuroblastoma	136
7.1.3	Ganglioneuroblastomas	136
7.1.4	Rhabdomyosarcoma	137
7.1.5	Acute Lymphoblastic Leukaemia and LBL	139
7.1.6	Small Round Cell Tumours of Kidney	141
7.1.7	Hepatoblastoma	141
7.1.8	Pleuropulmonary Blastoma	142
7.1.9	Small-Cell Synovial Sarcoma	142
7.2	**Small Round Cell Tumours in Adults**	142
7.2.1	Desmoplastic Small Round Cell Tumour	143
7.2.2	Small-Cell Carcinoma of the Lung	144
7.2.3	Burkitt's Lymphoma	144
7.2.4	Lymphoglandular Bodies	145
7.2.5	Merkel Cell Carcinoma	146
7.2.6	Olfactory Neuroblastoma	147
	References	148

The term small round-cell tumour (SRCT) is a generic term for tumours composed of malignant round cells that are slightly larger or double the size of red blood cells in air-dried smears or measure less than 10 μm in diameter in alcohol-fixed smears, and have scanty cytoplasm. Their features, including cellularity, morphology, pattern of cell arrangement and smear background, often pose a diagnostic challenge in FNAC since similar features may reflect a variety of tumour types and subtypes. Within the group of tumours that express a dominant or occasional SRCT (excluding the central nervous system neoplasms) include Ewing's sarcoma and primitive neuroectodermal tumour (PNET; ES/PNET) and its variants, neuroblastoma, desmoplastic SRCT, rhabdomyosarcoma (RMS) (alveolar, solid and embryonal), small-cell osteosarcoma, chondrosarcoma (myxoid and mesenchymal), round-cell and myxoid liposarcoma, synovial sarcoma (monophasic undifferentiated), primitive malignant peripheral nerve sheath tumour (malignant small-cell schwannoma), Non Hodgkin lymphome (NHL), Merkel cell tumour of the skin and small-cell carcinoma including neuroendocrine carcinoma [1].

7.1 Small Round Cell Tumours of Childhood

Tumours of infancy and childhood are most commonly referred to as the SRCT group and include ES/PNET, neuroblastoma, RMS and malignant lymphoma. Other malignancies that may be considered in the differential diagnosis include small-cell osteogenic sarcoma, undifferentiated (anaplastic) hepatoblastoma, granulocytic sarcoma, blastemal-type Wilms' tumour, and desmoplastic small-cell tumour of the peritoneum [2]. Although challenging, FNAC of childhood SRCT can be diagnostic in the majority of cases, allowing specific therapy to be given to patients with unresectable SRCT without a tissue biopsy as well as documenting recurrent and/or metastatic disease [2]. SRCTs usually have characteristic cytomorphology. However, when these tumours are undifferentiated, morphological criteria may not be sufficient to arrive at a correct diagnosis. A variety of ancillary studies including electron microscopy, immunohistochemistry, DNA ploidy, cytogenetics and FISH may provide valuable additional information for the precise characterisation of these neoplasms. Some ancillary studies may also be used for assigning these cases to prognostically significant subgroups, helping to define the most suitable chemotherapeutic regimens. Since most of these special studies require only a small amount of cellular material, FNAC is ideally suited for obtaining samples for these procedures [3].

7.1.1 Ewing's Sarcoma/Primitive Neuroectodermal Tumour

ES/PNET is a family of malignant SRCTs that exhibits neuroepithelial differentiation, most often presenting as a soft-tissue or bone lesion in the trunk or axial skeleton, predominantly in older children and adolescents. Isolated cases of PNET have been observed in FNAC samples from visceral sites such as the ovary, testis, uterus, bladder, pancreas and kidney [4]. In some cases the primary diagnosis made by FNAC enables the paediatric oncologist to give specific therapy for the otherwise unresectable tumour and thus achieve remission [5]. Local recurrences may include the chest wall, pleura and pericardium, whilst metastatic disease may be found almost anywhere.

The cytological features of ES/PNET include malignant cells with a high N/C ratio, hyperchromatic nuclei without prominent nucleoli, distinctively smooth nuclear membrane contour, finely granular chromatin, one or two small nucleoli and scant, but almost always present, perinuclear clear cytoplasm, suggesting epithelial differentiation (Fig. 7.1). Cells are arranged singly or in cohesive clusters. Homer-Wright rosettes may be seen and there are no ganglion cells or neuropil. There is an absence of frequent mitotic figures, large nucleoli, nuclear pleomorphism, cellular debris, histiocytes and polymorphonuclear leukocytes [6]. Smears appear clean, with small, uniform cells having features suggesting a neuroendocrine epithelial tumour (Fig. 7.2). As regards the differentiation of Ewing's sarcoma, a few subtle differentiating features can be observed: the cells in Ewing's sarcoma have a finer nuclear chromatin in comparison to those of PNET tumour, and punched-out clear cytoplasmic vacuoles are present. PNET shows nuclear moulding, unipolar cytoplasmic tags and Homer-Wright rosettes [7].

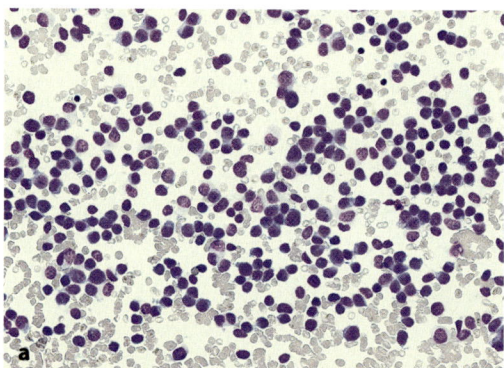

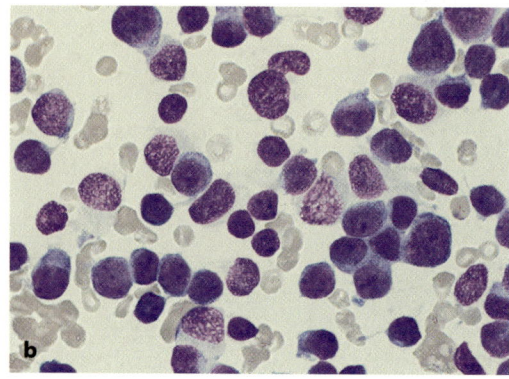

Fig. 7.1
FNAC bone lesion. Ewing's sarcoma/primitive neuroectodermal tumour (ES/PNET). **a** Low-power view revealing a small round-cell tumour (SRCT). **b** MGG stain.

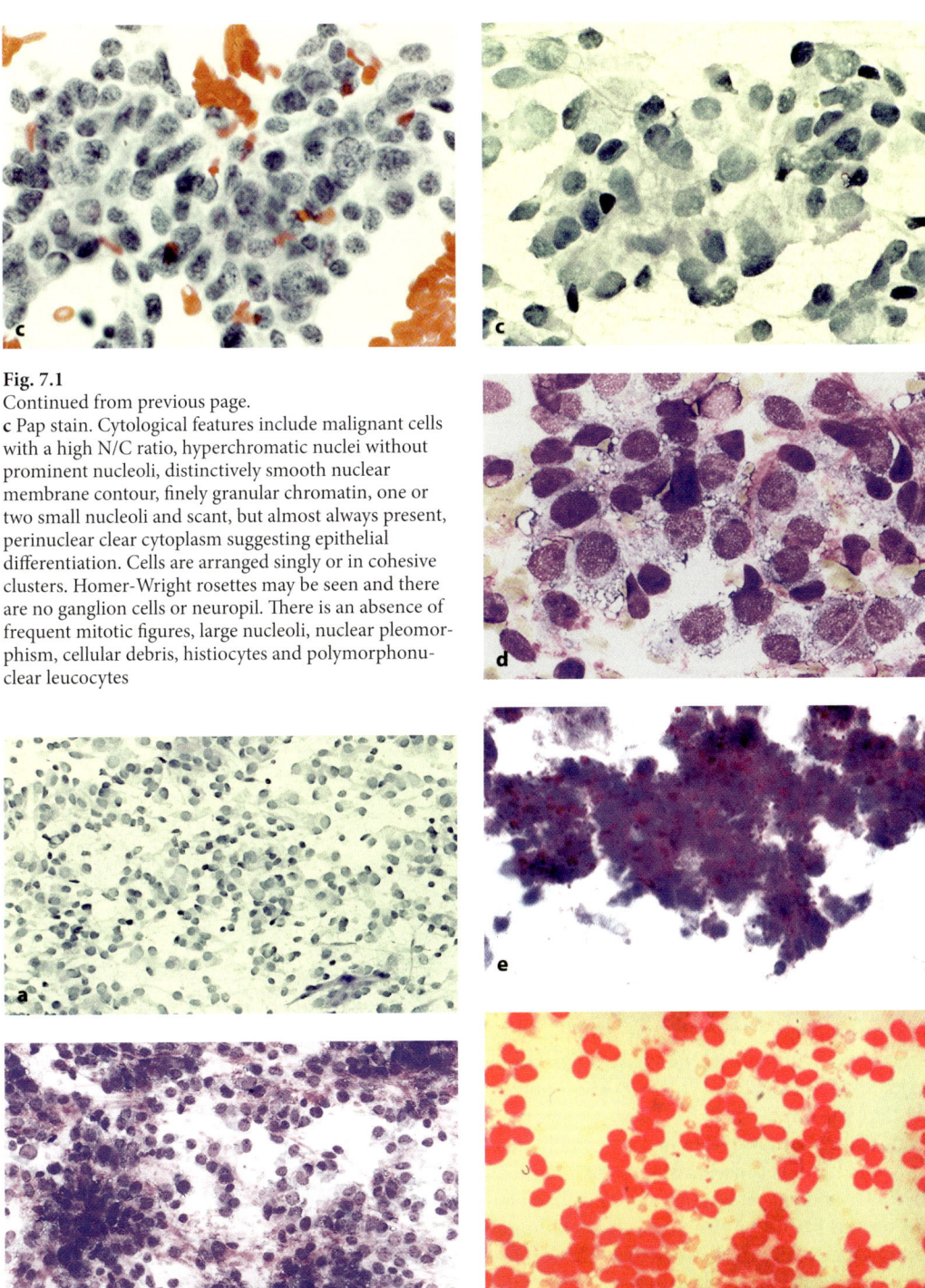

Fig. 7.1
Continued from previous page.
c Pap stain. Cytological features include malignant cells with a high N/C ratio, hyperchromatic nuclei without prominent nucleoli, distinctively smooth nuclear membrane contour, finely granular chromatin, one or two small nucleoli and scant, but almost always present, perinuclear clear cytoplasm suggesting epithelial differentiation. Cells are arranged singly or in cohesive clusters. Homer-Wright rosettes may be seen and there are no ganglion cells or neuropil. There is an absence of frequent mitotic figures, large nuclei, nuclear pleomorphism, cellular debris, histiocytes and polymorphonuclear leucocytes

Fig. 7.2
FNAC thigh lesion. ES/PNET. (see next page)

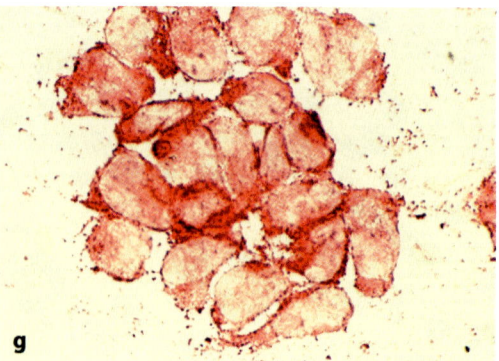

Fig. 7.2
Continued from previous page. FNAC thigh lesion. ES/PNET. **a** Smears appear clean, with small, uniform cells having features suggesting a neuroendocrine epithelial tumour. **b–d** As regards the differentiation of Ewing's sarcoma, a few subtle differentiating features can be observed: the cells in Ewing's sarcoma have a finer nuclear chromatin in comparison to those of the PNET tumour, and punched-out clear cytoplasmic vacuoles are present. PNET shows nuclear moulding, unipolar cytoplasmic tags and Homer-Wright rosettes. **e** PAS stain shows strong positivity for cytoplasmic glycogen. **f** Strongly positive for synaptophysin. **g** Strongly positive for CD99. Other small cell neoplasms, including rhabdomyosarcoma (RMS), blastemal Wilms' tumour and lymphoblastic lymphoma (LBL) have also shown positivity, but the staining reactions are usually weak and focal

Ancillary studies, including electron microscopy, immunocytochemistry and cytogenetics (t11;22) may be performed on FNAC material and thus exclude other SRCTs of childhood such as malignant lymphoma and RMS. CD99 immunostaining and/or molecular studies, particularly in the intermediate and atypical variants, may help to establish a definitive FNAC diagnosis, thus avoiding an open surgical biopsy [8] (Fig. 7.2g). Other small round cell neoplasms, including RMS, blastemal Wilms' tumour and lymphoblastic lymphoma (LBL) have also shown positivity, but the staining reactions are usually weak and focal [9]. The differential diagnosis between ES/PNET and neuroblastoma can be difficult based on the FNAC morphology alone, although morphological differences do exist. Clinical features (e.g. age, primary site, metastatic patterns), catecholamine levels, electron microscopy and cytogenetics are necessary to establish the correct diagnosis (see 7.1.2).

7.1.2 Neuroblastoma

Neuroblastoma is an SRCT that is characterised by rosettes and background filamentous/fibrillar material in FNAC material (Fig. 7.3) [10]. Cytological features in conjunction with immunocytochemistry and electron microscopy performed on the FNAC material enable making a diagnosis of primary or metastatic neuroblastoma [10]. It is possible to use the Southern blotting technique to demonstrate N-myc amplification in material obtained from FNAC [11]. N-myc amplification by interphase FISH and immunocytochemistry result in the molecular characterisation of neuroblastic tumours. Such analyses are of prognostic significance because they predict tumour behaviour and response to therapy according to International Neuroblastoma Staging System/International Neuroblastoma Risk Groups criteria [12]. Amplification of the transcription factor N-myc is an important molecular diagnostic tool in stratifying treatment for neuroblastoma [13].

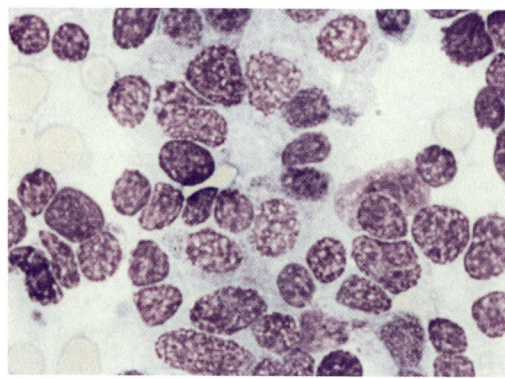

Fig. 7.3
FNAC paraspinal mass. Neuroblastoma. Homer-Wright rosette.

7.1.3 Ganglioneuroblastomas

Ganglioneuroblastomas show the characteristic Homer-Wright rosettes, ganglion cells and fibrillary material [14].

7.1.4 Rhabdomyosarcoma

RMS accounts for approximately 4% of all childhood malignancies. RMSs are classified into embryonal, alveolar and pleomorphic subtypes. Embryonal RMS, including the botryoid variant, typically occurs in young children, alveolar RMS typically occurs in older children and young adults, and pleomorphic RMS occurs in older adults, although it has been reported in children. The tumour may present clinically as a primary or metastatic. Cellular features that, according to the degree of differentiation, can be categorised as early, intermediate or late rhabdomyoblasts, may help differentiation into histological subtypes [15]. The distinction between RMS and the other small round cell tumours of childhood has therapeutic implications. Chemotherapy for RMS may be given before local treatment and prevent mutilating surgery and high-dose irradiation. FNAC can confirm the diagnosis and neoadjuvant treatment can start without delay [16].

The cytological features of RMS include two main cell types: a predominantly primitive, small round cell with scant cytoplasm and a large cell with abundant cytoplasm, sometimes tadpole or ribbon shaped. The tumour cells are often enclosed in a background of eosinophilic substances (Fig. 7.4). The primitive, uniform population of tumour cells can be arranged as single cells and cohesive aggregates. The cells are predominantly small and lymphocyte-like, round/polygonal, with uniform nuclei and scant to moderate amounts of cytoplasm. The nuclear chromatin is most often finely granular and hyperchromatic, while nucleoli are inconspicuous. Binucleated and multinucleated cells are found frequently. Intracytoplasmic vacuoles are common, ranging in frequency from occasional to numerous [17]. The finding of cells with more abundant cytoplasm, eccentrically located nuclei and bi/multinucleated tumour cells in a background of eosinophilic substance helps in the differential diagnosis. The lack of cytological features proving rhabdomyoblastic differentiation, such as cross-striation, necessitates the use of additional methods in the cytological diagnosis of embryonal RMS [18, 19]. Ultrastructural analysis and immunocytochemistry in the demonstration of desmin in FNAC is helpful in reaching a diagnosis.

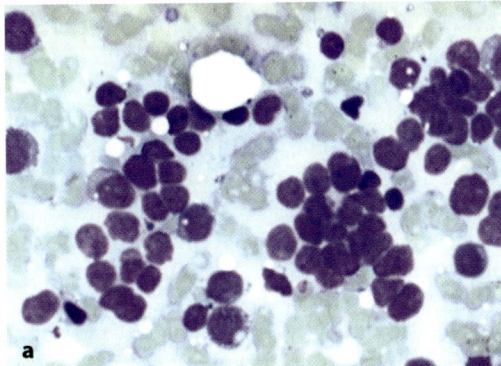

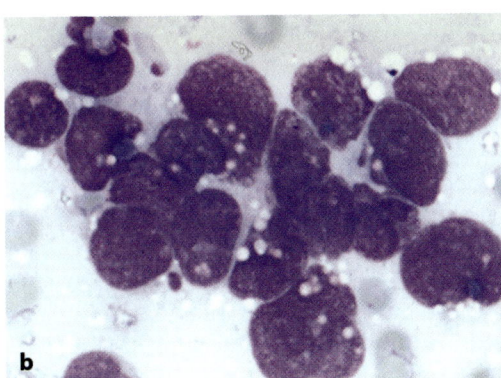

Fig. 7.4
FNAC neck mass. Embryonal RMS. **a** A predominantly primitive, small round cell population with scant cytoplasm arranged as single cells and cohesive aggregates. The cells are predominantly small and lymphocyte-like, round/polygonal, with uniform nuclei and scant to moderate amounts of cytoplasm. **b** The nuclear chromatin is most often finely granular and hyperchromatic, while nucleoli are inconspicuous. Binucleated and multinucleated cells are found frequently. Intracytoplasmic vacuoles are common, ranging from occasional to numerous. A reliable subclassification into alveolar and embryonal RMS cannot be made from FNAC smears

In an attempt to distinguish between embryonal and alveolar RMS on FNAC material, Pohar Marinsek et al. analysed a large series of cases aimed at identifying the morphological characteristics and architectural patterns of each RMS subtype [20]. Among the alveolar RMS subtypes, they identified two major architectural patterns: one containing completely dissociated cells and one containing many chance formations (Fig. 7.5). Among the embryonal type, the predominant architectural pattern contained large tissue fragments with abundant eosinophilic material and various numbers of dissociated cells. The pattern of only dissociated cells was similar to that seen in the alveolar type. The relative proportion of poorly to better and well-differentiated rhabdomyoblasts varied in both types and in all patterns. RMS exhibits a variety of morphological patterns of cellular morphology and architectural features, even within the same histological subtype. The authors conclude that a reliable subclassification into alveolar and embryonal RMS cannot be made from FNAC smears [20]. The embryonal type can be suggested in cases containing large tissue fragments with abundant eosinophilic material and small, tightly packed cells with oval nuclei. However, all cases suspected to be RMS must always be confirmed immunocytochemically since they could be confused with some benign and malignant tumours with similar morphology [21]. Myogenin and MyoD1, which are myogenic transcriptional regulatory proteins, which are expressed early in skeletal muscle differentiation, are considered sensitive and specific markers for RMS and are more specific than desmin and muscle-specific actin and more sensitive than myoglobin [22, 23]. It has been shown that 5-year survival is better for younger-age children with localised disease, with orbital and genitourinary tumour sites and tumours that have an embryonal histology (67%). A poor prognosis is associated with diagnosis during infancy and adolescence, metastatic disease at the time of presentation, alveolar histology (49%) and tumours of the extremities, retroperitoneum and trunk [24]. Identification of the alveolar subtype of RMS is important because the poor prognosis associated with this subtype necessitates a modified therapeutic regimen. At present, the diagnosis of alveolar subtype of RMS is made on the basis of histological findings and the extent of myogenin immunopositivity [25]. The absence of an alveolar pattern in the solid variant, the low degree of differentiation in certain embryonal RMSs and the increasing use of microbiopsy samples make the diagnosis of alveolar RMS difficult. Two specific translocations have been found in alveolar RMS, and fusion transcripts can be detected by reverse transcriptase-PCR. Molecular detection of these fusion transcripts via real-time reverse transcriptase-PCR analysis is a sensitive and specific method for the diagnosis of alveolar RMS. Immunohistochemical analysis of myogenin expression can be used to select cases for such molecular testing [25]. N-myc deregulation is a feature of RMS tumorigenesis, it defines groups of patients with a poor prognosis and is a potential target for novel therapies [13]. Increased copy number and overexpression of N-myc in RMS measured by using quantitative PCR, shows an increased copy number of N-myc to be significantly associated with adverse outcome [13].

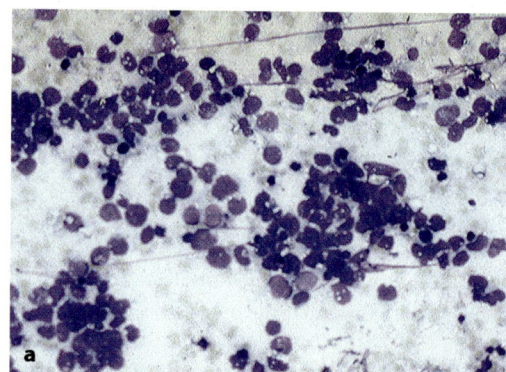

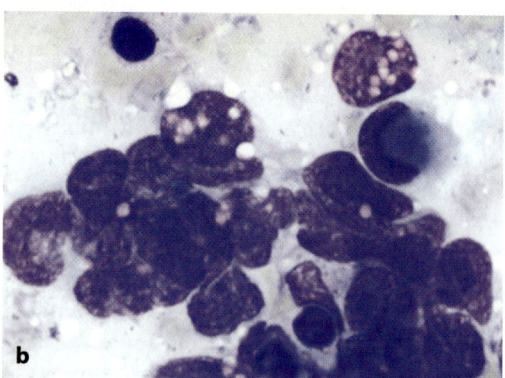

Fig. 7.5
FNAC inguinum. Alveolar RMS. (see next page)

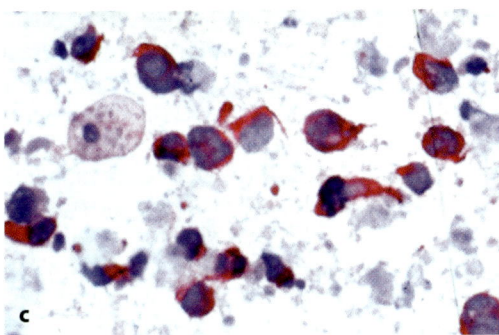

Fig. 7.5
Cont'd from prev page. Alveolar RMS.
a Small round cell population with scant cytoplasm arranged mainly as single dissociated cells and small chance formations. The cells are predominantly small and lymphocyte-like, round/polygonal, with uniform nuclei and scant to moderate amounts of cytoplasm.
b Larger cells with an abundant cytoplasm, sometimes tadpole- or ribbon-shaped. The tumour cells are often enclosed in a background of eosinophilic substance. Some cells may show myoid differentiation. **c** Desmin positivity in tumour cells. The finding of cells with more abundant cytoplasm, eccentrically located nuclei and bi/multinucleated tumour cells in a background of eosinophilic substance helps in the differential diagnosis. The lack of cytological features proving rhabdomyoblastic differentiation, such as cross-striation, necessitates the use of additional methods in the cytological diagnosis. A reliable subclassification into alveolar and embryonal RMS cannot be made from FNAC smears

7.1.5 Acute Lymphoblastic Leukaemia and LBL

Acute lymphoblastic leukaemia (ALL) and lymphoblastic lymphoma (LBL) are the most common malignancies in children and are also among the most curable. ALL is a heterogeneous disease with distinct biological and prognostic groupings. The identification of relevant prognostic factors for lymphoblastic malignant neoplasms, using a multiparametric approach including immunophenotyping, cytogenetic and molecular analysis and more traditional pathological criteria, provides information that allows each patient to receive appropriate treatment [26]. This has permitted tailoring therapy intensity to produce higher remission rates, even in unfavourable prognostic groups.

Diagnosis of ALL and LBL relies on traditional cytomorphological and immunohistochemical evaluation of the leukaemic blasts (Fig. 7.6). Immunophenotyping is important in characterising morphologically poorly differentiated acute leukaemias and in defining the prognostic categories of ALL [27]. Cytogenetic analysis identifies clonal numeric and/or structural chromosomal abnormalities that may be present, thus confirming the subtype classification [28]. Cytogenetic abnormalities have now emerged as the single most important prognostic factor for children with ALL. There are specific cytogenetic findings in the leukaemic blast cells that influence prognosis [29].

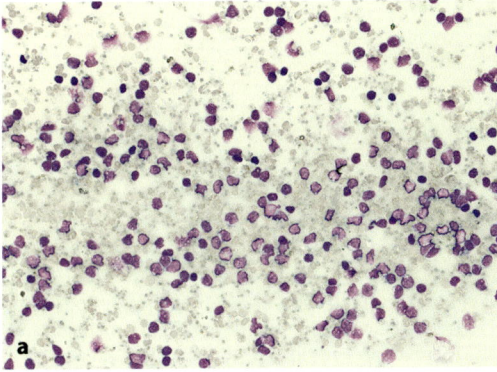

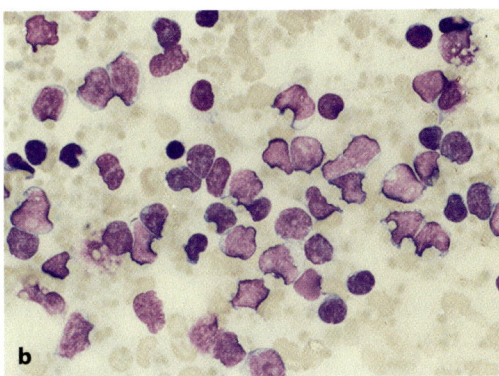

Fig. 7.6
FNAC lymph node. T-cell-type acute lymphoblastic leukaemia. (see next page)

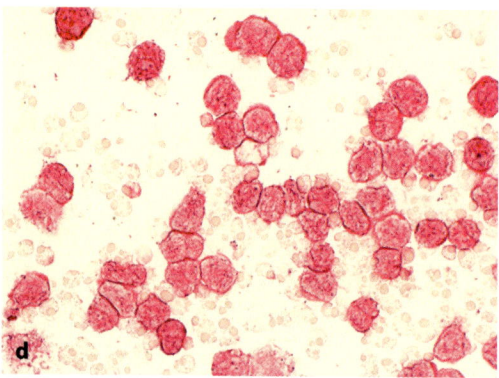

clear chromatin, small, inconspicuous nucleoli, irregular nuclear contours and scant basophilic cytoplasm. Frequent mitotic figures are seen (1–14 figures per 1,000 cells) [30]. The majority of LBLs are of the T-cell phenotype with considerable phenotypic variability. Burkitt's lymphoma (BL) and DLBL account for nearly all paediatric non-lymphoblastic B-cell lymphomas. Because clinical behaviour, prognosis and response to therapy might differ, diagnostic accuracy is important. Paediatric BLs and DLBLs have distinctive immunohistochemical profiles, and staining for c-myc, MIB-1 and bcl-2 might be useful in morphologically difficult cases [31, 32] (Fig. 7.7; see 7.2).

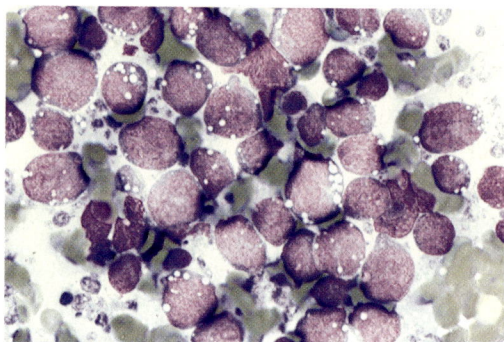

Fig. 7.6
Continued from previous page. FNAC lymph node. T-cell-type acute lymphoblastic leukaemia. **a** Diagnosis of ALL relies on traditional cytomorphological and immunohistochemical evaluation of the leukaemic blasts. **b** These are intermediate-sized cells (9.5–18.5 ìm) with fine nuclear chromatin, small, inconspicuous nucleoli, irregular nuclear contours and scant basophilic cytoplasm. **c** CD 3 positivity in blasts confirms a T-cell phenotype. The majority of LBLs are of the T-cell phenotype with considerable phenotypic variability.
d Terminal deoxynucleotidyl transferase (Tdt) positivity confirms the primitive nature of the cells. Cytogenetic abnormalities have now emerged as the single most important prognostic factor for children with ALL

Fig. 7.7
FNAC retroperitoneum. Burkitt lymphoma (BL) and DLBL account for nearly all paediatric non-lymphoblastic B-cell lymphomas. BL shows high cellularity and an individual cell pattern, abundant extracellular lymphoglandular bodies and prominent tingible body macrophages. Nuclei are intermediate in size and round with a finely dispersed chromatin pattern, cytoplasm is basophilic and scant with prominent vacuoles. Extracellular vacuoles and vacuoles within lymphoglandular bodies occur frequently

Morphological diagnoses of ALL and LBL are typically established by surgical tissue biopsy and/or bone marrow examination. The status of FNAC in the diagnosis and management of these lymphoblastic malignancies is controversial. Cellular aspirates (2×10⁷ cells) can be readily obtained for immunological, DNA/RNA flow cytometric and immunoglobulin and/or T-cell receptor gene rearrangement studies. Cytologically, FNAC material is characterised by intermediate-sized cells (9.5–18.5 μm) with fine nu-

When combined with immunological phenotyping, a definitive initial diagnosis of LBL and recurrent ALL is possible and preferable using FNAC only [30, 33, 34]. Flow cytometry may be a helpful tool in the identification of LBL and ALL [35, 36]. FNAC should be considered as part of the initial evaluation and management whenever a mass lesion appears in a child with a suspected lymphoblastic neoplasm. It can preclude the need for a surgical biopsy, particularly in those with a mediastinal mass and the superior mediastinal syndrome, sometimes clinically and morphologically mimicking thymoma, but also in cases where ALL and LBL present in unusual sites (e.g. LBL presenting as a localised intraosseous mass, which may mimic Ewing's sarcoma) [37–39].

7.1.6 Small Round Cell Tumours of Kidney

Some of the childhood tumours arising in the kidney may present on FNAC as SRCTs. Indications for FNAC of a kidney mass in children includes unresectable tumour, bilateral disease, initial presentation with metastatic disease, uncertainty regarding tumour site and documentation of recurrence [40]. Cytological findings observed in FNAC smears include: classical Wilms' tumour, anaplastic Wilms' tumour, clear-cell sarcoma of the kidney, malignant rhabdoid tumour of the kidney and congenital mesoblastic nephroma. FNAC of Wilms' tumour shows blastemal cells, small, round cells with slightly oval nucleoli and fine and evenly dispersed chromatin. Other features include tubular and glomerular differentiation, stromal components, rosette formation, striated muscle differentiation, anaplasia, inflammation and necrosis [41, 42]. The stromal component is seen in 94% of cases and the epithelial component in 76% [43]. Smears from malignant rhabdoid tumour of the kidney tend to be very cellular, containing round to polygonal cells that are arranged either singly or in irregularly shaped clusters. The cells do not differ much in shape and show clear, empty nuclei with prominent nucleoli; the cytoplasm is abundant and sometimes eosinophilic [44]. Cells from clear-cell sarcoma of the kidney are usually arranged in smaller discrete groups with fragile cytoplasm. The main feature of cytological interest is the presence of deep nuclear indentations and grooves in many of the tumour cells. Cytological features of clear-cell sarcoma of the kidney are distinct and different from those of other renal tumours in children. Its recognition in cytology is important because its behaviour is more aggressive than that of Wilms' tumour [45].

In congenital mesoblastic nephroma, cells tend to be spindly and very cohesive with minimal nuclear atypia and mitoses and with no evidence of epithelial, glomerular or tubular differentiation [46, 47]. A cytological diagnosis of mesoblastic nephroma is important because the tumour has an excellent prognosis and, unlike Wilms' tumour, requires only surgery. A definite diagnosis of a tumour type can be made on 93% of FNAC of renal tumours [43].

Differential diagnosis of SRCT in and around the kidney, apart from those mentioned earlier include neuroblastoma, ganglioneuroblastoma and adrenocortical carcinoma [48, 49]. Cell clusters with neuropil and cytoplasmic processes are diagnostic of neuroblastoma, ganglion cells of ganglioneuroblastoma and blastema with tubular differentiation of Wilms' tumour. FNAC from congenital mesoblastic nephroma and adrenal cortical carcinoma are considered as simulators/mimickers of SRCT because they have a superficial resemblance to it. Diagnostic morphological pitfalls for an incorrect diagnosis of neuroblastoma in the case of Wilms' tumour include nuclear moulding, pseudorosette formation and focal neuron-specific enolase positivity [40]. Immunocytochemistry performed for Wilms' tumour shows cytokeratin positivity in two-thirds of cases and vimentin positivity in all [40].

7.1.7 Hepatoblastoma

Hepatoblastoma represents the most common primary hepatic tumour in children. Cytological features of this tumour may be seen in FNAC and body-cavity effusions. FNAC samples show neoplastic cells with a high N/C ratio resembling immature hepatocytes, but smaller. Mixed embryonal and foetal subtypes of hepatoblastoma show cells to be rather uniform, arranged in three-dimensional clusters, loose sheets, cords, rosette or acinus-like structures, and occasional pseudopapillae or branched cords are seen [50]. Occasional cells have eccentrically placed nuclei and vacuolated cytoplasm. Numerous mitotic figures are present. Rare intranuclear inclusions may be noted. The anaplastic (small cell) hepatoblastoma shows tight clusters of small, round, primitive cells with hyperchromatic nuclei, high N/C ratios and prominent nuclear moulding. In addition, there may be numerous single cells with naked nuclei, often in an Indian-file configuration. This subtype of hepatoblastoma is the least common and is associated with the worst prognosis [51]. With knowledge of the cellular features and architectural patterns of hepatoblastoma, a reliable diagnosis can be obtained on FNAC samples in the majority of cases without the use of special techniques. Distinction between embryonal and foetal cells in some of the cases of epithelial hepatoblastoma may not be possible on FNAC [50]. The differential diagnosis of hepatoblastoma includes other childhood SRCTs and hepatocellular carcinoma [52].

7.1.8 Pleuropulmonary Blastoma

Pleuropulmonary blastoma is a rare malignant tumour of the intrathoracic cavity. FNAC smears are cellular with numerous small ovoid- to spindle-shaped cells with oval to elliptical nuclei exhibiting finely granular chromatin and inconspicuous nucleoli. The cytoplasm is scant and eosinophilic with indistinct borders. Focal chondroid material and blastema-like cells are noted. The differential diagnosis includes RMS, teratoma, neuroblastoma, malignant mesenchymoma and metastatic tumour [53].

7.1.9 Small-Cell Synovial Sarcoma

A small-cell variant of synovial sarcoma is another rare tumour that may be considered in the differential diagnosis of paediatric SRCTs. FNAC consists of numerous, small, round cells with very high N/C ratios. Ancillary studies demonstrate positive staining of the neoplastic cells for cytokeratin, epithelial membrane antigen (EMA) and CD99 [54]. Immunohistochemistry and identification of the SYT/SSX fusion transcript are useful for confirmation [55].

7.2 Small Round Cell Tumours in Adults

In a large series of intrathoracic/abdominal FNAC, Das et al. found that SRCTs represents 18.7% of cases [56]. These included neuroblastoma, hepatoblastoma, nephroblastoma, pulmonary blastoma, Ewing's sarcoma, NHL and small cell anaplastic carcinoma. Although the cell morphology on FNAC exhibits many overlapping features including small cells with round nuclei, slightly irregular nuclear membranes, fine chromatin and scant cytoplasm, there were morphological features that may be helpful in distinguishing different SCRT on the basis of cytomorphology. The frequencies of rosettes (60%) and filamentous/fibrillar matrix (100%) in neuroblastoma, acinar formation in hepatoblastoma (100%) and small cell anaplastic carcinoma (93.3%), tubule formation in nephroblastoma (100%), lipid vacuoles (69.6%), exclusive noncohesive cells (95.7%) and lymphoglandular bodies (LGBs; 87%) in NHL and nuclear moulding (100%) and paranuclear blue inclusions (60%) in small cell carcinoma were significantly higher as compared to other SRCTs. Various cytomorphological features, alone or in conjunction with immunotyping, ultrastructural and cytogenetic studies, as well as clinical/imaging findings are very useful in the diagnosis of specific types of SRCT. Immunophenotyping is often critical for the diagnosis. SCRTs may be successfully diagnosed by combining cytological examination with flow cytometry using a panel of markers (e.g.CD45, CD16/56 and CD99) [57] (Figs. 7.8 and 7.9).

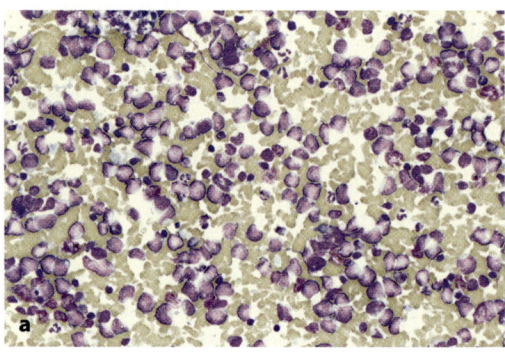

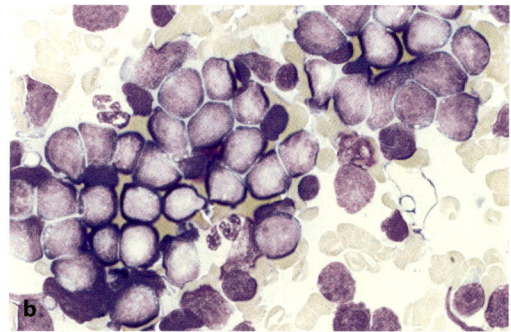

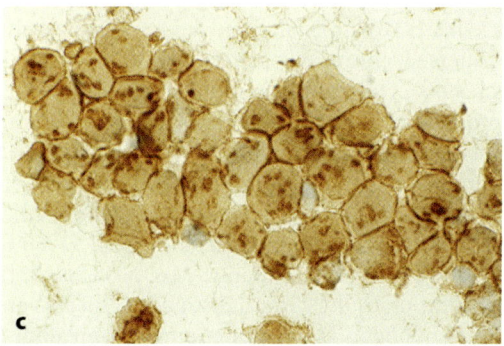

Fig. 7.8
FNAC lymph node. DLBL. **a** Low-power view revealing a discohesive population of small round cells. **b** High-power view showing lymphoid blasts and some apoptotic bodies. **c** CD 79a immunostaining shows tumour cells to be of the B-cell phenotype

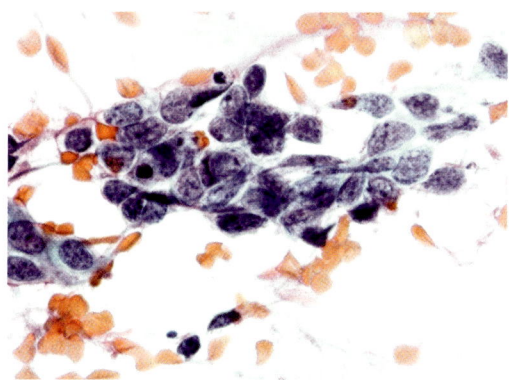

Fig. 7.9
FNAC lymph node. Small cell carcinoma. Nuclear moulding and paranuclear blue inclusions in small cell anaplastic carcinoma are significantly higher as compared to other SRCTs. The presence of evenly dispersed fine, granular chromatin, paranuclear blue inclusions, and nuclear fragments are statistically significant in differentiating small-cell carcinoma from NHL

7.2.1 Desmoplastic Small Round Cell Tumour

Desmoplastic SRCT (DSRCT) is a rare but well-defined high-grade malignant tumour that has a predilection for adolescent males and usually affects the abdominal or pelvic cavity [58]. It has distinct clinical, immunohistochemical and molecular features. The cytological features of DSRCT have been described on FNAC of primary and metastatic tumours [59]. The FNAC may be obtained from, amongst other tissues, the liver, flank soft tissue, abdomen, resected colon and ascitic fluid [60]. Specimens show moderate to high cellularity and tumour cells arranged singly and in clusters. Cytological features include: granular chromatin, small nucleoli, smooth to irregular nuclear membranes, nuclear moulding, scanty cytoplasm with cytoplasmic vacuoles, pseudorosettes and metachromatic stroma. Cytoplasmic densities may be observed in direct smears and ThinPrep slides [60–62]. Basic immunocytochemical stains show negativity for leukocyte-common antigen (LCA) and neuron-specific enolase (NSE) and positivity for cytokeratin cocktail (Cam 5.2), vimentin and desmin, the latter with characteristic paranuclear dot-like positivity [59].

Cytogenetically, DSRCTs present a reciprocal chromosomal translocation [t(11;22)(p13;q12)] that results in fusion of ES/PNET and Wilms' tumour (WT1) genes. A polyclonal antibody WT(C-19) resulting from this translocation may be used for immunostaining. All DSRCTs demonstrate strong WT1 nuclear immunoreactivity, with 71% of nephroblastomas and an occasional RMS also showing some WT1 immunoreactivity [63]. However, ES/PNET, neuroblastomas or rhabdoid tumours of the kidney are WT1 negative [63]. In nephroblastoma, differential diagnosis with DSRCT is not difficult since there are both clinical and morphological differences between the two conditions.

7.2.2 Small-Cell Carcinoma of the Lung

Small-cell carcinoma of the lung (SCCL) is a relatively common tumour in cytology FNAC practice, either in respiratory material or in lymph node FNAC (Fig. 7.9). The recognition of this entity is important given that when a diagnosis of SCCL is reached in a patient with a lung mass, surgical treatment is no longer considered and chemotherapy becomes the treatment of choice. FNAC of pulmonary hamartoma may be a potential pitfall in diagnosis of SCCL with a relatively high false-positive rate [64] (Fig. 7.10). Once the diagnosis of malignancy is established, FNAC is highly accurate in distinguishing SCCL from other neoplasms [65]. Cytological distinction of SCCL from NHL can be challenging. They may both present as SRCTs and be aggressive neoplasms that require prompt diagnosis and treatment. An immediate diagnosis can be obtained using FNAC from lymph nodes that are clinically or radiologically suspicious for tumour involvement. The presence of evenly dispersed, fine, granular chromatin, paranuclear blue inclusions and nuclear fragments are statistically significant in differentiating SCCL from NHL [66]. Paranuclear blue inclusions have been described as a feature of SCCL on air-dried cytological material stained with Romanowsky-type stains [67].

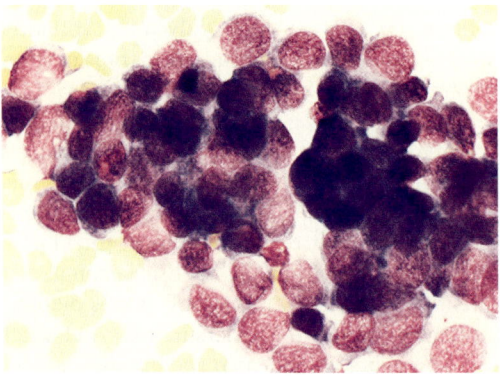

Fig. 7.10
FNAC lung. Hamartoma. FNAC of pulmonary hamartoma may be a potential pitfall in diagnosis of small-cell carcinoma, with a relatively high false positive rate

7.2.3 Burkitt's Lymphoma

Most NHLs that morphologically appear as SRCT may be diagnosed on cytomorphology and confirmed with immunocytochemistry (Figs. 7.11 and 7.12). BL often presents in the extranodal sites and is therefore not uncommonly subject to initial diagnosis by FNAC [68–72]. BL diagnosed by FNAC shows high cellularity and an individual cell pattern, abundant extracellular LGBs and prominent tingible body macrophages. Nuclei are intermediate in size and round with a finely dispersed chromatin pattern on MGG-stained smears. Cytoplasm is basophilic and scant with prominent vacuoles. Extracellular vacuoles and vacuoles within LGBs occur frequently (Fig. 7.7). Tumour cells show a proliferation index of at least 90%. BLs are characterised by the constitutive expression of c-Myc protein. In total, 50–60% of all BL cells carry mutant c-Myc proteins [73]. In addition to the clinical distinction, there is an immunophenotypic distinction between endemic and non-endemic BL. Endemic BLs shows a typical morphology and a homogeneous immunoprofile: CD10+, CD38+, CD77+, bcl-2-, and IgM+. Epstein-Barr virus DNA is present in all cases [74]. The immunoprofiles of the European BL are less homogeneous and inconsistent for CD10, CD38, CD77, IgM and bcl-2 expression; Epstein-Barr virus DNA is not detected. Other types of NHL, namely DLBL and its subtypes (Fig. 7.8) and the blastic type of Mantle Zone (MZ) lymphoma, may cause diagnostic dilemmas and should be considered in the differential diagnosis of adult SRCTs, particularly when occurring in extranodal sites [31, 32]. A growth fraction of nearly 100% and a monotonous proliferation of medium-sized cells and c-myc, should be of value in the diagnosis of BL, which is probably different from c-myc in DLBL [32]. Not all NHLs need a tissue biopsy to confirm diagnosis, particularly if ancillary studies are available [75] (Figs. 7.13 and 7.14).

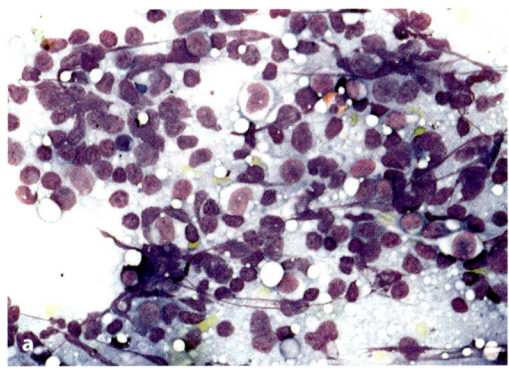

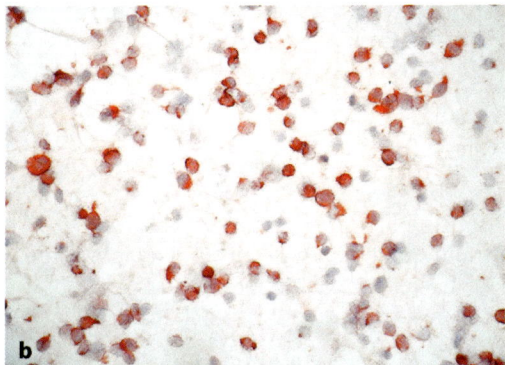

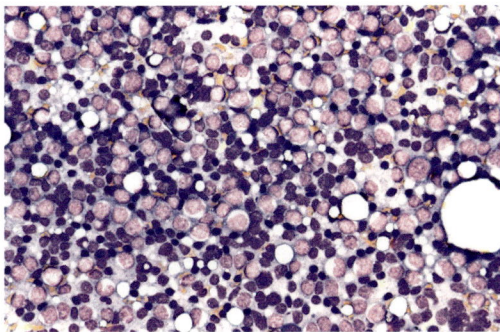

Fig. 7.13
FNAC lymph node. Follicular lymphoma. A two-cell monotonous cell population in a lymph node is suggestive of follicular lymphoma. Diagnosis must be confirmed with ancillary studies because of the morphological overlap with lymph node hyperplasia (see Fig. 7.14)

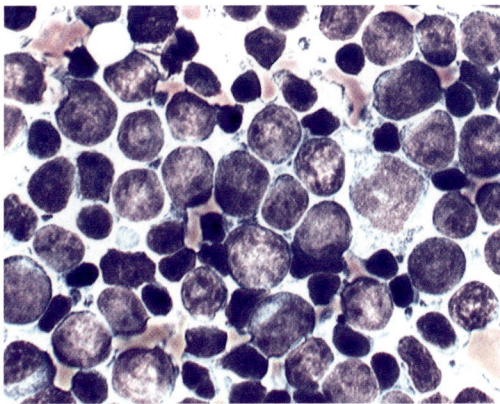

Fig. 7.11
FNAC lymph node. Peripheral T-cell lymphoma. **a** Low-power view revealing small- and medium-sized blue cells suggestive of lymphoma. **b** CD3 immunostaining confirms the T-cell phenotype

Fig. 7.14
FNAC lymph node. Lymph node hyperplasia. Florid lymph node hyperplasia may on occasion mimic a low-grade lymphoma. Ancillary studies are necessary if the lymph node is not excised

7.2.4 Lymphoglandular Bodies

Lymphoglandular bodies (LGB) (hyaline bodies or lymphoid globules, Soderstrom bodies), when found in cytology smears from FNAC, have long been accepted as being diagnostic of lymphoid tissue. However, Flanders et al. found LGBs in some non-lymphoid malignancies, namely in SCCL, non-SCC, ganglioneuroblastoma, melanoma and seminoma [76].

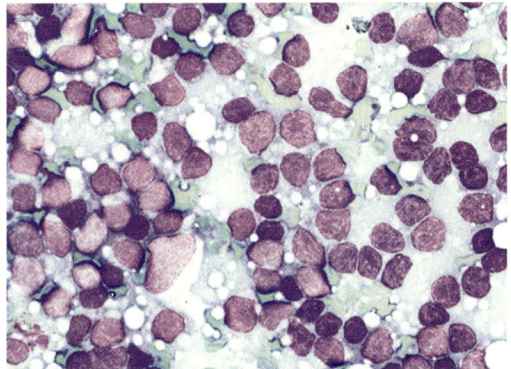

Fig. 7.12
FNAC lymph node. Chronic lymphocytic leukaemia. Chronic lymphocytic leukaemia can be difficult to diagnose morphologically if the clinical data are not available. Monotonous lymphoid cells with predominance of lymphocytes and prolymphocytes should raise suspicion of chronic lymphoid leukaemia

None of the smears obtained from carcinoma or sarcoma tissue had abundant LGBs (defined as >20 LGBs per high-power field) and most had hardly any lymphocytes [77]. Conversely, most, but not all NHLs have LGBs. When the number of LGBs was estimated to be abundant, the sensitivity for diagnosing a lymphoma was 54%; however, specificity was 100% [77]. In conclusion, although LGBs in the background of cytological smears taken from malignant tumours are useful in alerting the pathologist to the possibility of lymphoma, there are exceptions [78].

Case history 7.1: A 25-year-old female presented with several lymph nodes in the left neck and supraclavicular fossa. FNAC was requested. Cytology of the supraclavicular nodes showed dissociated cells, most of which were bare nuclei. Nuclei showed considerable pleomorphism and were multilobulated. A diagnosis of a high-grade NHL was given in the one-stop clinic and confirmed by immunocytochemistry (Fig. 7.15).

7.2.5 Merkel Cell Carcinoma

Merkel cell carcinoma of the skin is a rare, primary malignant skin neoplasm that can present as a cutaneous nodule. These neoplasms are seen primarily in the elderly and are located in the head and neck area or extremities, but may metastasise [79]. FNAC shows small- to intermediate-sized cells with a loosely cohesive pattern (Fig. 7.16). Nuclei are round with finely granular chromatin and multiple, small nucleoli. Cells have a thin rim of cytoplasm, and infrequent pseudorosette formations may be present. Immunocytochemistry is positive for cytokeratin, showing a paranuclear dot-like pattern, and neuron-specific enolase NSE, epithelial membrane antigen EMA, and S-100 protein are positive in varying degrees; leukocyte-common antigen LCA is negative. The diagnosis of Merkel's tumour of the skin by FNAC can be made by combining cytological features with ancillary studies and clinical information.

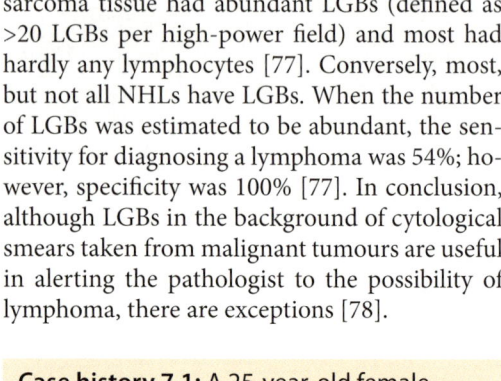
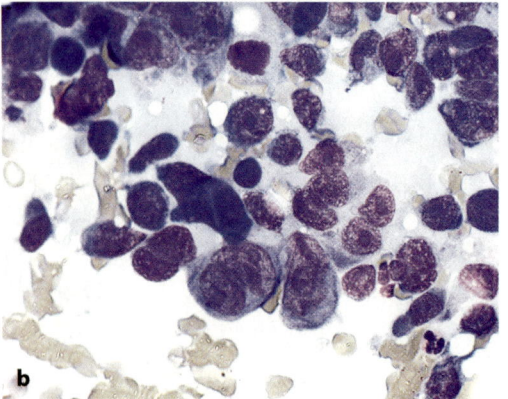
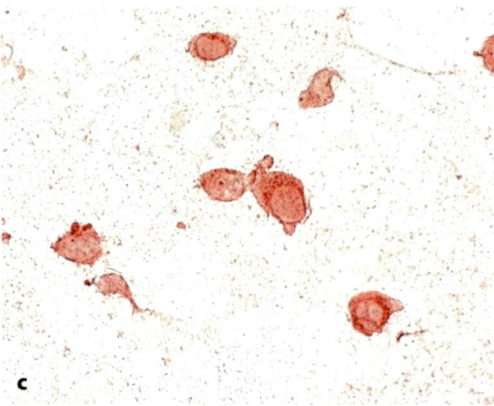

Fig. 7.15
FNAC neck. **a** A 25-year-old patient presented with a neck lymphadenopathy. **b** FNAC showed polymorphic population of lymphoid cells with prominent multinucleate giant cells. **c** Immunocytochemistry showed cells to be CD 30 and Alk-1 positive, confirming the diagnosis of anaplastic large cell lymphoma

7.2.6 Olfactory Neuroblastoma

Olfactory neuroblastoma is an uncommon tumour, presenting as a polypoid mass arising from the upper nasal cavity. FNAC is usually requested in cases of metastatic olfactory neuroblastoma, commonly presenting as ipsilateral cervical lymphadenopathy. FNAC shows well-preserved, small, monotonous cells with hyperchromatic nuclei, fibrillary cytoplasm and indistinct cell borders (Fig. 7.17). There are occasional pseudorosettes as well as rare true rosettes. Using immunocytochemistry, tumour cells are positive for cytokeratin, chromogranin and synaptophysin. Like adrenal neuroblastoma, olfactory neuroblastomas show distinctive cytological features, including a rosette or pseudorosette and fibrillary network. FNAC can accurately demonstrate these characteristic findings [80].

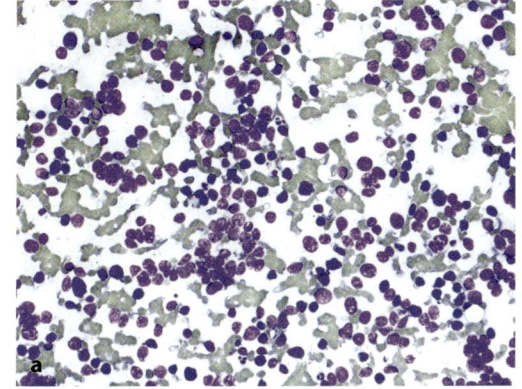
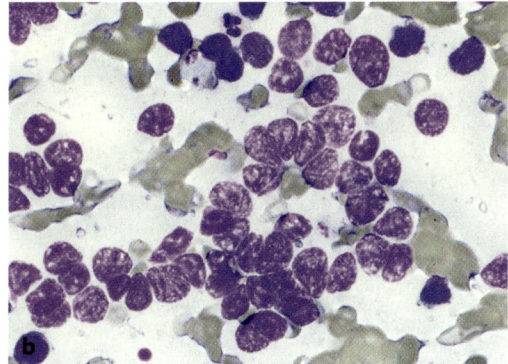
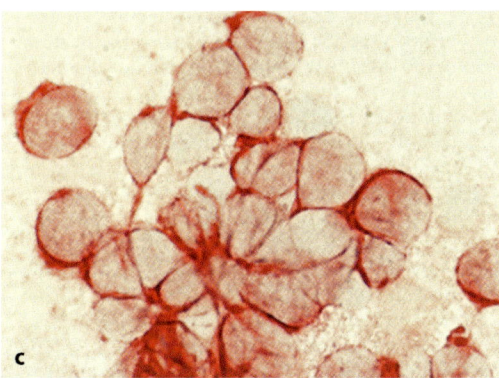

Fig. 7.16
FNAC subcutaneous mass. Merkel cell tumour. **a** Small- to intermediate-sized cells with a loosely cohesive pattern. **b** Nuclei are round with finely granular chromatin and multiple, small nucleoli. Cells have a thin rim of cytoplasm, and infrequent pseudorosette formations may be present. **c** Immunocytochemistry is positive for cytokeratin, showing a paranuclear punctate pattern

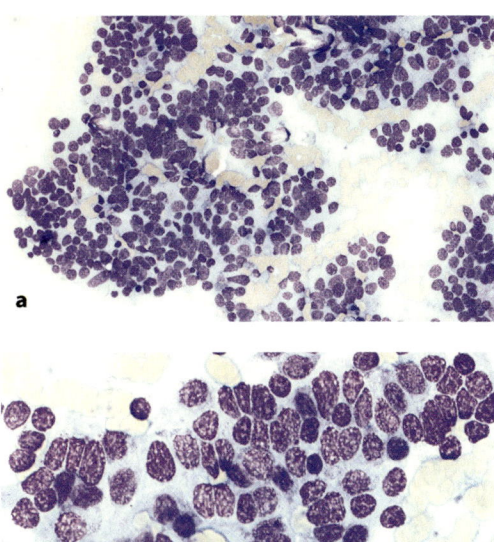

Fig. 7.17
FNAC neck node. Olfactory neuroblastoma. **a** Well-preserved, small, monotonous cells with hyperchromatic nuclei, fibrillary cytoplasm and indistinct cell borders. **b** There are occasional pseudorosettes as well as rare true rosettes. These tumour cells are immunopositive for cytokeratin, chromogranin and synaptophysin

References

1. Peydro-Olaya A, Llombart-Bosch A, Carda-Batalla C, Lopez-Guerrero JA. Electron microscopy and other ancillary techniques in the diagnosis of small round cell tumors. Semin Diagn Pathol 2003;20(1):25-45.
2. Silverman JF, Joshi VV. FNA biopsy of small round cell tumors of childhood: cytomorphologic features and the role of ancillary studies. Diagn Cytopathol 1994;10(3):245-55.
3. Akhtar M, Iqbal MA, Mourad W, Ali MA. Fine-needle aspiration biopsy diagnosis of small round cell tumors of childhood: A comprehensive approach. Diagn Cytopathol 1999;21(2):81-91.
4. Maly B, Maly A, Reinhartz T, Sherman Y. Primitive neuroectodermal tumor of the kidney. Report of a case initially diagnosed by fine needle aspiration cytology. Acta Cytol 2004;48(2):264-8.
5. Silverman JF, Berns LA, Holbrook CT, Neill JS, Joshi VV. Fine needle aspiration cytology of primitive neuroectodermal tumors. A report of these cases. Acta Cytol 1992;36(4):541-50.
6. Cohen MC, Pollono D, Tomarchio SA, Drut R. Cytologic characteristics of peripheral neuroectodermal tumors in fine-needle aspiration smears: a retrospective study of three pediatric cases. Diagn Cytopathol 1997;16(6):513-7.
7. Sahu K, Pai RR, Khadilkar UN. Fine needle aspiration cytology of the Ewing's sarcoma family of tumors. Acta Cytol 2000;44(3):332-6.
8. Guiter GE, Gamboni MM, Zakowski MF. The cytology of extraskeletal Ewing sarcoma. Cancer 1999;87(3):141-8.
9. Halliday BE, Slagel DD, Elsheikh TE, Silverman JF. Diagnostic utility of MIC-2 immunocytochemical staining in the differential diagnosis of small blue cell tumors. Diagn Cytopathol 1998;19(6):410-6.
10. Das DK, Sarin YK, Grover RK, Jain J, Khan VA, Chachra KL, et al. Neuroblastoma with concomitant giardiasis: report of a case with diagnosis by fine needle aspiration cytology. Acta Cytol 2001;45(5):740-4.
11. Barroca H, Carvalho JL, da Costa MJ, Cirnes L, Seruca R, Schmitt FC. Detection of N-myc amplification in neuroblastomas using Southern blotting on fine needle aspirates. Acta Cytol 2001;45(2):169-72.
12. Frostad B, Martinsson T, Tani E, Falkmer U, Darnfors C, Skoog L, et al. The use of fine-needle aspiration cytology in the molecular characterization of neuroblastoma in children. Cancer 1999;87(2):60-8.
13. Williamson D, Lu YJ, Gordon T, Sciot R, Kelsey A, Fisher C, et al. Relationship between MYCN copy number and expression in rhabdomyosarcomas and correlation with adverse prognosis in the alveolar subtype. J Clin Oncol 2005;23(4):880-8.
14. Kumar PV. Fine needle aspiration cytologic diagnosis of ganglioneuroblastoma. Acta Cytol 1987;31(5):583-6.
15. Akhtar M, Ali MA, Bakry M, Hug M, Sackey K. Fine-needle aspiration biopsy diagnosis of rhabdomyosarcoma: cytologic, histologic, and ultrastructural correlations. Diagn Cytopathol 1992;8(5):465-74.
16. Pohar-Marinsek Z, Anzic J, Jereb B. Topical topic: value of fine needle aspiration biopsy in childhood rhabdomyosarcoma: twenty-six years of experience in Slovenia. Med Pediatr Oncol 2002;38(6):416-20.
17. de Almeida M, Stastny JF, Wakely PE, Jr., Frable WJ. Fine-needle aspiration biopsy of childhood rhabdomyosarcoma: reevaluation of the cytologic criteria for diagnosis. Diagn Cytopathol 1994;11(3):231-6.
18. Seidal T, Walaas L, Kindblom LG, Angervall L. Cytology of embryonal rhabdomyosarcoma: a cytologic, light microscopic, electron microscopic, and immunohistochemical study of seven cases. Diagn Cytopathol 1988;4(4):292-9.
19. Atahan S, Aksu O, Ekinci C. Cytologic diagnosis and subtyping of rhabdomyosarcoma. Cytopathology 1998;9(6):389-97.
20. Pohar-Marinsek Z, Bracko M. Rhabdomyosarcoma. Cytomorphology, subtyping and differential diagnostic dilemmas. Acta Cytol 2000;44(4):524-32.
21. Imachi M, Tsukamoto N, Kamura T, Shigematsu T, Funakoshi K, Nakano H. Alveolar rhabdomyosarcoma of the vulva. Report of two cases. Acta Cytol 1991;35(3):345-9.
22. Cessna MH, Zhou H, Perkins SL, Tripp SR, Layfield L, Daines C, et al. Are myogenin and myoD1 expression specific for rhabdomyosarcoma? A study of 150 cases, with emphasis on spindle cell mimics. Am J Surg Pathol 2001;25(9):1150-7.
23. Tamiolakis D, Venizelos I, Nikolaidou S, Prassopoulos P, Alexiadis G, Simopoulos C, et al. Bilateral metastatic rhabdomyosarcoma to the breast in an adolescent female: touch imprint cytology and implication of MyoD1 nuclear antigen. Onkologie 2004;27(5):469-71.
24. Punyko JA, Mertens AC, Baker KS, Ness KK, Robison LL, Gurney JG. Long-term survival probabilities for childhood rhabdomyosarcoma. A population-based evaluation. Cancer 2005;103(7):1475-83.
25. Hostein I, Andraud-Fregeville M, Guillou L, Terrier-Lacombe MJ, Deminiere C, Ranchere D, et al. Rhabdomyosarcoma: value of myogenin expression analysis and molecular testing in diagnosing the alveolar subtype: an analysis of 109 paraffin-embedded specimens. Cancer 2004;101(12):2817-24.
26. Reddy KS, Perkins SL. Advances in the diagnostic approach to childhood lymphoblastic malignant neoplasms. Am J Clin Pathol 2004;122(Suppl):S3-18.
27. McKenna RW. Multifaceted approach to the diagnosis and classification of acute leukemias. Clin Chem 2000;46(8 Pt 2):1252-9.

28. Kebriaei P, Anastasi J, Larson RA. Acute lymphoblastic leukaemia: diagnosis and classification. Best Pract Res Clin Haematol 2002;15(4):597-621.
29. Robinson DL. Childhood leukemia: Understanding the significance of chromosomal abnormalities. J Pediatr Oncol Nurs 2001;18(3):111-23.
30. Jacobs JC, Katz RL, Shabb N, el-Naggar A, Ordonez NG, Pugh W. Fine needle aspiration of lymphoblastic lymphoma. A multiparameter diagnostic approach. Acta Cytol 1992;36(6):887-94.
31. Frost M, Newell J, Lones MA, Tripp SR, Cairo MS, Perkins SL. Comparative immunohistochemical analysis of pediatric Burkitt lymphoma and diffuse large B-cell lymphoma. Am J Clin Pathol 2004;121(3):384-92.
32. Nakamura N, Nakamine H, Tamaru J, Nakamura S, Yoshino T, Ohshima K, et al. The distinction between Burkitt lymphoma and diffuse large B-Cell lymphoma with c-myc rearrangement. Mod Pathol 2002;15(7):771-6.
33. Wakely PE, Jr., Kornstein MJ. Aspiration cytopathology of lymphoblastic lymphoma and leukemia: the MCV experience. Pediatr Pathol Lab Med 1996;16(2):243-52.
34. Tani E, Liliemark J, Svedmyr E, Mellstedt H, Biberfeld P, Skoog L. Cytomorphology and immunocytochemistry of fine needle aspirates from blastic non-Hodgkin's lymphomas. Acta Cytol 1989;33(3):363-71.
35. Henrique RM, Sousa ME, Godinho MI, Costa I, Barbosa IL, Lopes CA. Immunophenotyping by flow cytometry of fine needle aspirates in the diagnosis of lymphoproliferative disorders: A retrospective study. J Clin Lab Anal 1999;13(5):224-8.
36. Horii A, Yoshida J, Hattori K, Honjo Y, Mitani K, Takashima S, et al. DNA ploidy, proliferative activities, and immunophenotype of malignant lymphoma: application of flow cytometry. Head Neck 1998;20(5):392-8.
37. Ozdemirli M, Fanburg-Smith JC, Hartmann DP, Shad AT, Lage JM, Magrath IT, et al. Precursor B-Lymphoblastic lymphoma presenting as a solitary bone tumor and mimicking Ewing's sarcoma: a report of four cases and review of the literature. Am J Surg Pathol 1998;22(7):795-804.
38. Ozdemirli M, Fanburg-Smith JC, Hartmann DP, Azumi N, Miettinen M. Differentiating lymphoblastic lymphoma and Ewing's sarcoma: lymphocyte markers and gene rearrangement. Mod Pathol 2001;14(11):1175-82.
39. Friedman HD, Hutchison RE, Kohman LJ, Powers CN. Thymoma mimicking lymphoblastic lymphoma: a pitfall in fine-needle aspiration biopsy interpretation. Diagn Cytopathol 1996;14(2):165-9; discussion 169-71.
40. Ellison DA, Silverman JF, Strausbauch PH, Wakely PE, Holbrook CT, Joshi VV. Role of immunocytochemistry, electron microscopy, and DNA analysis in fine-needle aspiration biopsy diagnosis of Wilms' tumor. Diagn Cytopathol 1996;14(2):101-7.
41. Quijano G, Drut R. Cytologic characteristics of Wilms' tumors in fine needle aspirates. A study of ten cases. Acta Cytol 1989;33(2):263-6.
42. Dey P, Radhika S, Rajwanshi A, Rao KL, Khajuria A, Nijhawan R, et al. Aspiration cytology of Wilms' tumor. Acta Cytol 1993;37(4):477-82.
43. Sharifah NA. Fine needle aspiration cytology characteristics of renal tumors in children. Pathology 1994;26(4):359-64.
44. Barroca HM, Costa MJ, Carvalho JL. Cytologic profile of rhabdoid tumor of the kidney. A report of 3 cases. Acta Cytol 2003;47(6):1055-8.
45. Krishnamurthy S, Bharadwaj R. Fine needle aspiration cytology of clear cell sarcoma of the kidney. A case report. Acta Cytol 1998;42(6):1444-6.
46. Dey P, Srinivasan R, Nijhawan R, Rajwanshi A, Banerjee CK, Rao KL, et al. Fine needle aspiration cytology of mesoblastic nephroma. A case report. Acta Cytol 1992;36(3):404-6.
47. Drut R. Cytologic characteristics of congenital mesoblastic nephroma in fine-needle aspiration cytology: a case report. Diagn Cytopathol 1992;8(4):374-6.
48. Serrano R, Rodriguez-Peralto JL, De Orbe GG, Melero C, de Agustin P. Intrarenal neuroblastoma diagnosed by fine-needle aspiration: a report of two cases. Diagn Cytopathol 2002;27(5):294-7.
49. Ravindra S, Kini U. Cytomorphology and morphometry of small round-cell tumors in the region of the kidney. Diagn Cytopathol 2005;32(4):211-216.
50. Us-Krasovec M, Pohar-Marinsek Z, Golouh R, Jereb B, Ferlan-Marolt V, Cerar A. Hepatoblastoma in fine needle aspirates. Acta Cytol 1996;40(3):450-6.
51. Kaw YT, Hansen K. Fine needle aspiration cytology of undifferentiated small cell („anaplastic") hepatoblastoma. A case report. Acta Cytol 1993;37(2):216-20.
52. Weir EG, Ali SZ. Hepatoblastoma: cytomorphologic characteristics in serious cavity fluids. Cancer 2002;96(5):267-74.
53. Gelven PL, Hopkins MA, Green CA, Harley RA, Wilson MM. Fine-needle aspiration cytology of pleuropulmonary blastoma: case report and review of the literature. Diagn Cytopathol 1997;16(4):336-40.
54. Silverman JF, Landreneau RJ, Sturgis CD, Raab SS, Fox KR, Jasnosz KM, et al. Small-cell variant of synovial sarcoma: fine-needle aspiration with ancillary features and potential diagnostic pitfalls. Diagn Cytopathol 2000;23(2):118-23.

55. Kwon MS. Aspiration cytology of pulmonary small cell variant of poorly differentiated synovial sarcoma metastatic from the tongue: a case report. Acta Cytol 2005;49(1):92-6.
56. Das DK, Bhambhani S, Chachra KL, Murthy NS, Tripathi RP. Small round cell tumors of the abdomen and thorax. Role of fine needle aspiration cytologic features in the diagnosis and differential diagnosis. Acta Cytol 1997;41(4):1035-47.
57. Leon ME, Hou JS, Galindo LM, Garcia FU. Fine-needle aspiration of adult small-round-cell tumors studied with flow cytometry. Diagn Cytopathol 2004;31(3):147-54.
58. Insabato L, Di Vizio D, Lambertini M, Bucci L, Pettinato G. Fine needle aspiration cytology of desmoplastic small round cell tumor. A case report. Acta Cytol 1999;43(4):641-6.
59. Zeppa P, Lepore M, Vetrani A, Palombini L. Occult lymph node metastasis from desmoplastic small round cell tumor diagnosed by fine needle aspiration cytology. A case report. Acta Cytol 2003;47(3):501-5.
60. Crapanzano JP, Cardillo M, Lin O, Zakowski MF. Cytology of desmoplastic small round cell tumor. Cancer 2002;96(1):21-31.
61. Caraway NP, Fanning CV, Amato RJ, Ordonez NG, Katz RL. Fine-needle aspiration of intra-abdominal desmoplastic small cell tumor. Diagn Cytopathol 1993;9(4):465-70.
62. Setrakian S, Gupta PK, Heald J, Brooks JJ. Intra-abdominal desmoplastic small round cell tumor. Report of a case diagnosed by fine needle aspiration cytology. Acta Cytol 1992;36(3):373-6.
63. Barnoud R, Sabourin JC, Pasquier D, Ranchere D, Bailly C, Terrier-Lacombe MJ, et al. Immunohistochemical expression of WT1 by desmoplastic small round cell tumor: a comparative study with other small round cell tumors. Am J Surg Pathol 2000;24(6):830-6.
64. Hughes JH, Young NA, Wilbur DC, Renshaw AA, Mody DR. Fine-needle aspiration of pulmonary hamartoma: a common source of false-positive diagnoses in the College of American Pathologists Interlaboratory Comparison Program in Nongynecologic Cytology. Arch Pathol Lab Med 2005;129(1):19-22.
65. Delgado PI, Jorda M, Ganjei-Azar P. Small cell carcinoma versus other lung malignancies: diagnosis by fine-needle aspiration cytology. Cancer 2000;90(5):279-85.
66. De Las Casas LE, Gokden M, Mukunyadzi P, White P, Baker SJ, Hermonat PL, et al. A morphologic and statistical comparative study of small-cell carcinoma and non-Hodgkin's lymphoma in fine-needle aspiration biopsy material from lymph nodes. Diagn Cytopathol 2004;31(4):229-34.
67. Wittchow R, Laszewski M, Walker W, Dick F. Paranuclear blue inclusions in metastatic undifferentiated small cell carcinoma in the bone marrow. Mod Pathol 1992;5(5):555-8.
68. Geramizadeh B, Kaboli R, Vasei M. Fine needle aspiration cytology of Burkitt's lymphoma presenting as a breast mass. Acta Cytol 2004;48(2):285-6.
69. Das DK, Sheikh ZA, Jassar AK, Jarallah MA. Burkitt-type lymphoma of the breast: diagnosis by fine-needle aspiration cytology. Diagn Cytopathol 2002;27(1):60-2.
70. Myong NH, Cho KJ, Choi SW, Jang JJ. Abdominal Burkitt's lymphoma diagnosed by fine needle aspiration cytology--a case report. J Korean Med Sci 1990;5(2):97-9.
71. Rebelo MJ, Das DK, Khan VA, Chachra KL, Thusoo TK. Burkitt's type lymphoma as a jaw tumour in old age: diagnosed by fine needle aspiration cytology. Indian J Pathol Microbiol 1990;33(3):274-6.
72. Abaza NA, Iczkovitz ML, Henefer EP. American Burkitt's lymphoma manifested in a solitary submandibular lymph node. Oral Surg Oral Med Oral Pathol 1981;51(2):121-7.
73. Fest T, Guffei A, Williams G, Silva S, Mai S. Uncoupling of genomic instability and tumorigenesis in a mouse model of Burkitt's lymphoma expressing a conditional box II-deleted Myc protein. Oncogene 2005;24(18):2944-53.
74. Barth TF, Muller S, Pawlita M, Siebert R, Rother JU, Mechtersheimer G, et al. Homogeneous immunophenotype and paucity of secondary genomic aberrations are distinctive features of endemic but not of sporadic Burkitt's lymphoma and diffuse large B-cell lymphoma with MYC rearrangement. J Pathol 2004;203(4):940-5.
75. Kocjan G. Cytological and molecular diagnosis of lymphoma. J Clin Pathol 2005;58:561-567.
76. Flanders E, Kornstein MJ, Wakely PE, Jr., Kardos TF, Frable WJ. Lymphoglandular bodies in fine-needle aspiration cytology smears. Am J Clin Pathol 1993;99(5):566-9.
77. Bangerter M, Herrmann F, Griesshammer M, Gruss HJ, Hafner M, Heimpel H, et al. The abundant presence of Soderstrom bodies in cytology smears of fine-needle aspirates contributes to distinguishing high-grade non-Hodgkin's lymphoma from carcinoma and sarcoma. Ann Hematol 1997;74(4):175-8.
78. Francis IM, Das DK, al-Rubah NA, Gupta SK. Lymphoglandular bodies in lymphoid lesions and non-lymphoid round cell tumours: a quantitative assessment. Diagn Cytopathol 1994;11(1):23-7.
79. Collins BT, Elmberger PG, Tani EM, Bjornhagen V, Ramos RR. Fine-needle aspiration of Merkel cell carcinoma of the skin with cytomorphology and immunocytochemical correlation. Diagn Cytopathol 1998;18(4):251-7.
80. Chung J, Park ST, Jang J. Fine needle aspiration cytology of metastatic olfactory neuroblastoma: a case report. Acta Cytol 2002;46(1):40-5.

Chapter 8

Diagnostic Dilemmas in FNAC Cytology: Soft-Tissue Lesions

Contents

8.1	Introduction	151
8.2	Spindle-Cell Lesions	153
8.2.1	Spindle-Cell Lesions of the Lung	156
8.2.2	Spindle-Cell Lesions of the Salivary Gland	156
8.2.3	Spindle-Cell Lesions of the Breast	157
8.2.4	Myofibrosarcoma	157
8.3	Myxoid and Chondroid Lesions	157
8.3.1	Low-Grade Fibromyxoid Sarcoma	159
8.3.2	Leiomyosarcoma	160
8.3.3	Ossifying Fibromyxoid Tumour	161
8.3.4	Myxoid Mucinous Neoplasms	161
8.3.5	Intramuscular Myxoma	162
8.3.6	Chondrosarcoma	162
8.3.7	Chondroblastoma	162
8.4	Pseudosarcomatous Lesions	162
8.4.1	Nodular Fasciitis	165
8.4.2	Nodular Myositis	165
8.4.3	Proliferative Fasciitis and Myositis	165
8.4.4	Fibromatoses	166
8.4.5	Fibrous histiocytoma	167
8.4.6	Pseudoangiomatous Stromal Hyperplasia	167
8.4.7	Pleomorphic Lipoma	168
8.4.8	Atypical Lipoma	168
8.4.9	Spindle-Cell Lipoma	169
8.4.10	Ancient Schwannoma	169
8.4.11	Angioleiomyoma	169
8.4.12	Calcifying Aponeurotic Fibroma	169
8.4.13	Lipomatous Haemangiopericytoma	169
8.5	Tumours of Low or Borderline Malignancy	169
8.5.1	Dermatofibrosarcoma Protuberans	170
8.5.2	Haemangiopericytoma	170
8.5.3	Acral Myxoinflammatory Fibroblastic Sarcoma	171
8.6	Soft-Tissue Deposits of Non-Sarcomatous Lesions	171
8.6.1	Malignant Lymphoma and Leukaemia	171
8.6.2	Calcinosis Cutis	171
8.7	Sarcomas Mimicking Other Lesions	171
8.7.1	Epithelioid Sarcoma	171
8.7.2	Metastatic Soft-Tissue Sarcomas	172
8.7.3	Well-Differentiated Liposarcoma	172
8.8	Rare and Difficult Sarcomas	172
8.8.1	Alveolar Soft-Part Sarcoma	172
8.8.2	Angiosarcoma	172
8.8.3	Kaposi's Sarcoma	174
8.8.4	Clear-Cell Sarcoma of Soft Parts	175
8.8.5	Haemangioendothelioma	175
8.8.6	Giant-Cell Fibroblastoma	175
8.8.7	Rhabdomyosarcoma	175
8.8.8	Synovial Sarcoma	176
References		177

8.1 Introduction

In the last few years, the primary diagnosis of soft-tissue lesions has emerged as an important new target for FNAC. Until recently, FNAC, as a diagnostic modality for the evaluation of soft-tissue neoplasms and non-neoplastic soft-tissue mass lesions, was uncommon and controversial. This procedure contrasts with more traditional diagnostic methods such as marginal excision, incision (open) biopsy, or even core biopsy (CB) to obtain tissue for diagnosis [1]. Soft-tissue masses that present for FNAC are most commonly found in the extremities, the trunk, the head and neck and the retroperitoneum [2, 3]. Soft-tissue tumours are relatively rare and often difficult to correctly diagnose using FNAC. Most practicing pathologists are inexperienced with the wide array of soft-tissue neoplasms and their morphological heterogeneity, making them susceptible to misdiagnosis. A close clinicopathological cooperation is essential. FNAC should be performed on the most accessible part, avoiding penetration of the deep portions of the tumour. Needles of 0.7 mm (22 guage) size are recommended. For deep lesions, needles with a stylet should be used. The method is most effective when an experienced pathologist performs the aspiration [4]. After the FNAC, tattooing of the aspiration channel is recommended and, if a sarcoma, the channel should be surgically removed together with the tumour [5]. Material from the FNAC can be used for additional examinations such as electron microscopy, immunohistochemistry, DNA cytometry and chromosomal analysis (e.g. cytogenetic analysis on aspirated material confirms t(11;22) in Ewing's sarcoma and t(X;18) in synovial sarcomas [6] using FISH) [7]. Those techniques are of great importance in the differential diagnosis, particularly with regard to paediatric SRCTs.

In the hands of experienced cytopathologists, FNAC in conjunction with ancillary techniques has a diagnostic accuracy approaching 95% for the diagnosis of soft-tissue malignancy [8]. Gonzales-Campora advocates a six-tier structured approach to the smear pattern in soft-tissue tumours. First, in myxoid-rich matrix tumours, special attention should be paid to lipoblasts, ganglion type, stellate cells and metachromatic fibrillary matrix [9]. Second, in round-cell tumours the following cytological findings are of special interest: atypical rhabdomyoblasts, atypical lipoblasts, neuroblast rosettes, cytoplasmic glycogen, melanin pigment, islets of mature cartilage, hyaline cytoplasmic inclusions and fragments of connective tissue closely associated with round cells [9]. Third, in spindle tumours the most important cytological findings are: biphasic cellularity, elongated, buckled or wavy and tapered nuclei, nuclear palisades, straight, elongated, blunt-ended nuclei, melanotic pigment, storiform pattern, tissue fragments with collagen fibres or degenerated elastin, intracytoplasmic hyaline globules and scattered spindle cells in a background of red blood cells [9]. Fourth, in allomorphic tumours, specific typing is often difficult, if not impossible, since cells display few or no differential features [9]. Fifth, in epithelial-like cell tumours the cytological findings of major diagnostic interest are: melanin deposits, crystalline inclusions, intracytoplasmic lumina, anisonucleosis and nuclear cytoplasmic inclusions [9]. Finally, in mature-like cell tumours, the architectural pattern resembles that of mature tissues. Although cytological analysis of primary soft-tissue tumours is hampered by the paucity of diagnostic findings, the establishment of clinicocytological correlation, taking into account architectural patterns, cytological details and clinical characteristics of the lesion, allows precise diagnosis of a significant number of tumours [9].

The use of FNAC of soft-tissue mass lesions can be used for the initial diagnosis of primary benign and malignant soft-tissue masses, for the confirmation of metastatic tumours to soft tissue and for the documentation of locally recurrent soft-tissue neoplasms [10, 11]. The sensitivity, specificity and positive predictive value of FNAC in diagnosis of soft-tissue tumours is reported to be 91.5%, 92.5% and 95.5%, respectively [11]. With a specificity of more than 90%, FNAC is of particular value in any subcutaneous lesion of less than 5 cm, in all paediatric tumours and whenever direct incision biopsy is particularly contraindicated [4]. FNAC has been shown to have a diagnostic yield nearly identical with CB while avoiding significant clinical complications [8, 12]. CBs may have the advantage of subtyping selected sarcomas diagnosed by FNAC. Unsatisfactory FNAC should be evaluated further by a repeat aspirate or CB [12]. However, FNAC is capable of specifically subtyping a large percentage of primary and metastatic soft-tissue tumours either if cellular material is in the form of a cell block or flow cytometry is obtained in addition to cell smears [1].

Although the majority of sarcomas can be defined as low-grade or high-grade malignant in FNAC [5], FNAC has limitations related to the accurate histological grading and subtyping of certain subgroups of sarcomas. Dey et al. found that only 46.8% were correctly categorised [11]. It may also be difficult to accurately distinguish between low-grade sarcomas and benign or borderline cellular lesions, especially in the spindle-cell sarcoma subgroup [7]. Although the specific diagnosis for sarcomas is challenging and FNAC usually does not provide a specific diagnosis (only in 20.9% of cases), it evaluates effectively lesions in 86.5%, confirming its usefulness as a screening tool for sarcomas [2, 13]. This compares favourably with histology where the analysis of problem-prone diagnostic situations by the consultative (expert) second opinions in soft-tissue pathology showed that the essential agreement between the original histological diagnosis and the second opinion was achieved in 68% of cases, with minor discrepancies in 7% and major discrepancies in 25% [14]. The major discrepancies in histopathology could be divided into four groups: benign mesenchymal lesions diagnosed as sarcomas (45%), sarcomas diagnosed as benign tumours (23%), non-mesenchymal lesions diagnosed as sarcomas (20%) and major grading discrepancies (12%). Problematic lesions were lipoma and fasciitis and their variants and desmoplastic neurotropic melanoma [14]. The lack of familiarity with rare or unusual lesions is probably the most significant factor in explaining diagnostic discrepancies [14].

Cytological diagnosis should be based on a correct evaluation of clinical data (age, localisation, size, effect on bone, nerve and vessel involvement), radiological information, cytological findings (architectural pattern, cell and stroma characteristics) and the results of special staining techniques. The final cytology report should aim at least to classify the tumour in one of three basic categories: benign, malignant and inconclusive or undetermined [4, 15, 16]. In order to facilitate the evaluation of FNAC smears from soft-tissue tumours and to suggest cytological criteria for diagnoses, Akerman and Domanski classify FNAC material according to their principal microscopic appearances [17]. For malignancy grading, the following parameters are used: cellularity, pleomorphism, chromatin pattern, nucleolar structure, mitotic figures and necroses [5]. Lin et al. found that pleomorphism and abundant single cells were parameters associated with high-grade tumours [18]. The combination of absence of pleomorphism, rare single cells, a tight cluster arrangement, fine chromatin pattern and absence of macronucleoli is seen only in benign cases. Assessment of background material is helpful in differential diagnosis and classification. Necrosis is only found in high-grade cases [18]. FNAC was found to be most accurate for subtyping of skeletal osteosarcoma, paediatric small round cell bone/soft-tissue sarcomas, synovial sarcoma, skeletal chondrosarcoma and adult myxoid soft-tissue sarcomas [6]. In general, although almost always recognised as sarcoma, subtyping of adult pleomorphic soft-tissue sarcomas has not been possible but has not influenced therapy; all were considered high-grade sarcomas for treatment purposes [6].

8.2 Spindle-Cell Lesions

Spindle-cell proliferations are a frequent cause of diagnostic pitfalls in FNAC. Cases that may be cytologically regarded as a low-grade sarcoma may histologically prove to be nodular fasciitis and an inflammatory pseudotumour [19]. Cases diagnosed by FNAC as spindle-cell lesion, undetermined if benign or malignant, and malignant fibrous histiocytoma (MFH) may histologically be a leiomyosarcoma (LMS). In the evaluation of FNAC smears dominated by spindle cells, cellularity, individual cells and cell patterns and background stromal features, together with a precise clinical history may allow a narrow differential diagnosis with a focus on whether the lesion is benign or malignant. Caution is warranted in the exact classification of spindle-cell tumours from FNAC as this may have a major impact on patient management [19].

Following on from the above, spindle-cell lesions can be broadly categorised on FNAC into low-grade and high-grade lesions. Liu et al. studied the key diagnostic cytological criteria for low- and high-grade spindle-cell lesions [20, 21]. From the low-grade spindle-cell lesions, they reviewed synovial sarcoma, benign neural tumours, reparative lesions and other benign and additional malignant low-grade spindle-cell lesions [21]. Statistical analysis selected high cellularity, short spindle cells, small nucleoli and absence of tissue culture appearance as the main criteria for malignant neoplasms. Tissue fragments and high cellularity were selected as the primary criteria and absence of long filamentous cells and of myxoid background as the secondary criteria for synovial sarcomas. Fibrillary ground substance and absence of ovoid/round nuclei were the key criteria for benign neural tumours. The presence of a tissue culture appearance was the major criterion for reparative lesions [21] (Fig. 8.1 and 8.2; Case history 8.1).

Case history 8.1: A 45-year-old male patient presented with a lump in the jugulodigastric area, which he had noticed while shaving and was not sure how long it may have been there. It was painless, firm and mobile. FNAC yielded myxoid material. Microscopic features were typical of benign nerve sheath tumour (Fig. 8.2)

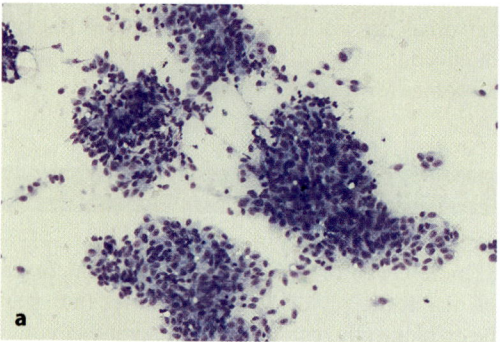

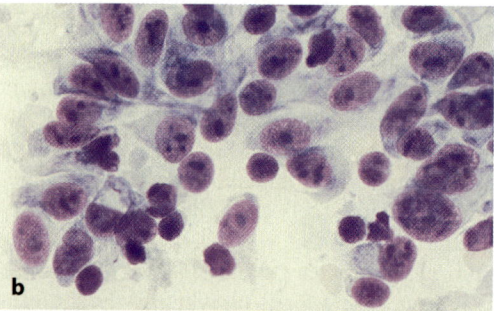

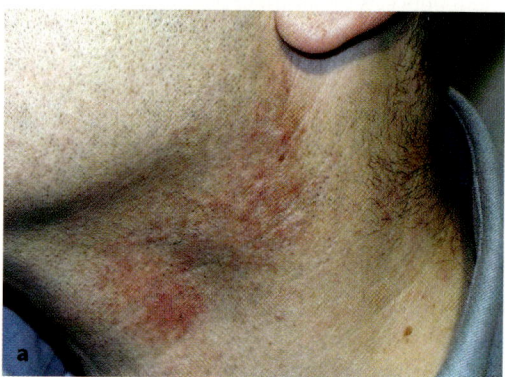

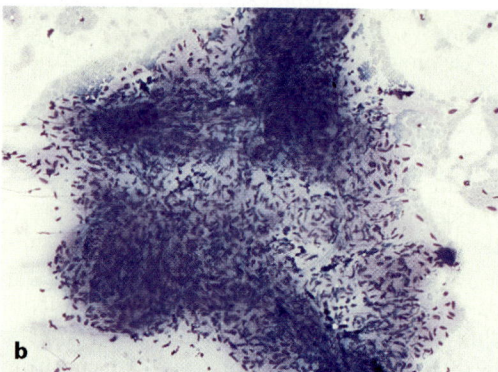

Fig. 8.2
FNAC jugulodigastric node. Schwannoma. **a** See Case history 8.1. **b** Low-power view showing fibrillary ground substance and spindle cells in bundles.

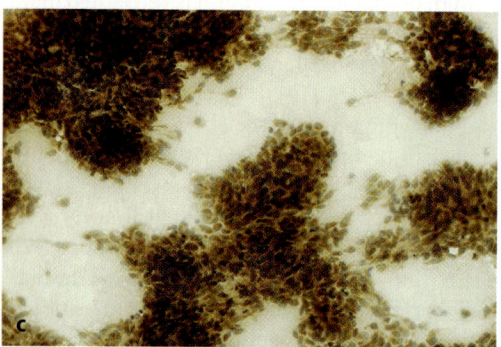

Fig. 8.1
FNAC thigh. Synovial sarcoma. **a** Low-power view showing high cellularity and tissue fragments of spindle cells. **b** High-power view showing haphazardly arranged short spindle cells with ovoid/round nuclei and prominent, small, multiple nucleoli. **c** BCL2 positivity in tumour cells

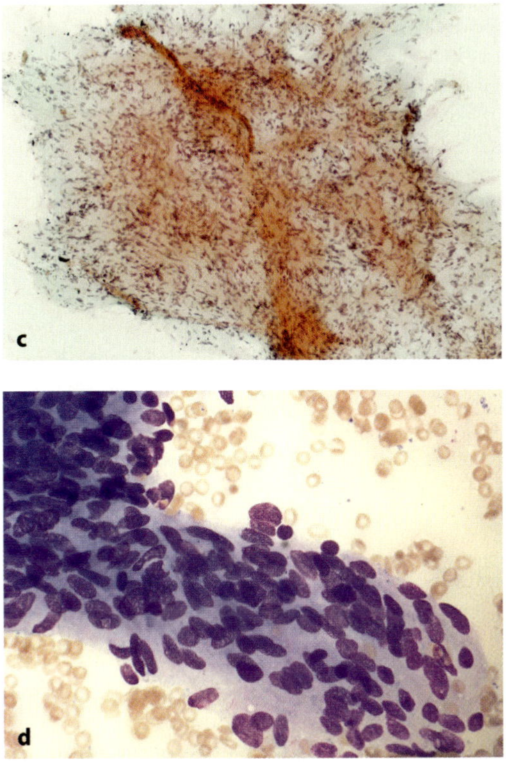

Fig. 8.2
c Same case. Alcohol-fixed preparations may not show fibrillary background material so prominently. **d** High-power view showing elongated oval nuclei immersed in the fibrillary background material giving the appearance of a wavy bundle

Similarly, in order to identify primary diagnostic cytological criteria for various high-grade spindle-cell neoplasms, namely osteosarcoma, malignant melanoma, chondrosarcoma, leiomyosarcoma (LMS), angiosarcoma and liposarcomas, Liu et al. tried to identify the variables predictive of each diagnostic category [20]. The statistical analysis selected positive expression of osteoid, osteoclastic giant cells and low cellularity as the primary criteria associated with osteosarcomas (Fig. 8.3). The analysis selected the presence of melanin as the major criterion for malignant melanomas, cells lying in lacunae for chondrosarcomas, fishhook nuclei for LMSs, intracytoplasmic iron deposits for angiosarcomas and lipoblast-like cells for liposarcomas [20] (Fig. 8.4).

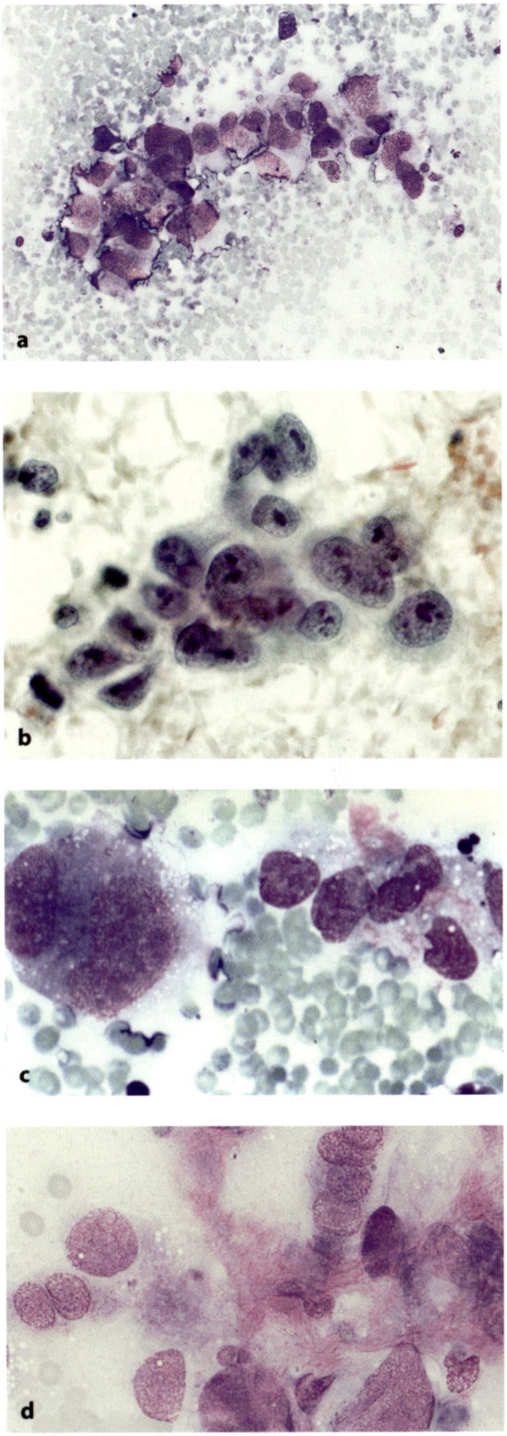

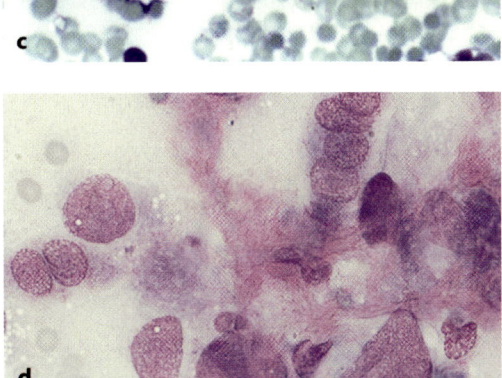

Fig. 8.3
FNAC bone. Osteosarcoma. (see next page)

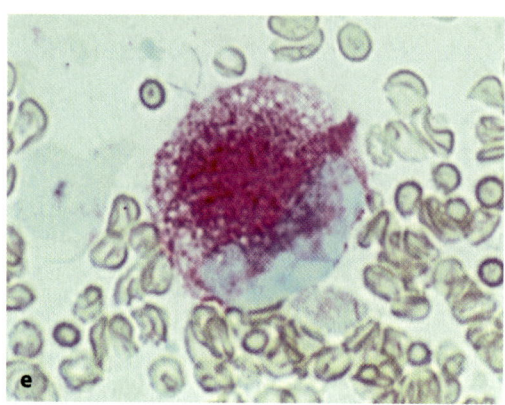

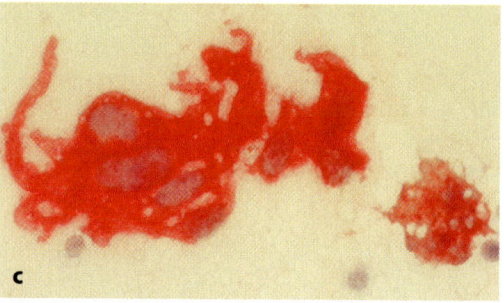

c

Fig. 8.4
FNAC breast. Angiosarcoma. **a** Low-power view showing cellular aggregates of spindle cells with ill-defined outlines. **b** High-power view showing oval nuclei, elonglated cytoplasm with occasional intracytoplasmic vacuoles. Haemosiderin may be seen within the cells. **c** CD34 positivity in tumour cells

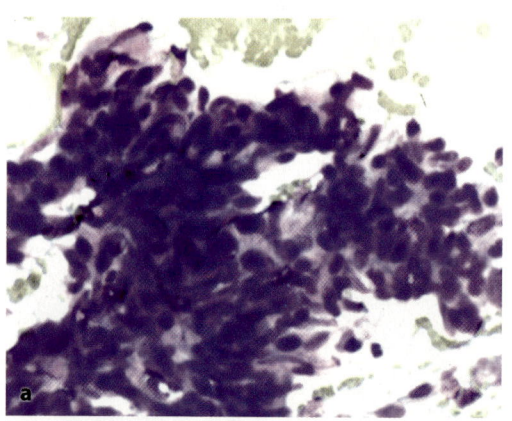

e

Fig. 8.3
Continued from previous page. FNAC bone. Osteosarcoma. **a** Low cellularity with a cluster of highly pleomorphic cells with eccentric nuclei. **b** Pap stain showing nuclear detail with prominent irregular nucleoli.
c Osteoclastic giant cells. **d** Intercellular matrix.
e Positive expression of osteoid in malignant cells with alkaline phosphatase staining

8.2.1 Spindle-Cell Lesions of the Lung

Spindle-cell lesions of the lung may also pose diagnostic dilemma on FNAC. They may represent reactive processes (granuloma, organising pneumonia and inflammatory pseudotumour), benign neoplasms (hamartomas, solitary fibrous tumours [22] and schwannoma), malignant tumours (carcinomas with spindle-cell or sarcomatoid features, spindle-cell carcinoid tumour, LMS and synovial sarcoma) and secondary tumours (melanomas, LMSs, meningioma, sarcomatoid renal cell carcinoma and uterine malignant mixed Mullerian tumour) [23].

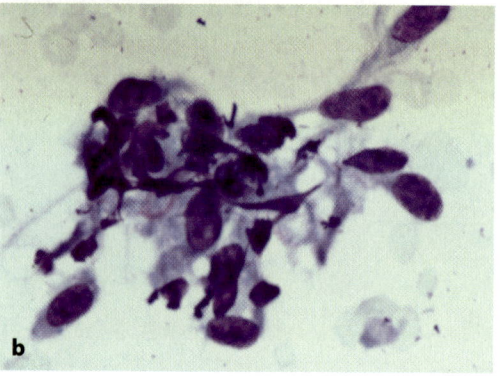

a

b

8.2.2 Spindle-Cell Lesions of the Salivary Gland

Spindle-cell lesions of the salivary gland represent 3.0% of all salivary gland FNAC findings [24]. Such smears may be classified into three categories: (1) reactive or inflammatory conditions, including granulation tissue and granulomatous sialadenitis; (2) benign neoplasms including Schwannoma, fibromatosis, lipoma and pleomorphic adenoma; (3) malignant neoplasms, including metastatic melanoma, RMS and metastatic osteosarcoma [24] (Fig. 8.5). Benign peripheral nerve sheath tumours should always be considered in the differential diagnosis of pleomorphic adenoma [25]. Kapila et al. recommend a diligent search for epithelial elements prior to diagnosing benign nerve sheath tumour in the head and neck region [25].

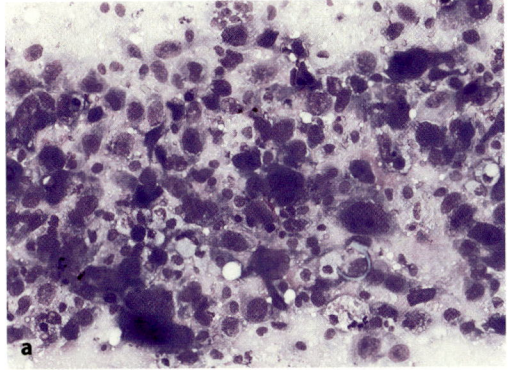

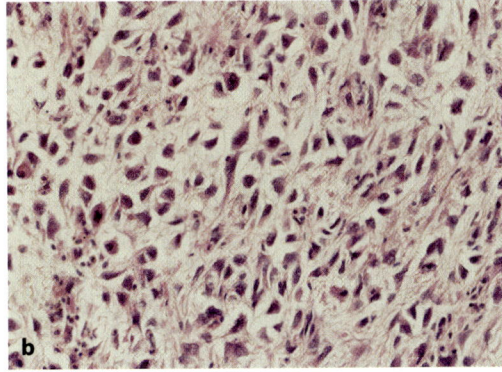

Fig. 8.5
FNAC upper arm. Rhabdomyosarcoma, pleomorphic type. **a** Cytology shows pleomorphic, dissociated tumour cells with large nuclei, prominent nucleoli and spindle-shaped cytoplasm in which there are sometimes signs of rhabdoid differentiation. **b** Histological section of the same tumour

8.2.3 Spindle-Cell Lesions of the Breast

Spindle-cell lesions of the breast are described in Chap. 9 (Fig. 8.4).

8.2.4 Myofibrosarcoma

Low- and intermediate-grade myofibrosarcomas are fascicular spindle-cell neoplasms resembling fibrosarcoma or LMS [26]. They infiltrate deep soft tissue with disproportionate involvement of head and neck sites and can recur locally but infrequently metastasise. Their differential diagnosis includes benign myofibroblastic proliferations such as fasciitis and fibromatosis as well as other types of spindle-cell sarcoma. High-grade (pleomorphic) myofibrosarcomas are an ultrastructurally defined subset of MFH, which they resemble in morphology and behaviour. Inflammatory myofibroblastic tumour and infantile fibrosarcoma are neoplasms that have myofibroblastic features and have been included in this category, but they have distinctive genetic findings.

8.3 Myxoid and Chondroid Lesions

A subgroup of lesions that yield a large amount of chondromyxoid and myxoid stroma on FNAC deserves special consideration. The most common malignant neoplasms showing this change are: extraskeletal chondrosarcoma, myxoid liposarcoma, myxoid malignant fibrous histiocytoma MFH and chordoma (Figs. 8.6 and 8.7). The benign entities are ganglion cyst, myxoma and neurofibroma [27] (Fig. 8.8). Layfield et al. performed a logistic regression analysis to identify the variables predictive of myxoid MFH, chordoma, myxoid chondrosarcoma and myxoid liposarcoma [28]. The statistical analysis selected pleomorphic giant cells and the presence of fibroblast-like cells as most predictive of MFH, physalipherous cells as most closely associated with chordoma, chondroid fragments as most predictive of chondrosarcoma, and lipoblasts as most predictive of liposarcoma [28].

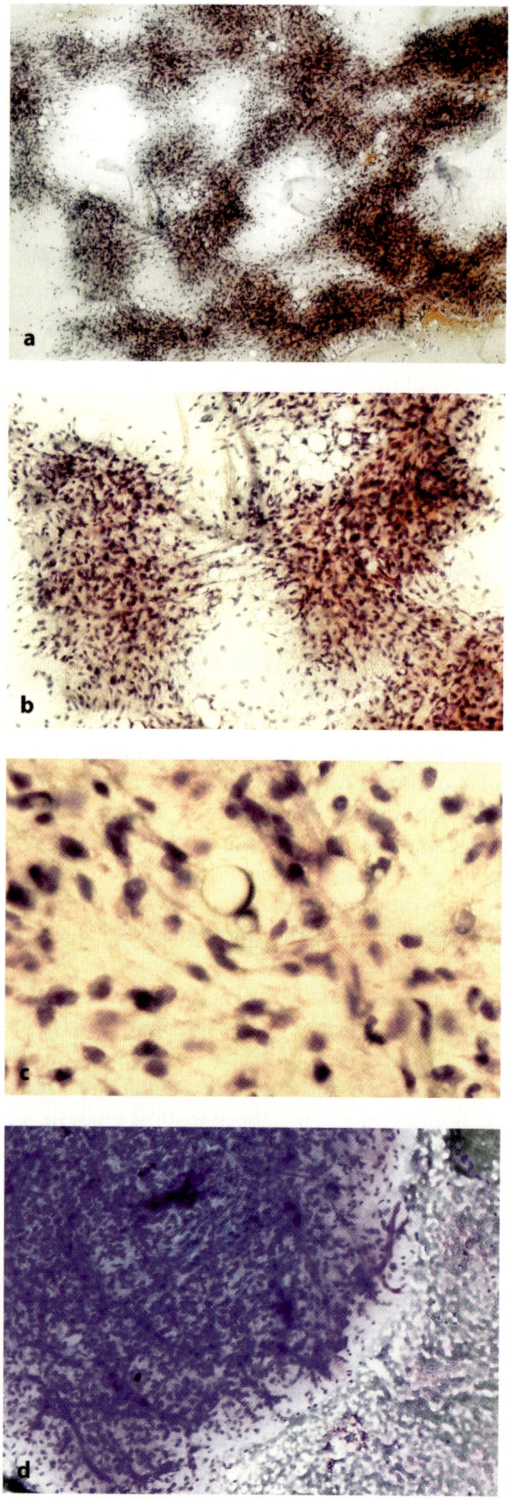

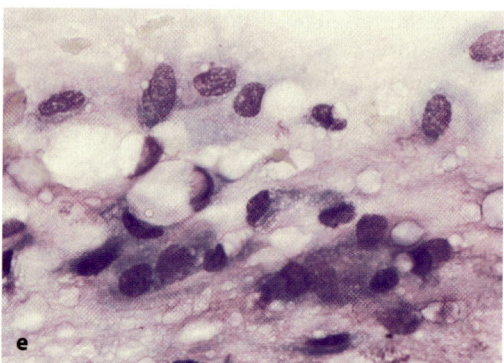
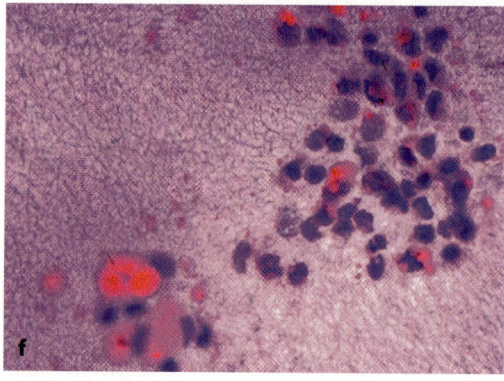

Fig. 8.6
FNAC retroperitoneum. Myxoid liposarcoma. **a** Low-power view showing cellular tissue fragments. **b** Fragments are connected by capillaries in a "chicken wire" manner. **c** Lipoblasts are prominent amongst the tumour cells. **d** Air-dried, MGG-stained smears showing myxoid background material. **e** Lipoblasts may also be seen on MGG-stained preparations. **f** Oil red O stains fat in the cytoplasm of lipoblasts

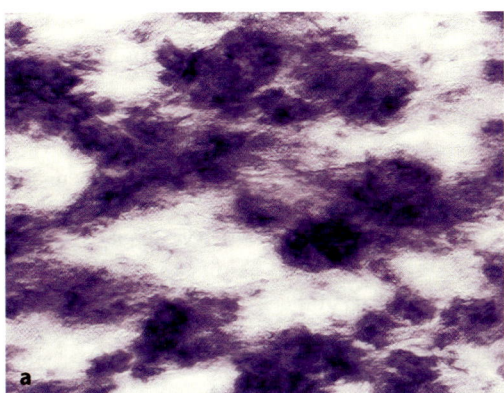

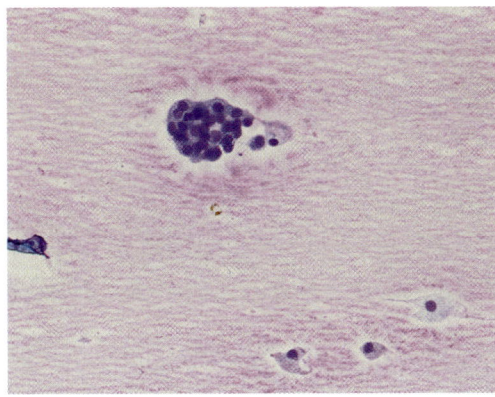

Fig. 8.8
FNAC nodule hand. Ganglion cyst. Smears contain amorphous myxoid background and macrophages

8.3.1 Low-Grade Fibromyxoid Sarcoma

First described in 1987, this is a rare sarcoma that is characterised by a bland and deceptively benign histological appearance but with aggressive behaviour. FNAC shows abundant myxoid background with occasional thick bands of collagen (Fig. 8.9). Tumour cells present in the myxoid background are spindle shaped, with focally mild nuclear enlargement, hyperchromasia and pleomorphism. Clinical and radiological correlation is necessary to make the correct diagnosis [29–31].

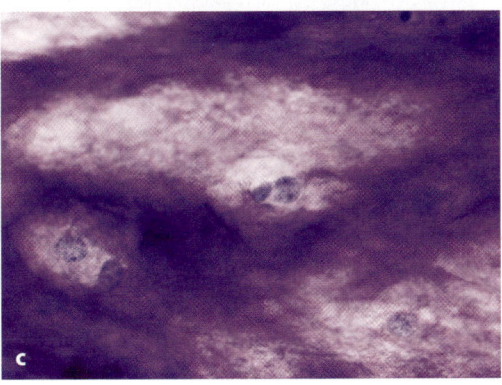

Fig. 8.7
FNAC pelvic mass. Extraskeletal chondrosarcoma. **a** Aspirate has a pinkish, granular, myxoid background. **b** Tumour cells are immersed in the chondromyxoid matrix and are difficult to visualise. **c** They have granulated, dark blue cytoplasm and oval-round, lobulated, slightly indented, hyperchromatic nuclei. Grooved nuclei, arranged in a cordlike pattern suggest chondroid differentiation

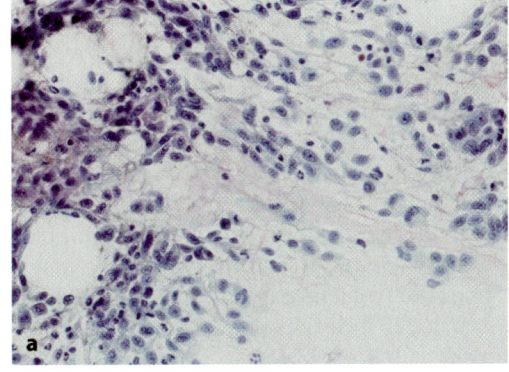

Fig. 8.9
FNAC thigh. Fibromyxoid sarcoma. (see next page)

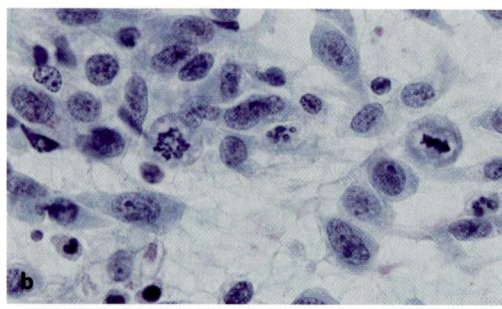

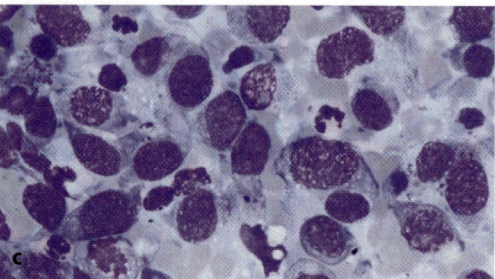

Fig. 8.9
Continued from previous page. FNAC thigh. Fibromyxoid sarcoma. **a** Tumour cells present in the myxoid background. **b** Individual cells are spindle shaped, with focally mild nuclear enlargement, hyperchromasia, pleomorphism and mitoses. **c** MGG-stained appearance of the same cells. Clinical and radiological correlation is necessary to make the correct diagnosis

8.3.2 Leiomyosarcoma

Leiomyosarcoma LMS variants may contain myxoid features. Histological variants of LMS are: classical/usual, epithelioid and myxoid. Klijanienko et al. reviewed the original cytology reports and found that 71.8% of LMSs were originally diagnosed as other types of malignancies [32]. The cytological features of classical variants of LMS have a various proportion of spindle-shaped, cohesive and small- or large-sized cells arranged in parallel alignment. Large spindle, round, binucleated, giant cells with intracytoplasmic granulations are frequently seen. Blunt-ended nuclei, intranuclear inclusions and mitotic figures are occasionally seen, as well as stromal fragments. The epithelioid variant of LMS is composed of an admixture of small and large, spindle-shaped and round cells, also arranged in parallel alignment. However, tumour cells with granular cytoplasm, blunt-ended nuclei, intranuclear inclusions, mitotic figures and fibrous or myxoid stroma are not observed. The myxoid variant of LMS shows large amounts of background myxoid matrix containing large spindle shaped and giant cells (Fig. 8.10). Entities such as leiomyoma, malignant peripheral nerve sheath tumour, monophasic synovial sarcoma and MFH should be considered in the differential diagnosis of LMS of the classical type. Epithelioid leiomyoma may share similar cytological features with epithelioid LMS (Fig. 8.11). The cytological features of the myxoid variant of LMS can be easily confused with other types of benign and malignant mesenchymal tumours depicting degenerative myxoid changes and/or a myxoid matrix component [32].

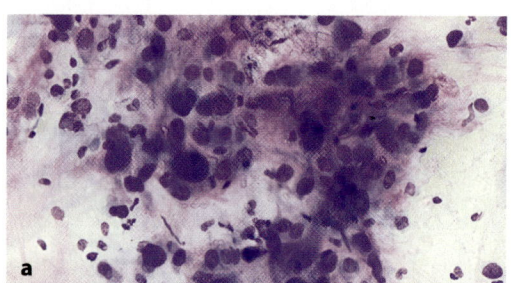

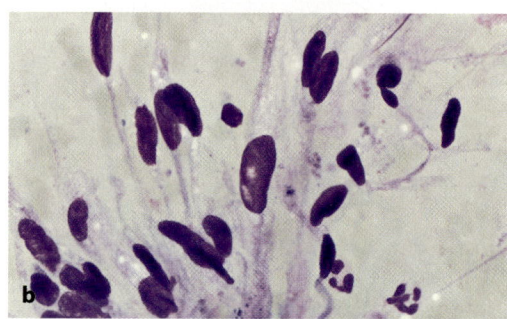

Fig. 8.10
FNAC abdomen. Leiomyosarcoma. **a** The myxoid variant of leiomyosarcoma exhibits large amounts of background myxoid matrix containing large spindle-shaped and giant cells. **b** Spindle-shaped, cohesive, small- or large-sized cells arranged in parallel alignment. Blunt-ended nuclei, intranuclear inclusions and mitotic figures are occasionally seen, as well as stromal fragments. These cytological features can easily be confused with other types of benign and malignant mesenchymal tumours depicting degenerative myxoid changes and/or a myxoid matrix component

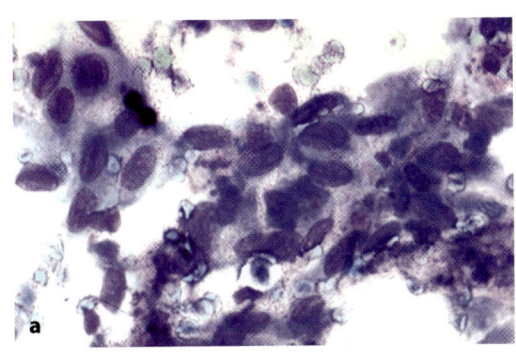

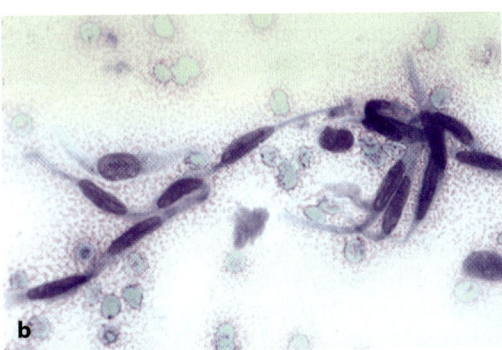

Fig. 8.11
EUS-FNAC tumour in the stomach wall. Epithelioid leiomyoma. **a** Features are similar to epithelioid leiomyosarcoma. The tumour is composed of an admixture of small and large, spindle-shaped and round cells, also arranged in parallel alignment. **b** Tumour cells with blunt-ended nuclei and spindle shaped cytoplasm

8.3.3 Ossifying Fibromyxoid Tumour

Ossifying fibromyxoid tumour (OFMT) of soft tissue is an uncommon, recently described neoplasm. It is usually, but not universally, a benign neoplasm and cases of metastatic so-called malignant OFMT have been reported [33]. Patients present with a subcutaneous well-circumscribed nodular soft-tissue mass. X-ray and CT imaging reveals an incomplete shell of calcification surrounding the nodular mass along with foci of ossification within it. FNAC shows round to polygonal- to spindle-shaped neoplastic cells arranged in clusters, cords and small aggregates, lying discretely in a mucoid background [33]. Some osteoid-like material is also seen. FNAC of OFMT at a prethyroidal location may be misinterpreted as follicular neoplasia [34]. OFMT should be considered as a possibility in FNAC of myxoid soft-tissue tumour, especially where there is radiological evidence of ossification.

8.3.4 Myxoid Mucinous Neoplasms

A myxoid or mucinous background in cytological smears characterises a diagnostically important group of lesions involving the sacrum, spinal canal and parasacral soft tissues. This group of myxoid/mucoid neoplasms includes chordoma, myxopapillary ependymoma, metastatic mucinous adenocarcinoma and extraskeletal myxoid chondrosarcoma. Despite the similarity of the background substance, each neoplasm within this differential diagnosis has a characteristic composite set of morphological and immunophenotypic features. Because many of these masses are not easily surgically biopsied, FNAC is often used for their diagnosis. A panel of antibodies, including cytokeratin, glial fibrillary acid protein (GFAP), S-100 protein and CEA, can be used as an aid to the diagnosis. Layfield evaluated cytological features, including the presence of rosette like structures, physalipherous cells, gland like structures, chondroid fragments, signet-ring and goblet cells, as well as the character of the myxoid/mucinous background substance and found that physalipherous cells are highly specific for chordoma [35], a fibrillary myxoid stroma containing cells with elongated cytoplasmic processes and cells lying in a rosette like pattern around central cores of myxoid to fibrillary stroma are highly characteristic of myxopapillary ependymoma [36, 37]. Fragments of a myxoid/chondroid matrix with lacunar-like spaces strongly support the diagnosis of myxoid chondrosarcoma, whilst goblet or signet-ring cells with a single distinct vacuole favour mucinous adenocarcinoma [36].

8.3.5 Intramuscular Myxoma

Intramuscular myxoma is a benign tumour that involves the muscles of the thigh, upper arm and forearm. Magnetic resonance imaging reveals a well-defined, sharply demarcated tumour with a low signal intensity relative to muscle. FNAC yields clear, tenacious and viscous material. Smears contain a few spindle and histiocytoid cells in an abundant mucoid background [38]. Spindle cells exhibit long cytoplasmic processes that in areas intertwine to form fibrillary tangles. Nuclei are oval to spindle shaped with fine chromatin and inconspicuous nucleoli. Capillaries are sparse with simple (non-plexiform) branching. The differential diagnosis of myxoid lesions of the extremities includes benign entities such as myxoid schwannoma and neurofibroma, mesenchymal repair and ganglion cyst, as well as malignant neoplasms such as myxoid liposarcoma, fibrosarcoma, and extraskeletal chondrosarcoma. The findings of Caraway et al. revealed that although the cytological features are suggestive of intramuscular myxoma, a definitive diagnosis is often difficult owing to scant cellularity and lack of distinctive cytological features [38]. The authors suggest using the magnetic resonance imaging findings as an adjunct to the cytological features to more confidently suggest a diagnosis of intramuscular myxoma [38].

8.3.6 Chondrosarcoma

Chondroid change may be seen in conventional chondrosarcoma, chondroblastic osteosarcoma, extraskeletal myxoid chondrosarcoma, chondroma and chondroblastoma [39]. On FNAC, tumour cells in conventional chondrosarcoma are embedded in a pink, amorphous, chondroid matrix. They are larger than chondroma cells and have vacuoles and small, pink, chondroid-substance-like granules. Chondroblastic osteosarcoma contains extremely pleomorphic chondrocytes, osteoid matrix and osteoblastic cells, and may be morphologically confused with chondrosarcoma. Clinical and radiological correlation is essential in these cases. Extraskeletal myxoid chondrosarcoma has a pinkish, granular, myxoid background (Fig. 8.7). Tumour cells have granulated, dark blue cytoplasm and oval-round, lobulated, slightly indented, hyperchromatic nuclei. Grooved nuclei arranged in a cord-like pattern suggest chondroid differentiation. FNAC can be diagnostic of extraskeletal myxoid chondrosarcoma even in the absence of obvious chondroid differentiation [40]. FNAC is efficient for the diagnosis of chondrosarcoma and its variants as long as a pathologist familiar with bone pathology and cytology correlates it with radiological and clinical findings.

8.3.7 Chondroblastoma

Chondroblastoma is a benign tumour arising in the epiphysis of long bones. The extraskeletal presentation is most unusual: chondroid matrix surrounding individual round to oval mononuclear cells, calcifications among cells and multinucleate osteoclasts are the decisive cytological features, seen better in MGG than in Pap-stained smears [41]. The single polygonal or round cells have a uniform, sometimes eccentric nucleus, microvacuolated cytoplasm and haemosiderin pigment. Nuclear grooves and mitoses may be seen [42].

8.4 Pseudosarcomatous Lesions

Pseudosarcomatous lesions are benign tumours of the musculoskeletal system that are likely to be misdiagnosed as malignant, based on clinical and morphological features [43]. These include soft-tissue tumours that are considered to be reactive or reparative lesions such as nodular fasciitis, proliferative fasciitis [44, 45], proliferative myositis [46], intravascular fasciitis, myositis ossificans [47, 18], atypical fibroxanthoma, juvenile xanthogranuloma, pigmented villonodular synovitis, fibrous hamartoma of infancy [47] and pseudomalignant osseous tumour of soft tissues (Figs. 8.12–8.15). Also included in the pseudosarcoma category are benign neoplasms, which show cytological atypia. The latter include lipoma, leiomyoma, angiomyolipoma, spindle-cell lipoma and benign peripheral nerve-sheath tumours (e.g. ancient neurilemmoma).

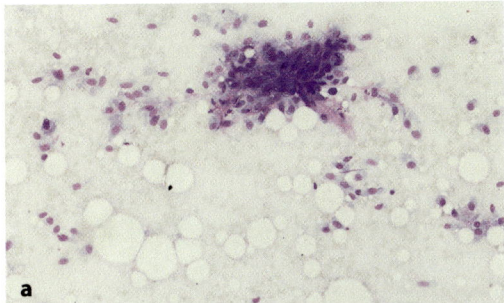

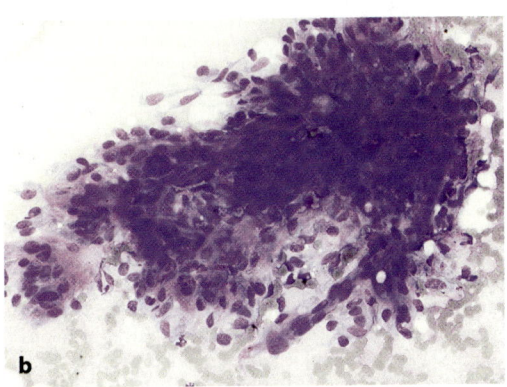

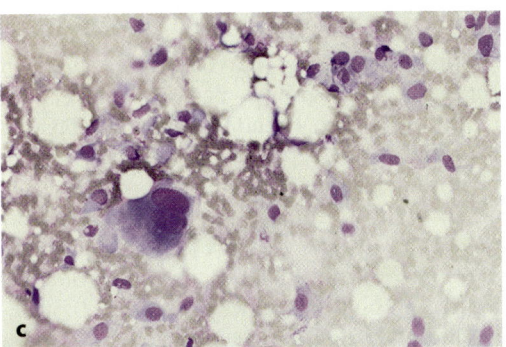

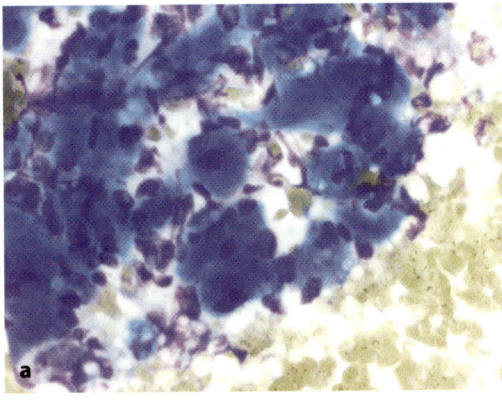

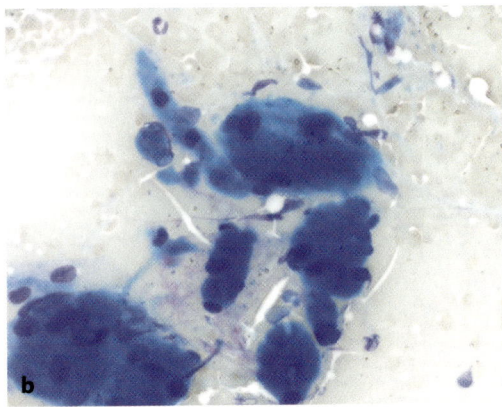

Fig. 8.13
FNAC nodule in the thigh. Nodular myositis. **a** Fragments of striated muscle including degenerating and regenerative myocytes. **b** High-power view. The lesion may include a mixed inflammatory background and necrotic debris

Fig. 8.12
FNAC forearm. Nodular fasciitis. **a** Uniform fibroblast-like spindle cells (singly and in groups). **b** Collagen, myxoid material. **c** Admixed large cells with abundant cytoplasm, one to two eccentric nuclei, macronucleoli and abundant cytoplasm (ganglion-cell-like cells). Nodular fasciitis with its hypercellular smears containing overlapping, relatively isomorphic spindle cells, may be mistaken cytologically for sarcoma

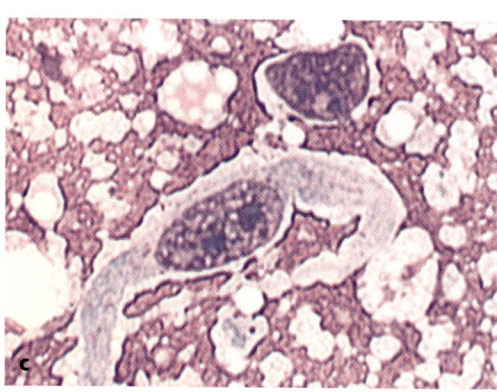

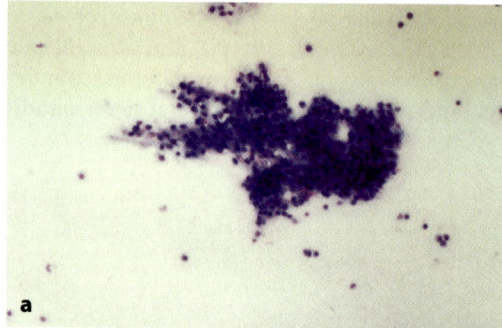

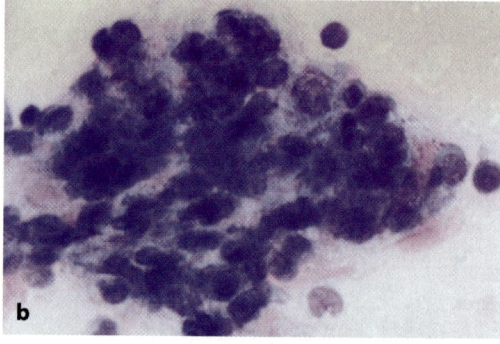

Fig. 8.15
FNAC knee. Pigmented villonodular synovitis. **a** Low-power view showing one of the numerous aggregates of cells found in synovial fluid. **b** Higher-power view of pigmented synovial cells. They display a heterogeneous immunophenotype indicating functional properties of both macrophages and fibroblasts

Fig. 8.14
FNAC arm. Twelve-year-old child. Proliferative fasciitis. **a** Lesion consists of admixtures of large polygonal- to spindle-shaped cells. **b** Ganglion-cell-like fibroblasts with vesicular nuclei and prominent inclusion-like nucleoli. **c** The lesions may be initially diagnosed as sarcomas, most commonly RMS. (Case courtesy of Dr T Levine)

The pseudosarcomas have several features in common: rapid growth, pain and tenderness, infiltrative growth extending along fascial planes or subcutaneous septa or radiating into lobules of adipose tissue [49]. Another common denominator is the pleomorphic pattern of proliferating fibroblasts and myofibroblasts, the presence of more or less ganglion-cell-like large cells, mono- or binucleated with prominent nucleoli and a high mitotic rate. In order to avoid a false diagnosis of sarcoma Akerman emphasises several factors: (1) awareness of the existence of these lesions, (2) combined evaluation of clinical and morphological data (3) rapid growth, often noted by the patients, is rare in sarcomas except in some cases of RMS (similarly, the pain and tenderness are not typical for sarcoma), (4) the appearance of the lesion at low power and (5) at high power, in spite of the cellular pleomorphism, the nuclei are cytologically benign and atypical mitoses are never seen [50]. In cases of doubt, immunocytochemistry and DNA ploidy analysis may be helpful. These lesions may be tetraploid but are never aneuploid. A wait and see policy regarding the clinical follow-up of pseudosarcomatous lesions may be prudent, as many of them regress or disappear after the needling and there is no need for primary surgery.

8.4.1 Nodular Fasciitis

Nodular fasciitis can be cytologically and histologically be mistaken for a sarcoma. Typical cases are small palpable subcutaneous masses of less than 5 cm that evolve rapidly over days or weeks before diagnosis. The natural history of nodular fasciitis is unknown, since the diagnosis is usually based on excised lesions. FNAC features include uniform fibroblast-like spindle cells (occurring singly and in groups), collagen, myxoid material and admixed large cells with abundant cytoplasm, one to two eccentric nuclei, macronucleoli and abundant cytoplasm (ganglion-cell like cells) (Fig. 8.12). The most common sites are the arm (forearm), thigh, trunk and head and neck, but it can be found in other areas (e.g. breast) [51–54]. The lesions range from 0.5 to 5.0 cm [55] in diameter. Nodular fasciitis occurs most commonly in young adults between the ages of 20 and 29 years. However, the other variants of nodular fasciitis, including proliferative myositis and intravascular fasciitis, occur in older people and more commonly in men [56]. Nodular fasciitis, with its hypercellular smears containing overlapping, relatively isomorphic spindle cells, may be mistaken cytologically for sarcoma, particularly if occurring in a non-typical site such as the hand [57]. The lesion should be managed non-surgically. If resolution does not occur within a few weeks, surgery can then be performed [55].

8.4.2 Nodular Myositis

Nodular myositis is a lesion that may be a precursor of generalised polymyositis, including polymyositis associated with graft vs. host disease, or it may remain a localised process. FNAC from localised nodular myositis demonstrates fragments of striated muscle including degenerating and regenerative myocytes, a mixed inflammatory background and necrotic debris (Fig. 8.13). Cytological identification of this lesion can be therapeutically important, particularly in post-bone-marrow transplant patients [58].

8.4.3 Proliferative Fasciitis and Myositis

Proliferative fasciitis and myositis can also occur in children between the ages of 2.5 months and 13 years [59]. Like proliferative fasciitis and myositis in adults, these lesions consist of admixtures of large polygonal to spindle, ganglion-cell-like fibroblasts with vesicular nuclei and prominent inclusion-like nucleoli (Fig. 8.14). The lesions may be initially diagnosed as sarcomas, most commonly RMS [59]. There are some histological differences from adult-type proliferative fasciitis and myositis. Childhood lesions are generally well circumscribed, lobulated, extremely cellular with less collagen production and often associated with acute inflammation and microscopic foci of necrosis. Immunocytochemical comparison with adult proliferative fasciitis and myositis shows similar immunoprofiles; the ganglion-like cells stain for vimentin and actin and focally with KP1, suggesting myofibroblastic and histiocytic features. None of the lesions stains for keratin, desmin or S-100 protein. Recognition of this cellular variant of proliferative fasciitis and myositis is important to prevent misdiagnosis as a sarcoma and unnecessary, excessive therapy [59].

8.4.4 Fibromatoses

Fibromatoses form a spectrum of clinicopathological entities that are characterised by the infiltrative proliferation of fibroblasts that lack malignant cytological features [60]. Fibromatoses present as nodular soft-tissue masses almost anywhere in the body and thus are often amenable to FNAC (e.g. in the abdominal wall - musculoaponeurotic fibromatosis or extra-abdominal desmoid, plantar surface - Ledderhose's disease, the shoulder, the breast and the sternocleidomastoid muscle -fibromatosis coli) (Fig. 8.16). The FNAC findings may be misinterpreted as either nodular fasciitis or a low-grade sarcoma [60]. The FNAC diagnosis of musculoaponeurotic fibromatosis in a patient with familial polyposis coli suggests the diagnosis of Gardner's syndrome. Cytologically, the aspirates consist of groups of loosely cohesive, bland-appearing, spindle-shaped cells having oval to elongated nuclei and cytoplasmic tags. Individual spindle cells and rare inflammatory cells are also present. The aspirate of fibromatosis coli may contain degenerating skeletal muscle cells. In fibromatosis of the breast, numerous spindle cells are admixed with epithelial cells and may be mistaken for cellular fibroadenoma, phyllodes tumour or metaplastic carcinoma [61]. FNAC is a useful procedure for the initial and recurrent diagnosis of fibromatoses and in the separation of fibromatoses from other benign and malignant soft-tissue lesions [60]. In fibromatosis of the breast, clinical and mammographic suspicion of carcinoma and fibroadenoma are often present [61]. Differential diagnosis includes mesenchymal repair, fasciitis and spindle-cell types of sarcoma (Fig. 8.17 and 8.18).

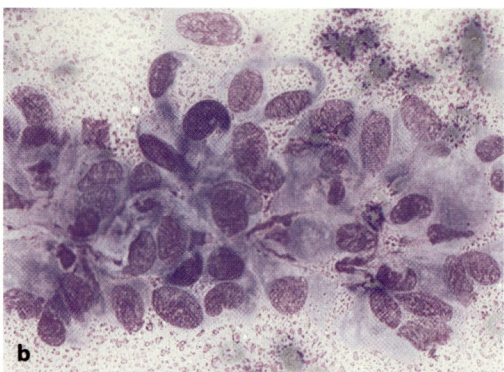
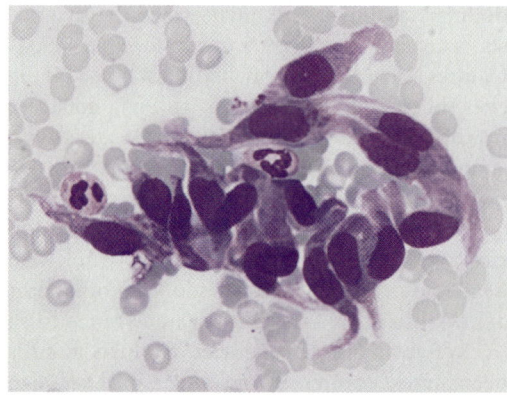

Fig. 8.16
FNAC neck. Fibromatosis coli. **a** Groups of loosely cohesive, bland-appearing, spindle-shaped cells. **b** Higher-power view showing cells with oval to elongated nuclei and cytoplasmic tags. Individual spindle cells and rare inflammatory cells may also be present. Differential diagnosis includes mesenchymal repair, fasciitis and spindle-cell types of sarcoma

Fig. 8.17
FNAC scar tissue. Mesenchymal repair. Fibroblasts may be clustered together and give an impression of malignant spindle-cell tumour

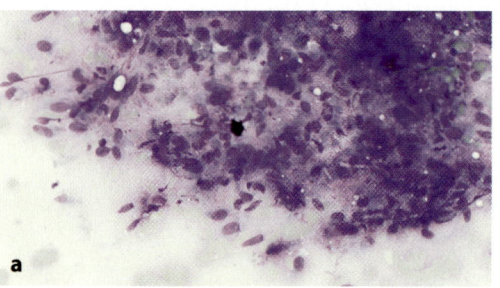
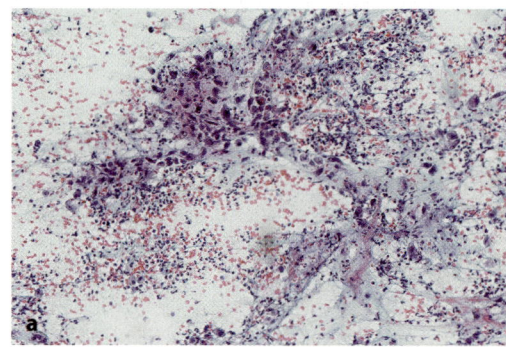

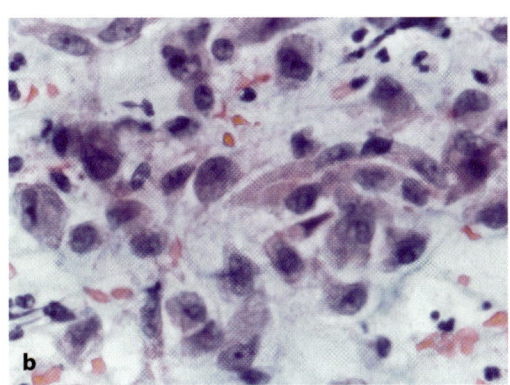

Fig. 8.18
FNAC operation site. Suture granuloma. **a** Cellular smears containing fibroblasts, macrophages, endothelial cells and inflammatory cells. **b** High-power view of these cells may give an impression of pleomorphism and lead to an erroneous diagnosis of malignancy

8.4.5 Fibrous histiocytoma

Fibrous histiocytoma (FHC) may occasionally pose diagnostic problems, a fact that is reflected in a false-positive rate of 8.3% of cases in some series [62]. Smears from FHC are homogenous, composed of histiocytic cells with finely vacuolated cytoplasm, small regular spindle cells and giant cells in 47% of cases. Histiocytic cells are attached to vascular structures in 25% of cases. Slight nuclear atypia may be seen in some cases. Numerous siderophages and/or abundant inflammatory background or myxoid background may be seen. A storiform pattern, round cells, prominent atypia, necrosis, or mitotic figures are not seen. FHC should be differentiated from other benign, low- and intermediate-grade spindle-cell neoplasms such as low-grade fibrosarcoma, dermatofibrosarcoma protuberans, nodular fasciitis, spindle-cell malignant melanoma and monophasic synovial sarcoma. Some cases may be misinterpreted as malignant, especially in cases of recurrence or in patients with a history of cancer [62].

8.4.6 Pseudoangiomatous Stromal Hyperplasia

Pseudoangiomatous stromal hyperplasia (PASH) of the breast is a stromal proliferation that should not be mistaken for sarcoma. It is described in Chap. 9 [63].

Case history 8.2: A 64-year-old patient with a history of carcinoma of the prostate presented with a lump in the left supraclavicular fossa, thought clinically to be a lymph node. FNAC yielded fatty material. Microscopy revealed features mature fat, consistent with a lipoma (Fig. 8.19).

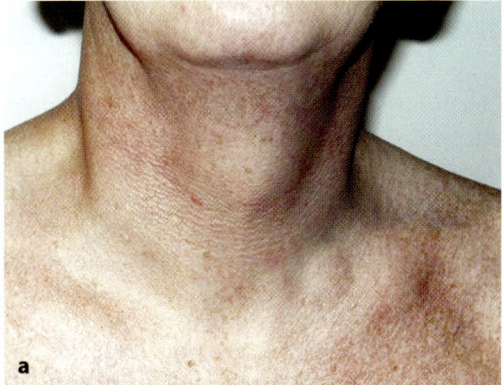

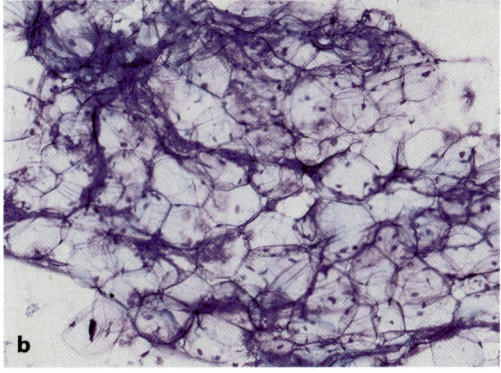

Fig. 8.19
FNAC supraclavicular fossa. Case history 8.2. (see next page)

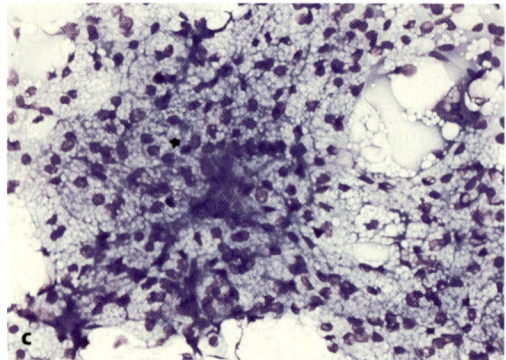

Fig. 8.19
Continued from previous page. FNAC supraclavicular fossa. Case history 8.2. **a** Patient with a left supraclavicular fossa node. **b** Mature fat cells consistent with a lipoma. **c** Another case. Lipomas may sometimes consist of foetal-like fat cells

8.4.7 Pleomorphic Lipoma

This is an unusual pseudosarcomatous condition, most commonly seen in the head and neck regions of middle-aged men [64]. It has a characteristic morphology: the FNAC is focally cellular containing round to oval, hyperchromatic cells, rare multinucleated cells and fragments of mature adipose tissue. On initial evaluation, the smear pattern may suggest a malignant neoplasm [65]. However, the characteristic pattern, including floret cells may be recognised on cytology. The atypical cellular features of the aspirate can cause difficulty in diagnosing this entity. Awareness of this entity, along with clinical correlation, is crucial in arriving at the correct diagnosis [65]. Despite its pleomorphic appearance, it follows a benign course and does not recur or metastasise if completely excised.

8.4.8 Atypical Lipoma

Atypical lipoma as a concept was introduced in 1975 and refers to the well-differentiated liposarcomas of lipoma-like type occurring in the subcutis, which behaves like a benign neoplasm. Patients present with well-defined subcutaneous nodules (e.g. in the supraclavicular region). FNAC shows fragments of mature fat tissue and numerous dispersed, large, hyperchromatic, often bizarre, nuclei (Fig. 8.20). Lipoma with atypical cells may be cytologically mistaken for liposarcoma. A correct cytological diagnosis of atypical lipoma can be established if cytomorphological features are correlated with clinical data [66]. Cytological and histological concordance may be achieved in 96% of lipomas and in 85% of atypical lipomatous tumours and liposarcomas [67]. Clinical and radiological correlation is essential (Fig. 8.21).

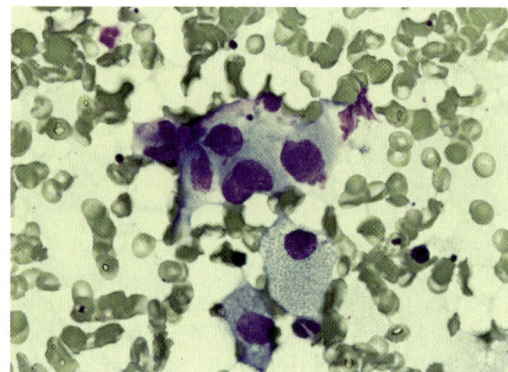

Fig. 8.20
FNAC trunk. Atypical lipoma. Atypical cells and macrophages containing fat in an otherwise typical lipoma

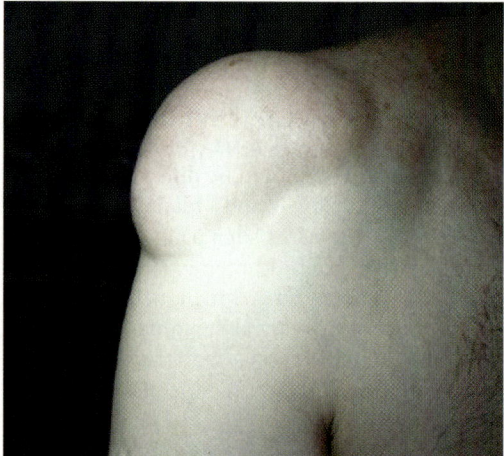

Fig. 8.21
Shoulder mass, 75-year-old man. Lesion is clinically well defined, present for many years, painless and mobile. Excision confirmed cytological diagnosis of lipoma

8.4.9 Spindle-Cell Lipoma

Spindle-cell lipoma is a relatively uncommon, benign tumour that usually presents in the subcutaneous fat of adult men. The cytological features are poorly defined, and aspirates may cause diagnostic problems because spindle-cell lipoma shares some features with other fatty/spindle-cell or myxoid lesions, benign as well as malignant. FNAC is characterised by a mixture of mature adipocytes, uniform spindle cells and collagen bundles and/or fibres in varying proportions [68]. The presence of a myxoid matrix and of mast cells is less specific and occurs less frequently. Comparison of these features and the clinical data helps to exclude low-grade liposarcoma as well as other spindle-cell and myxoid lesions.

8.4.10 Ancient Schwannoma

Prior to the realisation that the observed atypia was a regressive phenomenon, many of FNAC smears from ancient schwannoma were erroneously diagnosed as sarcomas. FNAC shows many of the same features as FNAC of regular schwannoma: aggregates of spindle cells with indistinct cytoplasm and elongated nuclei with blunt point ends. The feature unique to these lesions is nuclear pleomorphism, which is identified in all aspirates [69]. Nuclear inclusions are frequently identified, as is the evidence of cystic degeneration and xanthomatous changes. The FNAC features of ancient schwannoma are important to note because of the potential to confuse this lesion with a sarcoma on FNAC.

8.4.11 Angioleiomyoma

Angioleiomyoma presents in the skin or subcutaneous tissue of the lower extremities, the shoulder and the lower arm, often as a painful or tender mass. FNAC shows moderate or sparse cellularity composed of uniform spindle cells. These may be admixed with smooth muscle cells, fragments of collagenous tissue in varying proportions and with macrophages and fat cells. Smears from angioleiomyoma are not sufficiently characteristic to permit a definitive diagnosis, but together with typical clinical data (painful or tender nodule) may help to exclude other skin or subcutaneous lesions [70].

8.4.12 Calcifying Aponeurotic Fibroma

This is a rare benign soft-tissue proliferation that occurs in the distal extremities in children. Clinically and radiographically it may be a suspected sarcoma. Cytological examination reveals benign-appearing spindle cells, chondroid cells, multinucleated giant cells and calcific debris [71]. These features recapitulate the classical histological features of calcifying aponeurotic fibroma. Conservative excision is usually performed.

8.4.13 Lipomatous Haemangiopericytoma

This is a rare benign soft-tissue tumour that clinically may mimic soft-tissue sarcoma. Despite the fact that lipomatous haemangiopericytoma shares most of the histological features with solitary fibrous tumour, it may be occasionally misdiagnosed as myxoid liposarcoma or some other type of spindle-cell sarcoma. Cytological evaluation of lipomatous haemangiopericytoma can be difficult due to its rarity and to its similarity with other spindle-cell or fatty tumours [72].

8.5 Tumours of Low or Borderline Malignancy

A subset of low-grade fibrosarcomas is composed of CD34-positive spindle cells. These include dermatofibrosarcoma, its morphologic variants its associated fibrosarcoma, solitary fibrous tumour, haemangiopericytoma and its malignant counterparts and some cases of myxoinflammatory fibroblastic sarcoma. Dermatofibrosarcoma and related lesions are characterised by a t(17;22)(q22;q13) rearrangement, which results in fusion of the genes COL1A (17q21-22) and PDGFB1 (22q13) [73].

8.5.1 Dermatofibrosarcoma Protuberans

Dermatofibrosarcoma protuberans is a nodular cutaneous mesenchymal tumour of intermediate malignancy with a characteristic tendency for recurrence. Metastases are unusual. This tumour usually occurs in the trunk and extremities and, infrequently, on the face and scalp (Fig. 8.22). FNAC smears are surprisingly homogeneous and composed of numerous fibroblast-like cells arranged as single cells or in clusters of spindle cells arrayed in a storiform pattern [74, 75]. Fibrillary stromal fragments, naked nuclei and slight to moderate cytological atypia, mitotic figures, myxoid background, mast cells and dispersed adipocytes may be seen [75]. Giant cells, necrosis, or marked cytological atypia are not seen. Dermatofibrosarcoma protuberans shares morphological characteristics with some of the low-grade spindle-cell neoplasms. It should be differentiated from other benign low- and intermediate-grade spindle neoplasm such as low-grade fibrosarcoma, low-grade malignant peripheral nerve sheath tumour, benign peripheral nerve sheath tumour, nodular fasciitis and FHC [76].

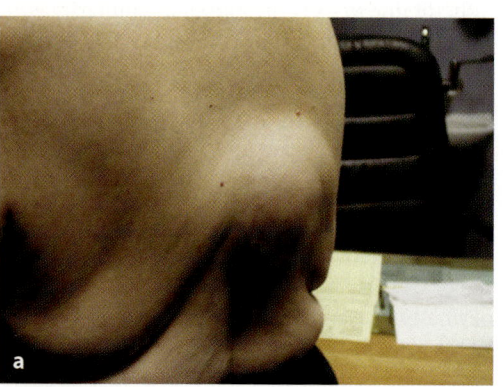

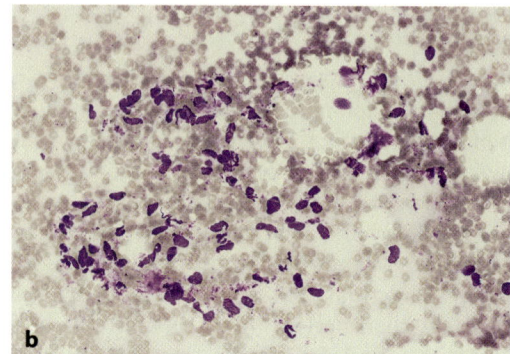

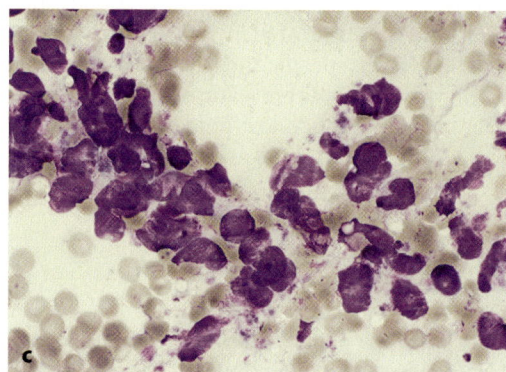

Fig. 8.22
FNAC trunk. Dermatofibrosarcoma protuberans. **a** Recurrence of the tumour on the trunk of the 64-year-old female patient. **b** FNAC smears are composed of numerous fibroblast like cells arranged as single cells or in clusters of spindle cells arrayed in a storiform pattern. **c** Fibrillary stromal fragments, naked nuclei and slight to moderate cytological atypia, mitotic figures, myxoid background, mast cells and dispersed adipocytes may be seen

8.5.2 Haemangiopericytoma

Haemangiopericytoma is a relatively rare neoplasm that accounts for approximately 2.5% of all soft-tissue tumours. FNAC may be performed on lesions arising in the lower extremities, trunk and breast as well from metastases. Aspirates are cellular, composed of single and tightly packed clusters of oval- to spindle-shaped cells aggregated around branched capillaries. Basement membrane material is observed in 67% of cases [77]. The nuclei are uniform and oval, with finely granular chromatin and inconspicuous nucleoli. No mitotic figures or areas of necrosis are identified. Haemangiopericytomas show a spindle-cell pattern in cytological preparations and must be distinguished from more common spindle-cell lesions. Immunohistochemistry and electron microscopy performed on FNAC samples may be helpful in the differential diagnosis [78]. Prediction of the biological behaviour of Raemangiopericytoma based on cytologic features is not feasible.

8.5.3 Acral Myxoinflammatory Fibroblastic Sarcoma

Acral myxoinflammatory fibroblastic sarcoma (AMIFS) may be difficult to distinguish from other myxoid lesions on FNAC. Cytologically, AMIFS exhibits all of the characteristic features described in surgical biopsy specimens: myxoid material, spindle cells with bipolar cytoplasmic extensions, epithelioid cells with globules of extracellular material and ganglion-like and lipoblast-like giant cells. Only the inflammatory component may be scarce. Pohar-Marinsek et al. conclude that cytomorphology of AMIFS may be characteristic enough to enable a definitive diagnosis from FNAC, provided all the distinctive features are sampled [79].

8.6 Soft-Tissue Deposits of Non-Sarcomatous Lesions

8.6.1 Malignant Lymphoma and Leukaemia

Malignant lymphoma and leukaemia infrequently involve soft tissue and may be diagnosed on FNAC. Patients may have superficial or deep soft-tissue masses. The involved sites include the extremities, trunk and head. Occasionally, FNAC represents the initial diagnosis of malignant lymphoma, more frequently they are from a recurrent malignant lymphoma or leukaemia. In the majority of cases, it is possible to determine a specific diagnosis and subtype of soft-tissue malignant lymphoma or leukaemia using FNAC [80]. (see chapter 5.3.1)

8.6.2 Calcinosis Cutis

Calcinosis cutis is an uncommon condition since calcific deposits in patients with end-stage renal disease are now somewhat rare due to improvements in disease management. Since calcific deposits may clinically resemble a tumour, it is feasible to investigate them using FNAC. The mass may enlarge to nearly four times its original size and be clinically suspicious of malignancy. FNAC preparations show abundant calcium, indicative of soft-tissue calcinosis.

8.7 Sarcomas Mimicking Other Lesions

8.7.1 Epithelioid Sarcoma

Epithelioid sarcoma is a rare aggressive soft-tissue malignant tumour generally arising in the distal extremities of young adults. Although it has characteristic morphological and immunohistochemical features, it can be confused histologically and cytologically with a variety of benign and malignant lesions, including a granulomatous process, synovial sarcoma, melanoma, SqCC and adenocarcinoma [81]. The cytological features include: predominantly dissociated epithelioid-like cells with eccentrically placed nuclei and mild to moderate pleomorphism and a plasmacytoid appearance [82]. Well-defined cytoplasm with intercellular spaces between malignant cells is frequently seen. A granuloma-like structure may be seen [81]. Although clearly malignant, the cytological features are difficult to differentiate morphologically from melanoma, epithelioid LMS, schwannoma or adenocarcinoma [83]. The immunocytochemical stains show diffuse cytoplasmic positivity for cytokeratins (CAM 5.2) and both cytoplasmic and cell membrane positivity for vimentin, while they are immunonegative for S-100 protein and HMB 45 [82]. Epithelioid sarcoma may be difficult to differentiate from an extraskeletal osteosarcoma in cases with abundant hyalinised collagen on FNAC [84].

8.7.2 Metastatic Soft-Tissue Sarcomas

Metastatic soft-tissue sarcomas may involve lymph nodes and be diagnosed with FNAC. The most common type of sarcoma to involve the lymph node is embryonal RMS, followed by synovial sarcoma, LMS, fibrosarcoma, malignant peripheral nerve sheath tumour and RMS [85]. FNAC is helpful in the early diagnosis, staging and management of metastatic sarcomas. Importantly, it avoids the need for a lymph node biopsy in the majority of cases.

8.7.3 Well-Differentiated Liposarcoma

Well-differentiated liposarcoma may be difficult to diagnose on FNAC. Cytological criteria for the evaluation of FNAC samples of possible liposarcoma include the following: a complex capillary network, increased cellularity, the presence of a metachromatic stroma for myxoid liposarcoma and the identification of lipoblasts (Fig. 8.6). Complex capillary networks are identified in 75%; usually in myxoid liposarcomas and some well-differentiated neoplasms. Increased cellularity is seen in 58%, metachromatic stroma in 25% and lipoblasts in 33% of cases [86]. The cytological diagnosis of well-differentiated liposarcoma should be accepted with caution, and the sites should be taken into consideration. Deep-seated tumours with large, bizarre giant cells should have wide excision as they recur more frequently [87].

8.8 Rare and Difficult Sarcomas

8.8.1 Alveolar Soft-Part Sarcoma

Alveolar soft-part sarcoma is a rare soft-tissue tumour. It has a characteristic histology, with typical ultrastructural features demonstrating unique crystalloids. It occurs predominantly in adolescents and young adults, in whom the most common location is within the fascial planes of skeletal muscle of the lower extremity. FNAC smears exhibit single and small groups of polyhedral malignant cells with granular cytoplasm, anisokaryosis and prominent central nucleoli. The delicate cytoplasm has a tendency to rupture, with the resulting presence of many bare nuclei. Binucleated and occasional multinucleated cells are present. The characteristic crystals may be observed in Pap-stained smears within the cytoplasm and in the background near the tumour cells [88]. Electron microscopy confirms the diagnosis, demonstrating membrane-bound, rhomboid crystalloids with a lattice-like ultrastructure. The differential diagnosis includes renal cell carcinoma, paraganglioma, granular cell tumour, clear cell sarcoma and epithelioid sarcoma [89].

8.8.2 Angiosarcoma

Angiosarcoma is an uncommon soft-tissue neoplasm with a predilection for skin and superficial soft tissues, but it may occur at unusual sites (e.g. the parotid gland and lung) [90] (Fig. 8.23) The morphological features that may be identified on FNAC include: hypocellular aspirates with predominantly single cells and clusters in a background of moderate to abundant amounts of blood [69]. Scattered inflammatory cells, primarily neutrophils, may be seen in the background. The individual tumour cells are polymorphous: oval, round or spindled, with eccentric, round- to spindle-shaped nuclei and moderate to abundant amounts of pale blue-grey, vacuolated cytoplasm. The cells range from two to nine times the size of the background red blood cells. Malignant cells may contain intracytoplasmic haemosiderin deposits; show small or sometimes large nucleoli and nuclear hyperchromasia. Mitotic figures, erythrophagocytosis, acinar-like or vascular structures and necrosis are not commonly seen. The presence of scarce single pleomorphic cells in a bloody background should raise the diagnostic possibility of angiosarcoma. In the epithelioid variant of angiosarcoma, the cells are morphologically similar and composed of round to oval and polygonal, epithelial-like cells, frequently arranged in clusters and showing erythrophagocytosis and prominent nuclear grooves [91, 92]. A definitive diagnosis of angiosarcoma is often difficult due to the paucity of diagnostic cells unless intracytoplasmic haemosiderin deposits can be identified. The tumour may be mistaken for granulation tissue on FNAC [93]. Epithelioid angiosarcomas are often confused with carcinomas, melanomas and other epithelioid sarcomas, both cytologically and histologically. Multiple aspirations are often needed in order to obtain diagnostic material. In the setting of radiotherapy, it may be impossible to distinguish angiosarcoma from radiation change, and biopsy is recommended [69]. Whenever FNAC suggests malignancy composed predominantly of epithelioid cells, , especially in the head and neck area, epithelioid angiosarcoma should be considered [92].

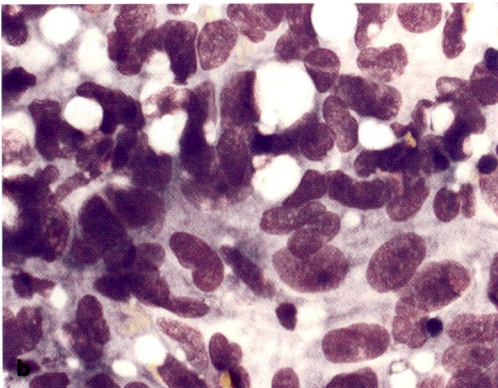

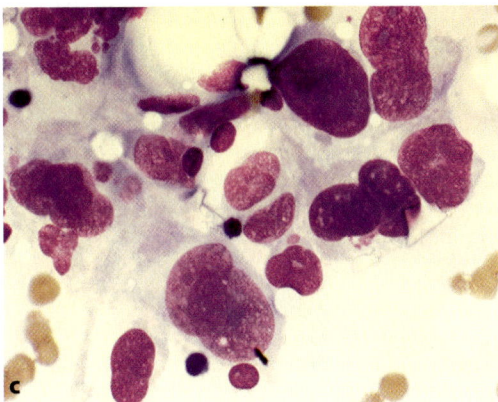

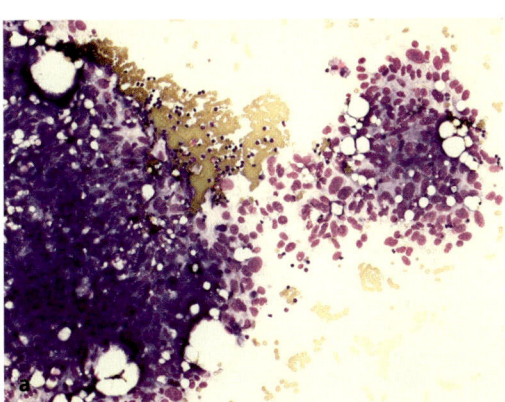

Fig. 8.23
FNAC scalp. Angiosarcoma. **a** Single cells and clusters in a background of moderate to abundant amounts of blood. **b** The individual tumour cells are polymorphous: oval, round or spindled, with eccentric, round- to spindle-shaped nuclei and moderate to abundant amounts of pale blue-grey, vacuolated cytoplasm.
c The cells range from two to nine times the size of the background red blood cells. Malignant cells may contain intracytoplasmic haemosiderin deposits; show small or sometimes large nucleoli and nuclear hyperchromasia. Mitotic figures, erythrophagocytosis, acinar like or vascular structures and necrosis are not commonly seen

Case history 8.3: Patient with a history of angiosarcoma of the scalp that had been treated by radiotherapy presented with enlarged neck nodes on the side that had been irradiated. FNAC was requested in order to distinguish between the reactive lymphadenopathy and possible tumour involvement. (Fig. 8.24)

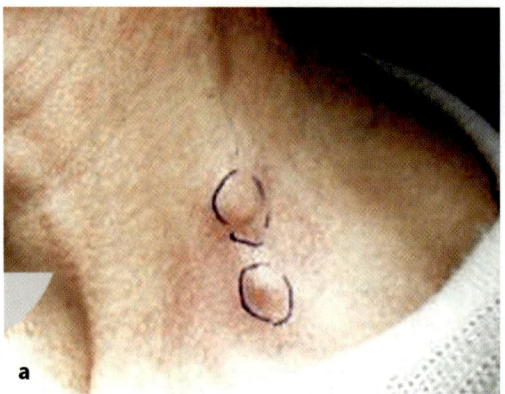

8.8.3 Kaposi's Sarcoma

Kaposi's sarcoma may be diagnosed by FNAC. Patients are usually HIV-positive or have a diagnosis of AIDS (Fig. 8.25). Aspirates are commonly obtained from enlarged lymph nodes or soft-tissue masses, but may be from oral cavity lesions, abdominal masses and other sites. The most characteristic cytological features are intact tissue fragments composed of overlapping spindle cells with nuclear distortion and ill-defined cytoplasmic borders. Smaller groups of loosely cohesive spindle-shaped cells and individual spindle cells with cytoplasm are also helpful features. Immunocytochemistry is often positive for Kaposi's sarcoma-associated herpesvirus (KSHV) and vascular markers (CD34). In the appropriate clinical setting, these cytological features on FNAC can be diagnostic of Kaposi's sarcoma [94].

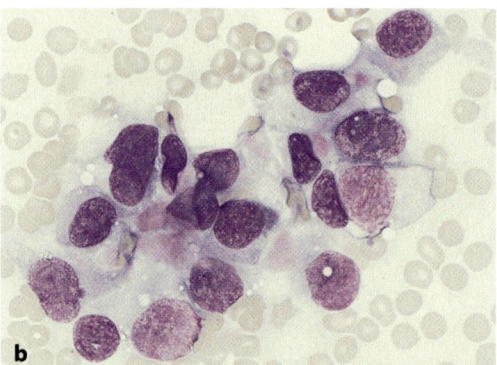

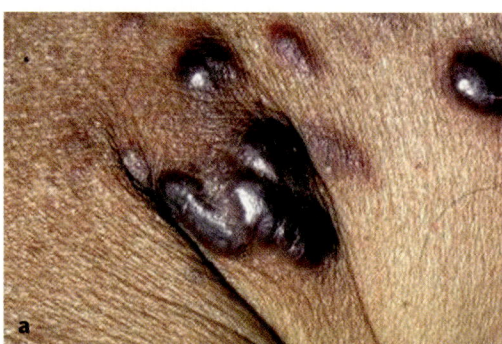

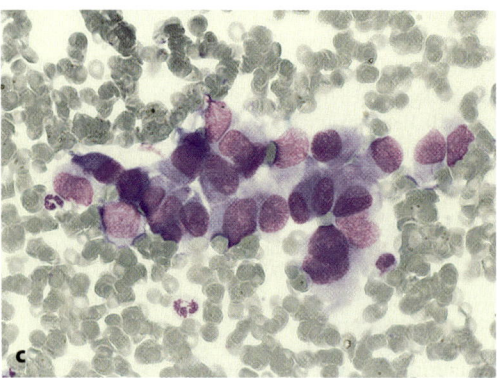

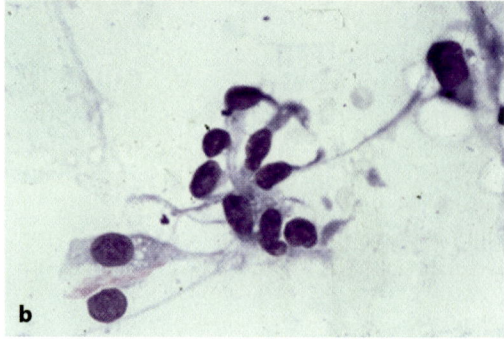

Fig. 8.24
FNAC neck nodes. Angiosarcoma. **a** A 65-year-old patient with neck nodes. In the setting of radiotherapy, it may be impossible to distinguish angiosarcoma from radiation change. **b** Epithelioid angiosarcomas are often confused with carcinomas, melanomas and other epithelioid sarcomas, both cytologically and histologically. **c** Whenever FNAC suggests malignancy composed predominantly of epithelioid cells, especially in the head and neck area, epithelioid angiosarcoma should be considered

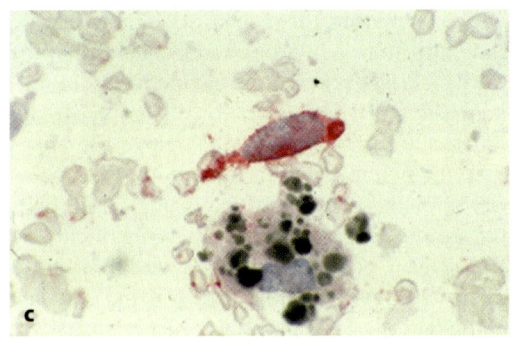

Fig. 8.25
FNAC lesion left shin. Kaposi's sarcoma. Patients are usually HIV-positive or have a diagnosis of AIDS. **a** The aspirates are commonly obtained from enlarged lymph nodes or soft-tissue masses but may be from oral cavity lesions, abdominal masses and other sites. **b** The most characteristic cytological features are intact tissue fragments composed of overlapping spindle cells with nuclear distortion and ill-defined cytoplasmic borders. Smaller groups of loosely cohesive spindle-shaped cells and individual spindle cells with cytoplasm are also helpful features. **c** Immunocytochemistry is positive for vascular markers. In the appropriate clinical setting, these cytological features on FNAC can be diagnostic of Kaposi's sarcoma

8.8.4 Clear-Cell Sarcoma of Soft Parts

Clear-cell sarcoma of soft parts (CCSSP) can be diagnosed on FNAC. Aspirates are markedly cellular, consisting predominantly of discohesive cells but also of clusters. The cytoplasm is eosinophilic and eccentric. The nuclei are round and contain macronucleoli. CCSSP should be considered when FNAC of a soft-tissue tumour shows uncharacteristically high cellularity and relatively uniform cells with macronucleoli [95]. Cohesion of some tumour cells does not rule out CCSSP. Melanin pigment and cytoplasmic clearing are infrequent and not necessary for the diagnosis. Sufficient material should always be taken for immunohistochemical studies, possibly on the cell block. A significant diagnostic pitfall is the potential of CCSSP to form microacinar structures mimicking adenocarcinoma, particularly in the metastatic to regional lymph nodes [96]. A rare case of the granular-cell variant of CCS-SP has been described [96]. Owing to the rarity of CCSSP, the diagnosis on cytological smears is extremely difficult and is aided substantially by the clinical data.

8.8.5 Haemangioendothelioma

Haemangioendothelioma may be diagnosed on FNAC. The aspirates are haemorrhagic; the smears show mostly dissociated and predominantly monomorphic tumour cells with focal rosette like clustering. A prominent cytological feature is the close association of tumour cells with endothelium-lined vascular structures, a pattern that can be seen in other sarcomas and sometimes in malignant epithelial tumours [97].

8.8.6 Giant-Cell Fibroblastoma

Giant-cell fibroblastoma is an unusual childhood tumour that occurs primarily in the superficial soft tissues. FNAC features include bland spindle- to oval-shaped cells entrapped in a metachromatic matrix, accompanied by rare multinucleated giant cells with wreath-like nuclei. Although a definitive diagnosis on FNAC is difficult, surgical resection of the mass establishes the diagnosis of giant cell fibroblastoma [98].

8.8.7 Rhabdomyosarcoma

RMS diagnosis on FNAC may present differential diagnostic problems [99–101]. Pohar-Marinsek and Bracko analysed several morphological features and identified architectural patterns and found that, among cases of alveolar RMS, there are two major architectural patterns: one containing completely dissociated cells and one containing many chance formations [102]. Among the embryonal type, the predominant architectural pattern contains large tissue fragments with abundant eosinophilic material and various numbers of dissociated cells. The pattern of only dissociated cells was similar to that one seen for the alveolar type (Figs. 7.4 and 7.5). The relative proportion of poorly to better- and well-differentiated rhabdomyoblasts varied in both types and in all patterns [102]. RMS exhibits a variety of morphological patterns of cellular morphology and architecture, even within the same histological subtype. Therefore, a reliable subclassification into alveolar and embryonal RMS cannot be made from FNAC smears [102]. All cases suspected to be RMS must always be confirmed by immunocytochemically since they could be confused with some benign and malignant tumours with similar morphology [103] (Fig. 8.5). (see also 7.1.4)

8.8.8 Synovial Sarcoma

Synovial sarcoma on FNAC material shows a typical pattern of a mixture of dispersed cells with the presence of stripped nuclei and cell tight tumour tissue fragments with irregular borders (Fig. 8.1). A branching network of vessels is often present in the fragments, imitating a true vascular tumour. Except in poorly differentiated synovial sarcomas, the tumour cells are small to medium in size, with rounded, ovoid or fusiform bland nuclei with inconspicuous nucleoli. In the biphasic variant, small glandular- or acinar-like structures are present, although not in all cases (Fig. 8.26). In the poorly differentiated type, however, the cellular pleomorphism is marked with the presence of cells with irregular nuclei and rhabdomyoblast-like cells, corresponding to the pleomorphic variant [104, 105]. Epithelial cells, squamous cells, round cells, mast cells, necrosis, comma-like nuclei, marked nuclear atypia, secretory mucin and rosette like structures are also occasionally observed [106]. The latter feature may be confused with neuroendocrine tumours [107]. Epithelial tumour cells with ovoid to round, mostly regular, centrally to eccentrically located nuclei, surrounded by scant to abundant cytoplasm may dominate in monophasic tumours and are admixed with spindle cells in a classical biphasic type. Multinucleated tumour giant cells are not observed. In biphasic synovial sarcoma, the neoplastic spindle cells are generally more numerous and frequent than the epithelial cells, making the distinction from monophasic synovial sarcoma or other spindle-cell soft-tissue tumours difficult. Despite the apparent distinction between the two types of synovial sarcoma, a spectrum of cytological findings can be seen in the monophasic type, including a secondary population of cells with morphology usually typical of biphasic synovial sarcoma [108]. The classical pattern is highly suggestive of synovial sarcoma of all three (monophasic, biphasic or poorly differentiated) subtypes. Cytogenetic results reveal a t(X; 18)(p11.2; q11.2) translocation, thus establishing the diagnosis of synovial sarcoma [109].

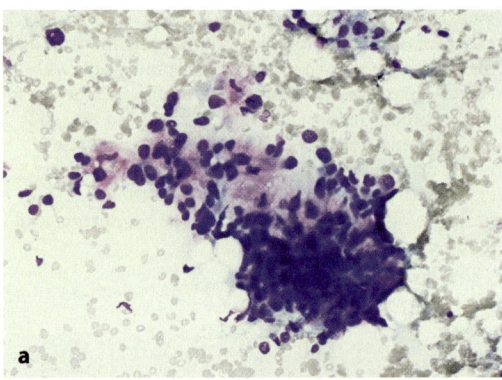

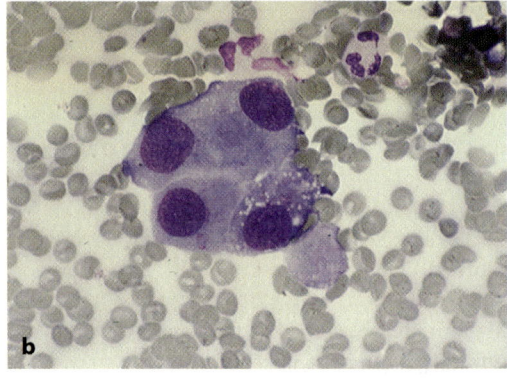

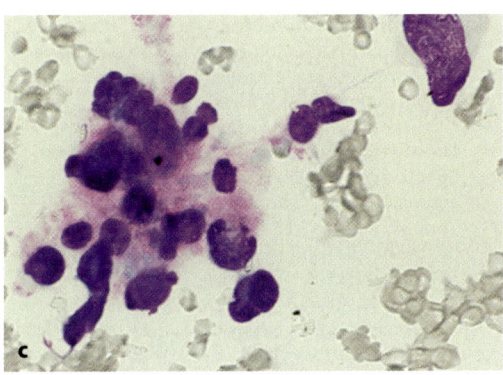

Fig. 8.26
FNAC chest wall. Synovial sarcoma. **a** Tumour cells are small to medium in size, with rounded, ovoid, or fusiform bland nuclei with inconspicuous nucleoli. **b** In the biphasic variant, small glandular- or acinar-like structures are present, although not in all cases. Epithelial tumour cells with ovoid to round, mostly regular, centrally to eccentrically located nuclei, surrounded by scant to abundant cytoplasm may dominate in monophasic tumours. **c** In the poorly differentiated type, the cellular pleomorphism is marked with the presence of cells with irregular nuclei and rhabdomyoblast-like cells, corresponding to the pleomorphic variant

References

1. Wakely PE, Jr., Kneisl JS. Soft tissue aspiration cytopathology. Cancer 2000;90(5):292-8.
2. Costa MJ, Campman SC, Davis RL, Howell LP. Fine-needle aspiration cytology of sarcoma: retrospective review of diagnostic utility and specificity. Diagn Cytopathol 1996;15(1):23-32.
3. Skoog L, Pereira ST, Tani E. Fine-needle aspiration cytology and immunocytochemistry of soft-tissue tumors and osteo/chondrosarcomas of the head and neck. Diagn Cytopathol 1999;20(3):131-6.
4. Gonzalez-Campora R. Fine needle aspiration cytology of soft tissue tumors. Acta Cytol 2000;44(3):337-43.
5. Willen H, Akerman M, Carlen B. Fine needle aspiration (FNA) in the diagnosis of soft tissue tumours; a review of 22 years experience. Cytopathology 1995;6(4):236-47.
6. Kilpatrick SE, Cappellari JO, Bos GD, Gold SH, Ward WG. Is fine-needle aspiration biopsy a practical alternative to open biopsy for the primary diagnosis of sarcoma? Experience with 140 patients. Am J Clin Pathol 2001;115(1):59-68.
7. Sapi Z, Antal I, Papai Z, Szendroi M, Mayer A, Jakab K, et al. Diagnosis of soft tissue tumors by fine-needle aspiration with combined cytopathology and ancillary techniques. Diagn Cytopathol 2002;26(4):232-42.
8. Singh HK, Kilpatrick SE, Silverman JF. Fine needle aspiration biopsy of soft tissue sarcomas: utility and diagnostic challenges. Adv Anat Pathol 2004;11(1):24-37.
9. Gonzalez-Campora R. Cytoarchitectural findings in the diagnosis of primary soft tissue tumors. Acta Cytol 2001;45(2):115-46.
10. Trovik CS, Bauer HC, Brosjo O, Skoog L, Soderlund V. Fine needle aspiration (FNA) cytology in the diagnosis of recurrent soft tissue sarcoma. Cytopathology 1998;9(5):320-8.
11. Dey P, Mallik MK, Gupta SK, Vasishta RK. Role of fine needle aspiration cytology in the diagnosis of soft tissue tumours and tumour-like lesions. Cytopathology 2004;15(1):32-7.
12. Bennert KW, Abdul-Karim FW. Fine needle aspiration cytology vs. needle core biopsy of soft tissue tumors. A comparison. Acta Cytol 1994;38(3):381-4.
13. Palmer HE, Mukunyadzi P, Culbreth W, Thomas JR. Subgrouping and grading of soft-tissue sarcomas by fine-needle aspiration cytology: a histopathologic correlation study. Diagn Cytopathol 2001;24(5):307-16.
14. Arbiser ZK, Folpe AL, Weiss SW. Consultative (expert) second opinions in soft tissue pathology. Analysis of problem-prone diagnostic situations. Am J Clin Pathol 2001;116(4):473-6.
15. Nagira K, Yamamoto T, Akisue T, Marui T, Hitora T, Nakatani T, et al. Reliability of fine-needle aspiration biopsy in the initial diagnosis of soft-tissue lesions. Diagn Cytopathol 2002;27(6):354-61.
16. Bezabih M. Cytological diagnosis of soft tissue tumours. Cytopathology 2001;12(3):177-83.
17. Akerman M, Domanski HA. The cytology of soft tissue tumours. Monogr Clin Cytol 2003;16:IX-X, 1-112.
18. Lin O, Zerbini MC, Latorre Mdo R, Saigo PE. Cytologic analyses of spindle-cell lesions of the thorax and retroperitoneum. Diagn Cytopathol 2002;27(6):343-9.
19. Powers CN, Berardo MD, Frable WJ. Fine-needle aspiration biopsy: pitfalls in the diagnosis of spindle-cell lesions. Diagn Cytopathol) 1994;10(3):232-40; discussion 241.
20. Liu K, Dodge RK, Layfield LJ. Logistic regression analysis of high grade spindle cell neoplasms. A fine needle aspiration cytologic study. Acta Cytol 1999;43(4):593-600.
21. Liu K, Dodge RK, Dodd LG, Layfield LJ. Logistic regression analysis of low grade spindle cell lesions. A cytologic study. Acta Cytol 1999;43(2):143-52.

22. Clayton AC, Salomao DR, Keeney GL, Nascimento AG. Solitary fibrous tumor: a study of cytologic features of six cases diagnosed by fine-needle aspiration. Diagn Cytopathol 2001;25(3):172-6.
23. Hummel P, Cangiarella JF, Cohen JM, Yang G, Waisman J, Chhieng DC. Transthoracic fine-needle aspiration biopsy of pulmonary spindle cell and mesenchymal lesions: a study of 61 cases. Cancer 2001;93(3):187-98.
24. Chhieng DC, Cohen JM, Cangiarella JF. Fine-needle aspiration of spindle cell and mesenchymal lesions of the salivary glands. Diagn Cytopathol 2000;23(4):253-9.
25. Kapila K, Mathur S, Verma K. Schwannomas: a pitfall in the diagnosis of pleomorphic adenomas on fine-needle aspiration cytology. Diagn Cytopathol 2002;27(1):53-9.
26. Fisher C. Myofibroblastic malignancies. Adv Anat Pathol 2004;11(4):190-201.
27. Wakely PE, Jr., Geisinger KR, Cappellari JO, Silverman JF, Frable WJ. Fine-needle aspiration cytopathology of soft tissue: chondromyxoid and myxoid lesions. Diagn Cytopathol 1995;12(2):101-5.
28. Layfield LJ, Liu K, Dodge RK. Logistic regression analysis of myxoid sarcomas: a cytologic study. Diagn Cytopathol 1998;19(5):355-60.
29. Estrada Villasenor EG, Delgado Cedillo EA, Linares Gonzalez LM, Rico Martinez G. Fine needle aspiration cytology of low grade fibromyxoid sarcoma. Report of a case with histologic correlation. Acta Cytol 2004;48(1):69-72.
30. Lindberg GM, Maitra A, Gokaslan ST, Saboorian MH, Albores-Saavedra J. Low grade fibromyxoid sarcoma: fine-needle aspiration cytology with histologic, cytogenetic, immunohistochemical, and ultrastructural correlation. Cancer 1999;87(2):75-82.
31. Silverman JF, Nathan G, Olson PR, Prichard J, Cohen JK. Fine-needle aspiration cytology of low-grade fibromyxoid sarcoma of the renal capsule (capsuloma). Diagn Cytopathol 2000;23(4):279-83.
32. Klijanienko J, Caillaud JM, Lagace R, Vielh P. Fine-needle aspiration of leiomyosarcoma: a correlative cytohistopathological study of 96 tumors in 68 patients. Diagn Cytopathol 2003;28(3):119-25.
33. Mohanty SK, Srinivasan R, Rajwanshi A, Vasishta RK, Vignesh PS. Cytologic diagnosis of ossifying fibromyxoid tumor of soft tissue: a case report. Diagn Cytopathol 2004;30(1):41-5.
34. Lax S, Langsteger W. Ossifying fibromyxoid tumor misdiagnosed as follicular neoplasia. A case report. Acta Cytol 1997;41(4 Suppl):1261-4.
35. Kay PA, Nascimento AG, Unni KK, Salomao DR. Chordoma. Cytomorphologic findings in 14 cases diagnosed by fine needle aspiration. Acta Cytol 2003;47(2):202-8.
36. Layfield LJ. Cytologic differential diagnosis of myxoid and mucinous neoplasms of the sacrum and parasacral soft tissues. Diagn Cytopathol 2003;28(5):264-71.
37. Pohar-Marinsek Z, Frkovic-Grazio S. Fine needle aspiration (FNA) cytology of primary subcutaneous sacrococcygeal myxopapillary ependymoma. Cytopathology 1998;9(6):415-20.
38. Caraway NP, Staerkel GA, Fanning CV, Varma DG, Pollock RE. Diagnosing intramuscular myxoma by fine-needle aspiration: a multidisciplinary approach. Diagn Cytopathol 1994;11(3):255-61.
39. Tunc M, Ekinci C. Chondrosarcoma diagnosed by fine needle aspiration cytology. Acta Cytol 1996;40(2):283-8.
40. Wadhwa N, Arora VK, Singh N, Bhatia A. Fine needle aspiration cytology of primary extraskeletal myxoid chondrosarcoma. A case report. Acta Cytol 2000;44(3):445-8.
41. Pohar-Marinsek Z, Us-Krasovec M, Lamovec J. Chondroblastoma in fine needle aspirates. Acta Cytol 1992;36(3):367-70.
42. Granados R, Martin-Hita A, Rodriguez-Barbero JM, Murillo N. Fine-needle aspiration cytology of chondroblastoma of soft parts: case report and differential diagnosis with other soft tissue tumors. Diagn Cytopathol 2003;28(2):76-81.
43. Dodd LG, Martinez S. Fine-needle aspiration cytology of pseudosarcomatous lesions of soft tissue. Diagn Cytopathol 2001;24(1):28-35.
44. Chow LT, Chow WH, Lee JC. Fine needle aspiration (FNA) cytology of proliferative fasciitis: report of a case with immunohistochemical study. Cytopathology 1995;6(5):349-57.
45. Anglo-Henry MR, Seaquist MB, Marsh WL, Jr. Fine needle aspiration of proliferative fasciitis. A case report. Acta Cytol 1985;29(5):882-6.
46. Jacobs JC. Aspiration cytology of proliferative myositis. A case report. Acta Cytol 1995;39(3):535-8.
47. Layfield LJ, Anders KH, Glasgow BJ, Mirra JM. Fine-needle aspiration of primary soft-tissue lesions. Arch Pathol Lab Med 1986;110(5):420-4.
48. Wakely PE, Jr., Almeida M, Frable WJ. Fine-needle aspiration biopsy cytology of myositis ossificans. Mod Pathol 1994;7(1):23-5.
49. Akerman M. Benign fibrous lesions masquerading as sarcomas. Clinical and morphological pitfalls. Acta Orthop Scand Suppl 1997;273:37-40.
50. Wong NL. Fine needle aspiration cytology of pseudosarcomatous reactive proliferative lesions of soft tissue. Acta Cytol 2002;46(6):1049-55.
51. Kaw YT, Cuesta RA. Nodular fasciitis of the orbit diagnosed by fine needle aspiration cytology. A case report. Acta Cytol 1993;37(6):957-60.
52. Abendroth CS, Frauenhoffer EE. Nodular fasciitis of the parotid gland. Report of a case with presentation in an unusual location and cytologic differential diagnosis. Acta Cytol 1995;39(3):530-4.
53. Matusik J, Wiberg A, Sloboda J, Andersson O. Fine needle aspiration in nodular fasciitis of the face. Cytopathology 2002;13(2):128-32.

54. Fernando SS, Gune S, George S, Van Gelderen P. Nodular fasciitis: a case with unusual clinical presentation initially diagnosed by aspiration cytology. Cytopathology 1993;4(5):305-9.
55. Stanley MW, Skoog L, Tani EM, Horwitz CA. Nodular fasciitis: spontaneous resolution following diagnosis by fine-needle aspiration. Diagn Cytopathol 1993;9(3):322-4.
56. Samaratunga H, Searle J, O'Loughlin B. Nodular fasciitis and related pseudosarcomatous lesions of soft tissues. Aust N Z J Surg 1996;66(1):22-5.
57. Plaza JA, Mayerson J, Wakely Jr PE. Nodular fasciitis of the hand: a potential diagnostic pitfall in fine-needle aspiration cytopathology. Am J Clin Pathol 2005;123(3):388-93.
58. Layfield LJ, Crim J, Gupta D. Fine-needle aspiration findings in nodular myositis: a case report. Diagn Cytopathol 2000;23(5):343-7.
59. Meis JM, Enzinger FM. Proliferative fasciitis and myositis of childhood. Am J Surg Pathol 1992;16(4):364-72.
60. Raab SS, Silverman JF, McLeod DL, Benning TL, Geisinger KR. Fine needle aspiration biopsy of fibromatoses. Acta Cytol 1993;37(3):323-8.
61. Lopez-Ferrer P, Jimenez-Heffernan JA, Vicandi B, Ortega L, Viguer JM. Fine-needle aspiration cytology of mammary fibromatosis: report of two cases. Diagn Cytopathol 1997;17(5):363-8.
62. Klijanienko J, Caillaud JM, Lagace R. Fine-needle aspiration of primary and recurrent benign fibrous histiocytoma: classic, aneurysmal, and myxoid variants. Diagn Cytopathol 2004;31(6):387-91.
63. Ng WK, Chiu CS, Han KC, Chow JC. Mammary pseudoangiomatous stromal hyperplasia. A reappraisal of the fine needle aspiration cytology findings. Acta Cytol 2003;47(3):373-80.
64. Yong M, Raza AS, Greaves TS, Cobb CJ. Fine-needle aspiration of a pleomorphic lipoma of the head and neck: a case report. Diagn Cytopathol 2005;32(2):110-3.
65. Thirumala S, Desai M, Kannan V. Diagnostic pitfalls in fine needle aspiration cytology of pleomorphic lipoma. A case report. Acta Cytol 2000;44(4):653-6.
66. Woyke S, Kapila K, Goswami KC. Atypical lipoma as a potential pitfall in the cytodiagnosis of subcutaneous tumors. A report of two cases. Acta Cytol 1997;41(3):897-902.
67. Einarsdottir H, Skoog L, Soderlund V, Bauer HC. Accuracy of cytology for diagnosis of lipomatous tumors: comparison with magnetic resonance and computed tomography findings in 175 cases. Acta Radiol 2004;45(8):840-6.
68. Domanski HA, Carlen B, Jonsson K, Mertens F, Akerman M. Distinct cytologic features of spindle cell lipoma. A cytologic-histologic study with clinical, radiologic, electron microscopic, and cytogenetic correlations. Cancer 2001;93(6):381-9.
69. Liu K, Layfield LJ. Cytomorphologic features of angiosarcoma on fine needle aspiration biopsy. Acta Cytol 1999;43(3):407-15.
70. Domanski HA. Cytologic features of angioleiomyoma: cytologic-histologic study of 10 cases. Diagn Cytopathol 2002;27(3):161-6.
71. Tai LH, Johnston JO, Klein HZ, Rowland J, Sudilovsky D. Calcifying aponeurotic fibroma features seen on fine-needle aspiration biopsy: case report and brief review of the literature. Diagn Cytopathol 2001;24(5):336-9.
72. Domanski HA. Fine-needle aspiration smears from lipomatous hemangiopericytoma need not be confused with myxoid liposarcoma. Diagn Cytopathol 2003;29(5):287-91.
73. Fisher C. Low-grade sarcomas with CD34-positive fibroblasts and low-grade myofibroblastic sarcomas. Ultrastruct Pathol 2004;28(5-6):291-305.
74. Filipowicz EA, Ventura KC, Pou AM, Logrono R. FNAC in the diagnosis of recurrent dermatofibrosarcoma protuberans of the forehead. A case report. Acta Cytol 1999;43(6):1177-80.
75. Klijanienko J, Caillaud JM, Lagace R. Fine-needle aspiration of primary and recurrent dermatofibrosarcoma protuberans. Diagn Cytopathol 2004;30(4):261-5.
76. Kocjan G, Sams V, Davidson T. Dermatofibrosarcoma protuberans as a diagnostic pitfall in fine-needle aspiration diagnosis of angiosarcoma of the breast. Diagn Cytopathol 1996;14(1):94-5.
77. Chhieng D, Cohen JM, Waisman J, Fernandez G, Cangiarella J. Fine-needle aspiration cytology of hemangiopericytoma: A report of five cases. Cancer 1999;87(4):190-5.
78. Geisinger KR, Silverman JF, Cappellari JO, Dabbs DJ. Fine-needle aspiration cytology of malignant hemangiopericytomas with ultrastructural and flow cytometric analyses. Arch Pathol Lab Med 1990;114(7):705-10.
79. Pohar-Marinsek Z, Flezar M, Lamovec J. Acral myxoinflammatory fibroblastic sarcoma in FNAB samples: can we distinguish it from other myxoid lesions? Cytopathology 2003;14(2):73-8.
80. Wakely P, Jr., Frable WJ, Kneisl JS. Soft tissue aspiration cytopathology of malignant lymphoma and leukemia. Cancer 2001;93(1):35-9.
81. Cardillo M, Zakowski MF, Lin O. Fine-needle aspiration of epithelioid sarcoma: cytology findings in nine cases. Cancer 2001;93(4):246-51.
82. Zeppa P, Errico ME, Palombini L. Epithelioid sarcoma: report of two cases diagnosed by fine-needle aspiration biopsy with immunocytochemical correlation. Diagn Cytopathol 1999;21(6):405-8.
83. Pohar-Marinsek Z, Zidar A. Epithelioid sarcoma in FNAB smears. Diagn Cytopathol 1994;11(4):367-72.
84. Kitagawa Y, Ito H, Sawaizumi T, Matsubara M, Yokoyama M, Naito Z, et al. Fine needle aspiration cytology of primary epithelioid sarcoma. A report of 2 cases. Acta Cytol 2004;48(3):391-6.

85. Khirwadkar N, Dey P, Das A, Gupta SK. Fine-needle aspiration biopsy of metastatic soft-tissue sarcomas to lymph nodes. Diagn Cytopathol 2001;24(4):229-32.
86. Nemanqani D, Mourad WA. Cytomorphologic features of fine-needle aspiration of liposarcoma. Diagn Cytopathol 1999;20(2):67-9.
87. Dey P. Fine needle aspiration cytology of well-differentiated liposarcoma. A report of two cases. Acta Cytol 2000;44(3):459-62.
88. Machhi J, Kouzova M, Komorowski DJ, Asma Z, Chivukala M, Basir Z, et al. Crystals of alveolar soft part sarcoma in a fine needle aspiration biopsy cytology smear. A case report. Acta Cytol 2002;46(5):904-8.
89. Shabb N, Sneige N, Fanning CV, Dekmezian R. Fine-needle aspiration cytology of alveolar soft-part sarcoma. Diagn Cytopathol 1991;7(3):293-8.
90. Mullick SS, Mody DR, Schwartz MR. Angiosarcoma at unusual sites. A report of two cases with aspiration cytology and diagnostic pitfalls. Acta Cytol 1997;41(3):839-44.
91. Klijanienko J, Caillaud JM, Lagace R, Vielh P. Cytohistologic correlations in angiosarcoma including classic and epithelioid variants: Institut Curie's experience. Diagn Cytopathol 2003;29(3):140-5.
92. Jeon YK, Kim HW, Choi HJ, Park IA. Fine needle aspiration cytology of epithelioid angiosarcoma. Report of a case with nuclear grooves and indentations. Acta Cytol 2004;48(2):223-8.
93. Carson KF, Hirschowitz SL, Nieberg RK, Sadeghi S. Pitfalls in the cytologic diagnosis of angiosarcoma of the breast by fine-needle aspiration: a case report. Diagn Cytopathol 1994;11(3):297-9; discussion 299-300.
94. Hales M, Bottles K, Miller T, Donegan E, Ljung BM. Diagnosis of Kaposi's sarcoma by fine-needle aspiration biopsy. Am J Clin Pathol 1987;88(1):20-5.
95. Tong TR, Chow TC, Chan OW, Lee KC, Yeung SH, Lam A, et al. Clear-cell sarcoma diagnosis by fine-needle aspiration: cytologic, histologic, and ultrastructural features; potential pitfalls; and literature review. Diagn Cytopathol 2002;26(3):174-80.
96. Creager AJ, Pitman MB, Geisinger KR. Cytologic features of clear cell sarcoma (malignant melanoma) of soft parts: a study of fine-needle aspirates and exfoliative specimens. Am J Clin Pathol 2002;117(2):217-24.
97. Jayaram G, Kapoor R, Saha MM. Hemangioendothelioma. Cytologic appearances in two cases presenting with multiple soft tissue and bone lesions. Acta Cytol 1987;31(4):497-501.
98. Maitra A, Timmons CF, Siddiqui MT, Saboorian MH. Fine-needle aspiration biopsy features in a case of giant cell fibroblastoma of the chest wall. Arch Pathol Lab Med 2001;125(8):1091-4.
99. Atahan S, Aksu O, Ekinci C. Cytologic diagnosis and subtyping of rhabdomyosarcoma. Cytopathology 1998;9(6):389-97.
100. Akhtar M, Ali MA, Bakry M, Hug M, Sackey K. Fine-needle aspiration biopsy diagnosis of rhabdomyosarcoma: cytologic, histologic, and ultrastructural correlations. Diagn Cytopathol 1992;8(5):465-74.
101. Pohar-Marinsek Z, Anzic J, Jereb B. Topical topic: value of fine needle aspiration biopsy in childhood rhabdomyosarcoma: twenty-six years of experience in Slovenia. Med Pediatr Oncol 2002;38(6):416-20.
102. Pohar-Marinsek Z, Bracko M. Rhabdomyosarcoma. Cytomorphology, subtyping and differential diagnostic dilemmas. Acta Cytol 2000;44(4):524-32.
103. Pohar-Marinsek Z, Srebotnik-Kirbis I. Desmin detection in FNAB samples of rhabdomyosarcoma: an immunocytochemical study. Cytopathology 2000;11(3):171-8.
104. Akerman M, Ryd W, Skytting B. Fine-needle aspiration of synovial sarcoma: criteria for diagnosis: retrospective reexamination of 37 cases, including ancillary diagnostics. A Scandinavian Sarcoma Group study. Diagn Cytopathol 2003;28(5):232-8.
105. Akerman M, Willen H, Carlen B, Mandahl N, Mertens F. Fine needle aspiration (FNA) of synovial sarcoma--a comparative histological-cytological study of 15 cases, including immunohistochemical, electron microscopic and cytogenetic examination and DNA-ploidy analysis. Cytopathology 1996;7(3):187-200.
106. Klijanienko J, Caillaud JM, Lagace R, Vielh P. Cytohistologic correlations in 56 synovial sarcomas in 36 patients: the Institut Curie experience. Diagn Cytopathol 2002;27(2):96-102.
107. Hummel P, Yang GC, Kumar A, Cohen JM, Winkler B, Melamed J, et al. PNET-like features of synovial sarcoma of the lung: a pitfall in the cytologic diagnosis of soft-tissue tumors. Diagn Cytopathol 2001;24(4):283-8.
108. Ewing CA, Zakowski MF, Lin O. Monophasic synovial sarcoma: a cytologic spectrum. Diagn Cytopathol 2004;30(1):19-23.
109. Saboorian MH, Ashfaq R, Vandersteenhoven JJ, Schneider NR. Cytogenetics as an adjunct in establishing a definitive diagnosis of synovial sarcoma by fine-needle aspiration. Cancer 1997;81(3):187-92.

Chapter 9

Diagnostic Dilemmas in FNAC Cytology: Difficult Breast Lesions

Contents

9.1	Fibroadenoma	182
9.2	Papillary Lesions	188
9.3	Apocrine Changes	193
9.4	Mucinous Lesions	195
9.5	Lobular Carcinoma	196
9.6	In Situ or Invasive Carcinoma?	198
9.7	Rare Lesions	202
9.7.1	Radial Scar/Complex Sclerosing Lesion	202
9.7.2	Collagenous Spherulosis	203
9.7.2	Ductal Adenoma	203
9.7.3	Gynaecomastia	203
9.7.5	Spindle-Cell and Mesenchymal Lesions of the Breast	204
9.7.6	Pseudoangiomatous Stromal Hyperplasia	205
9.7.7	Metaplastic Tumours	205
9.7.8	Secretory Carcinoma	205
9.7.9	Tumoral Calcinosis	205
9.7.10	Clear-Cell Hidradenoma	206
9.7.11	Tubular Adenoma	206
9.7.12	Adenomyoepithelioma	206
9.7.13	Squamous Cells	206
9.8	FNAC or core biopsy?	207
9.9	Radiation Changes	207
	References	207

FNAC forms part of the triple assessment of breast lesions. The NHS Breast-Screening Programme (NHSBSP) established guidelines for the reporting of cytological material from FNAC breast along these lines, recommending the use of five reporting categories for breast cytology: C1, unsatisfactory; C2, benign; C3, suspicious - probably benign; C4, suspicious - probably malignant; C5, malignant [1]. In 1996, the National Cancer Institute (NCI) also recommended five categories for the diagnosis of breast FNAC: benign, atypical, suspicious, malignant and unsatisfactory [2]. Application of the NHSBSP and NCI-supported diagnostic categories to FNAC of palpable and non-palpable breast lesions is useful in stratifying aspirates based on the likelihood of underlying malignancy. The subcategories diagnosed as atypical have similar probabilities of malignancy; this justifies their being grouped as a single category wherein tissue biopsy would be required to exclude carcinoma. Benign and inadequate FNAC diagnoses must be correlated with the clinical and imaging findings and in non-correlative cases the patient should undergo biopsy. FNAC is a sensitive and specific means with which to diagnose non-palpable breast lesions [3]. The evaluation of cytological criteria used to differentiate benign from malignant lesions (i.e. cellularity, loss of cohesion, myoepithelial cells, nuclear enlargement, nuclear overlap, prominent nucleoli) reveals significant overlap between benign and malignant cases, particularly in cases of fibroadenoma, tubular adenoma and proliferative breast disease [4].

Despite some of the shortcomings of the reporting categories described above, their constant use in daily practice has proved their value in describing the findings most accurately, if not always most helpfully. The latter relates to a grey zone that exists in FNAC of breast in cases where an unequivocal diagnosis cannot be made [5]. Instead, the categories of atypia probably benign (C3) and suspicious of malignancy (C4) provide a strategy for the classification of problematic or uncertain cases; this maintains the predictive value of the benign (C2) and malignant (C5) categories and allows separation of these difficult cases into clinically useful groups with differing probabilities of malignancy [6–11].

Deb et al. have audited the frequency of use and outcome of the equivocal/atypia probably benign (C3) and suspicious of malignancy (C4) categories for breast FNAC, according to the five categories of the NHSBSP guidelines for cytology reporting, 1992 [1, 6]. They found that 3.7% and 3.9% of cases were classified as equivocal (C3) and suspicious (C4), respectively, giving a total rate (C3+C4) of 7.6% [6]. Of the C3 cases, 68% were subsequently found to be benign and 32% were malignant. Of the C4 cases, 19% were subsequently benign and 81% malignant. The commonest benign lesions in both categories were fibroadenoma (7.6% of C3 and 19.8% of C4), fibrocystic change (14.3% of C3 and 12.5% of C4), radial scars (6.2% of C3 and 10.4% of C4) and papilloma (6.2% of C3 and 6.3% of C4). Of the malignant lesions (particularly those classified as C3), a high proportion were low-grade or special-type cancers. Similar findings were found by other centres. Kanoush et al. found 6% of cases to be cytologically atypical or suspicious. Of those, 52% yielded malignant findings on histology. Among the suspicious aspirates, 83% were ultimately diagnosed as malignant on histology [12]. Other authors also report a variable rate of cytologically atypical and suspicious smears, ranging from 6.9 to 20% [5, 13–15].

The causes of the equivocal diagnoses can be divided into three categories: (1) the inexperience of the aspirator, whereby the smears are either markedly limited in cellularity or obscured by blood and/or drying artefact; (2) inexperience of the pathologist, which includes cases that may be reclassified by the reviewing cytopathologist as benign or malignant; (3) the overlap of cytological features of benign and malignant lesions due to the nature of the lesion, justifying a biopsy [5]. FNAC of the breast accounted for 6% of surgical pathology and FNAC legal claims reviewed between 1995 and 1997. The majority of these claims were for false-negative breast FNAC resulting from sampling errors in women with a palpable breast mass [16]. Al Kaisi found that the true grey zone in breast cytology, accounted for 2% of all cases [5]. In this chapter, we shall concentrate on this grey zone and describe some of the more common areas of diagnostic dilemmas in breast FNAC.

9.1 Fibroadenoma

Fibroadenoma is a common benign breast lesion that is frequently sampled by FNAC. Although the cytological diagnosis is straightforward in most cases, cellular discohesion and atypia in fibroadenomas is common (27%) and may lead to falsely atypical or positive FNAC diagnoses [17]. Conversely, some adenocarcinomas mimic a fibroadenomatous pattern on FNAC, resulting in a false-negative diagnosis. Fibroadenomas constitute the largest single cause of equivocal diagnoses and the largest single cause of false-positive and false-negative diagnoses [18]. Fibroadenoma cytology may be highly cellular, showing marked discohesiveness and occasional nuclear atypia and prominent nucleoli (Fig. 9.1). It is sometimes composed of bland-appearing spindle/columnar cells that could represent either epithelial or stromal cells, mimicking a papillary carcinoma on ThinPrep samples [19] (Fig. 9.2). Simsir et al. analysed the spectrum of changes causing under- or overdiagnosis in atypical fibroadenomas [20]. The smears were assessed for cellularity, cellular discohesion, presence of dissociated intact cells and nucleoli, nuclear pleomorphism, oval bare nuclei and stromal fragments (Fig. 9.3). At excision, 88% of fibroadenomas classified as atypical on FNAC, were benign (fibroadenoma with ductal hyperplasia and lactational change, myxoid fibroadenoma, and other fibroepithelial lesions; Fig. 9.4). Differentiating between myxoid fibroadenoma and colloid carcinoma was difficult due to the abundance of extracellular mucin in which the dissociated epithelial cells were floating (Fig. 9.5). On excision, it was found that 8% of cases were carcinomas; the reasons for underdiagnosis were sampling and interpretative error, as discussed above (Fig. 9.6). The majority of fibroadenomas with atypia on FNAC are benign lesions (Fig. 9.7). Considering the grave consequences of a false-positive cytological diagnosis, it is wise to adopt a conservative approach in interpreting FNAC smears that overall display a fibroadenomatous pattern. Immunocytochemistry may be helpful to clarify whether the cells are epithelial or stromal in origin. At least occasional bipolar stromal cells may be seen in the background. The only appreciable difference between the benign and malignant conditions in these cases is a more significant nuclear atypia, which is barely discernible in the malignant cases. Closely associated pairs of stripped bipolar nuclei were found in 68% of benign lesions compared with only 3.8% of carcinomas, establishing their presence as a highly specific indicator of a benign process [21] (Fig. 9.8).

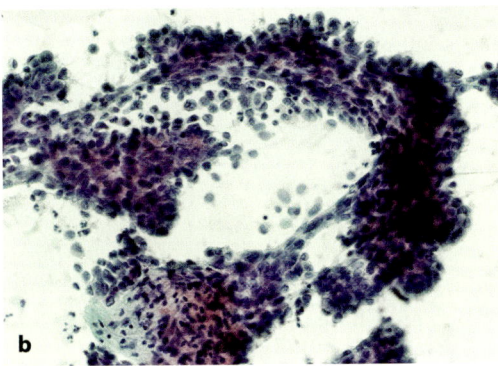

Fig. 9.2
FNAC breast. Fibroadenoma and a lookalike. **a** Sometimes samples are composed of bland-appearing spindle/columnar cells that could represent either epithelial or stromal cells, mimicking a papillary carcinoma. **b** Papillary carcinoma with dissociated cells and fibrovascular stalks

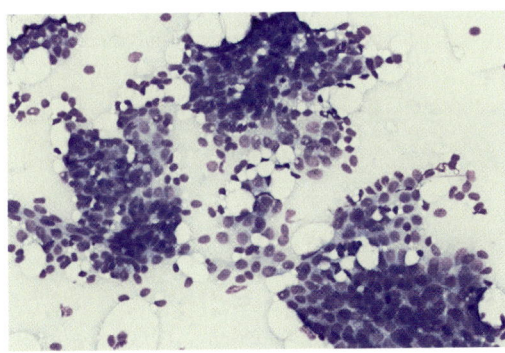

Fig. 9.1
FNAC breast. Fibroadenoma pitfall. Cytology preparations may be highly cellular showing marked discohesiveness

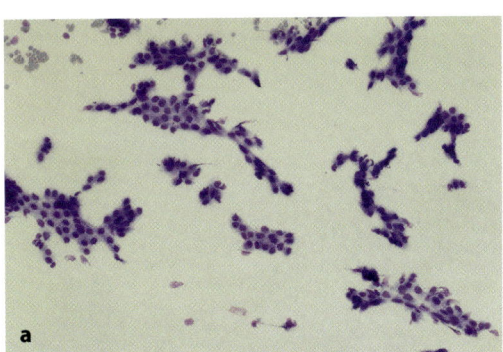

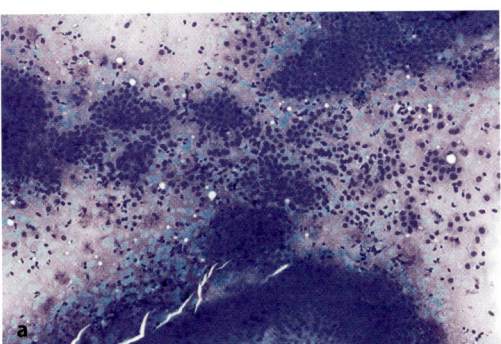

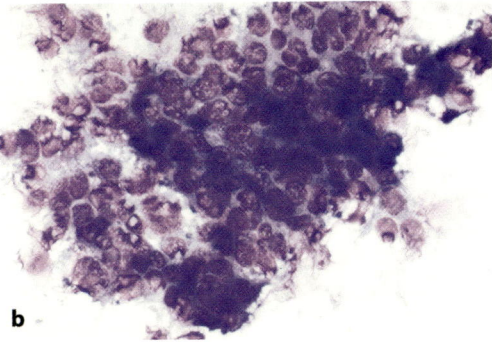

Fig. 9.3
FNAC breast. Preparation artefacts in fibroadenoma. **a** Cell discohesion and apparent lack of stromal and myoepithelial cells may be caused by preparation artefact and interpreted as malignant. **b** Air-drying may cause cell distortion and apparent coarseness of chromatin

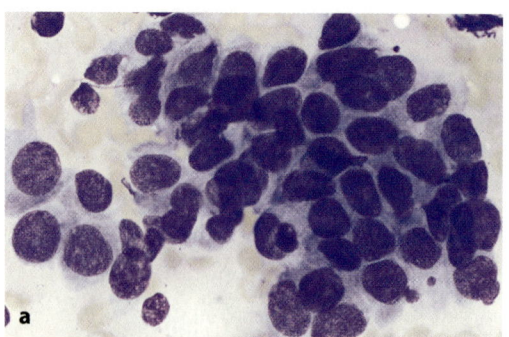

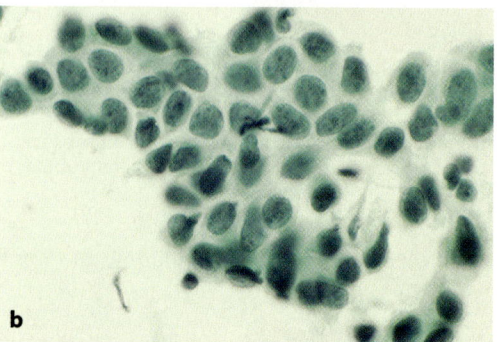

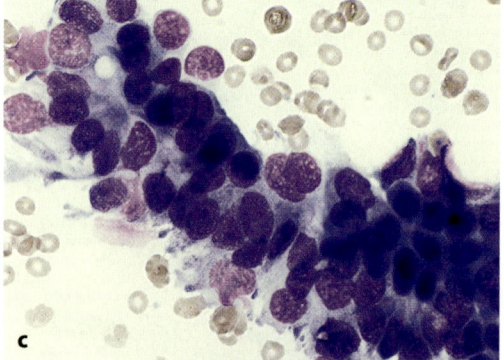

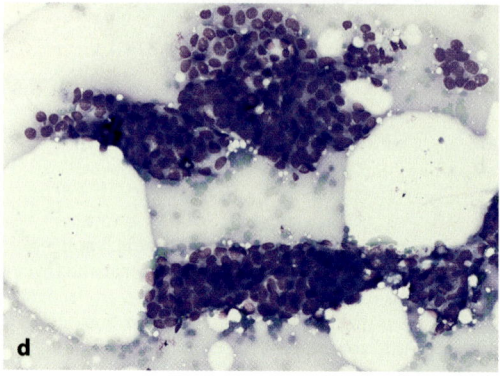

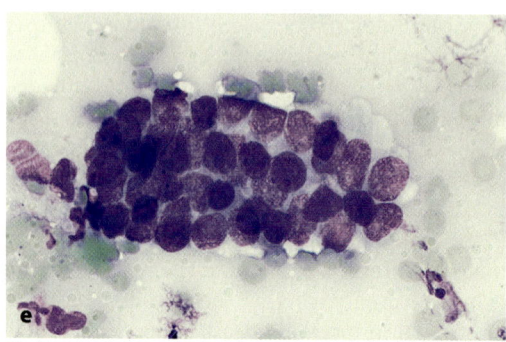

Fig. 9.4
FNAC breast. Fibroadenoma. Pregnancy and hormone-replacement therapy (HRT) may cause considerable epithelial hyperplasia in a fibroadenoma. **a** Nuclear enlargement, overlapping and crowding of epithelial cells. The myoepithelium is difficult to appreciate. Some cell dissociation at the edges of the cluster. **b** Same case. In other areas, myoepithelial cells are present but contribute to the apparent nuclear pleomorphism. Stromal cells are very few. **c** A 64-year-old patient on HRT. Striking epithelial hyperplasia, which may be mistaken for carcinoma. **d** Low-grade ductal carcinoma mimicking fibroadenoma. **e** Same case, high-power view revealing myoepithelial cells associated with the ductal epithelium

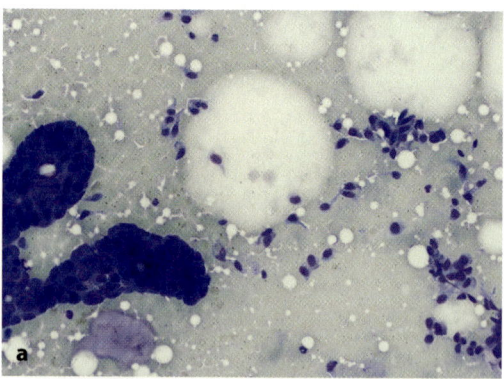

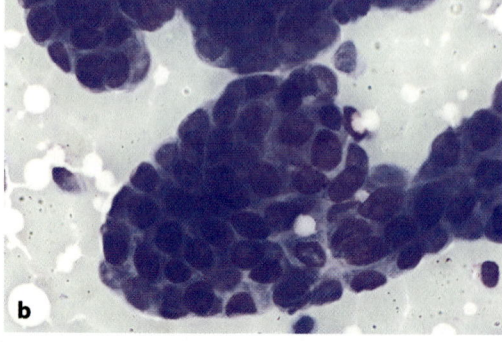

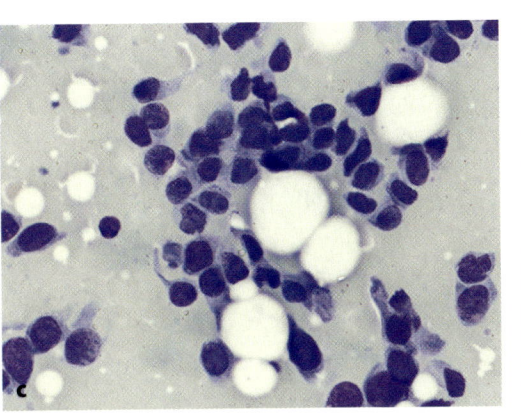
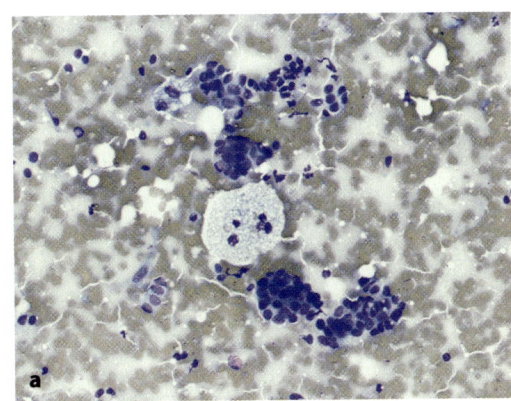
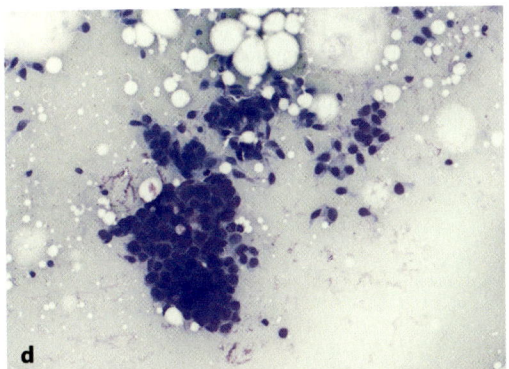
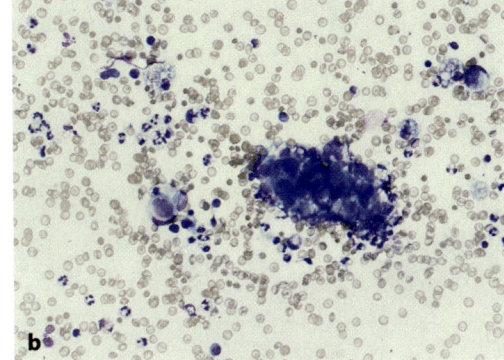
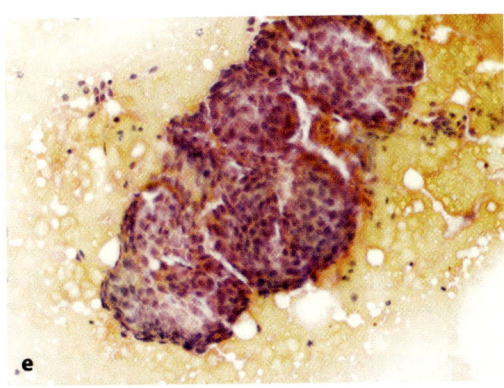
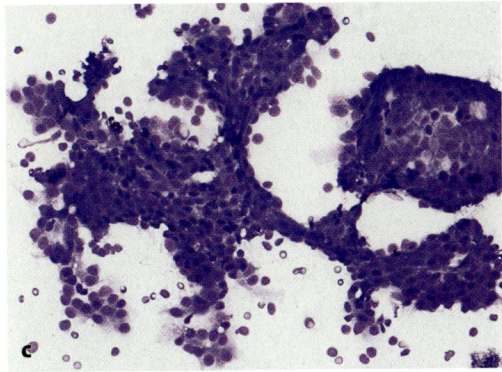

Fig. 9.5
FNAC breast. Diagnostic pitfall: mucinous carcinoma.
a Differentiating myxoid fibroadenoma from colloid carcinoma is difficult due to the abundance of extracellular mucin in which the dissociated epithelial cells are floating. **b** Epithelium of mucinous carcinoma may mimic the "staghorn" projections of fibroadenoma. **c** Dissociated epithelial cells should not be mistaken for stromal cells. **d** Low-power view may mimic that of fibroadenoma. **e** Pap stain of mucinous carcinoma may mimic fibroadenoma

Fig. 9.6
FNAC breast. Fibroadenoma and lookalikes. **a** Cystic change is not uncommon in fibroadenoma and may cause some rounding of the cytoplasmic edges in the clusters that are still monolayered. **b** Papillary carcinoma shows cystic and inflammatory background and three-dimensional cell clusters. **c** Tubular carcinoma may mimic architecture of fibroadenoma

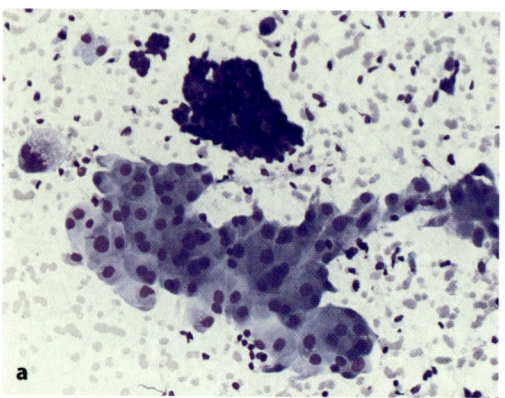

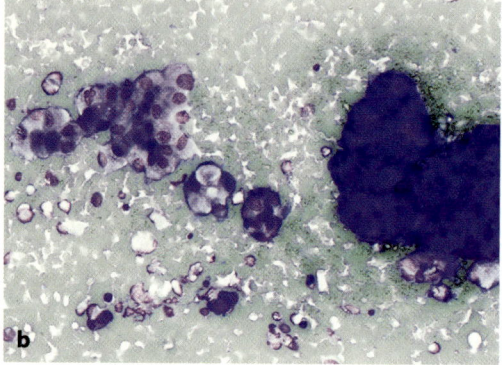

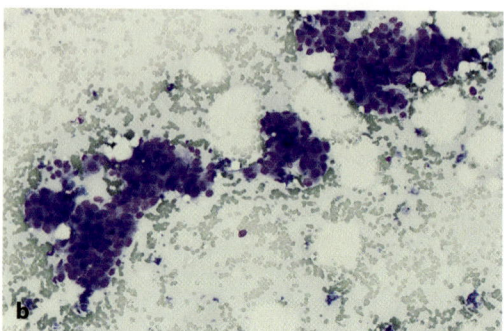

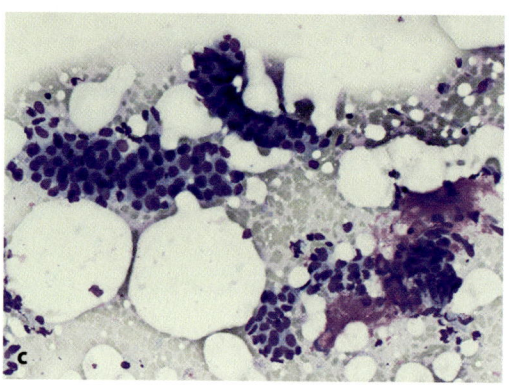

Fig. 9.7
FNAC breast. Apocrine change. **a** In most cases apocrine changes does not cause diagnostic difficulties. **b** Sometimes, apocrine changes may be misinterpreted as atypical hyperplasia or malignancy. This is particularly the case when clusters of apocrine cells appear three-dimensional

Fig. 9.8
FNAC breast. Invasive ductal carcinoma. **a** Tightly cohesive clusters with apparent bipolar nuclei in the background. The only appreciable difference between the benign and malignant conditions in these cases is a more significant nuclear atypia, which is barely discernible, in the malignant cases. Closely associated pairs of stripped bipolar nuclei were found in 68% of benign lesions compared with only 3.8% of carcinomas, establishing their presence as a highly specific indicator of a benign process. **b** Same case, different area shows cellular pleomorphism suggestive of malignancy. Clusters are still cohesive and there are further bare nuclei in the background. **c** Low-grade ductal carcinoma mimicking fibroadenoma

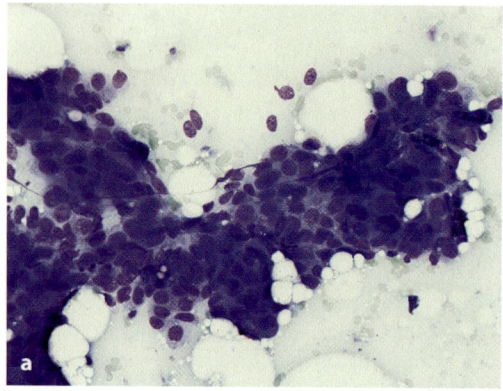

The differential diagnosis of fibroadenoma vs. phyllodes tumour (PT) by FNAC is not possible in the majority of cases. Cytological diagnosis of PT remains difficult, with significant overlap with fibroadenoma. PT are clinically significantly larger than fibroadenomas. Distinguishing criteria are: larger stromal fragments, numerous plump stromal bare nuclei and the higher ratio of stromal bare nuclei to epithelial bare nuclei in PT [22]. By applying these criteria, Veneti and Manek were able to improve the diagnosis of PT from the initial 38.9% to 83.3% of all cases [22]. However, hypercellular stromal fragments occur not only in PT, but also in fibroadenoma, and hence they cannot be used as the sole criterion for making a diagnosis (Fig. 9.9). The proportion of individual long spindle nuclei (>30%) amid the dispersed stromal cells in the background is another possible discriminator between the two lesions. Lesions in which long spindle nuclei constitute between 10% and 30% may represent either PT or fibroadenoma, and therefore such lesions should be categorised as indeterminate on FNAC [23]. Single columnar stromal cells with recognisable cytoplasm and multinucleated stromal giant cells are seen in some PT but not in fibroadenoma. The presence of hypercellular stromal fragments is the most useful feature in distinguishing PTs from fibroadenomas, and the presence of cytological atypia of the stromal cells was the most important feature in distinguishing malignant from benign PTs. Sampling error is the most common reason for cytological misdiagnosis of PTs. Scoyler et al. recommend that if hypercellular stromal fragments are identified in an FNAC specimen of a fibroepithelial lesion, the cytopathologist should raise the possibility of a PT and the surgeon treat the patient accordingly [24].

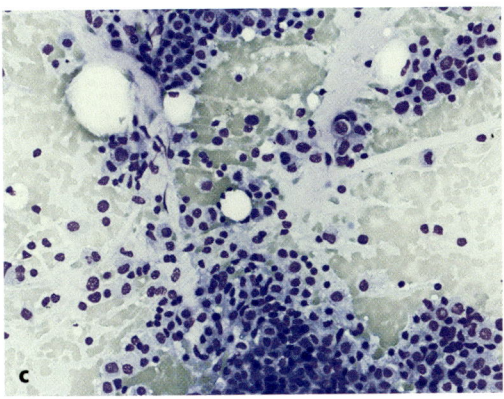

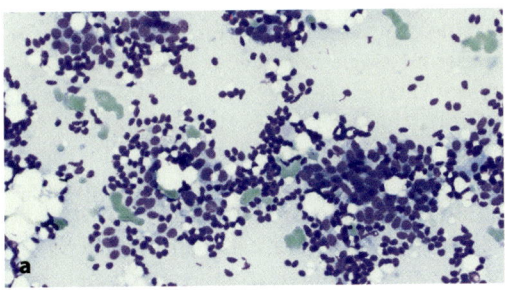

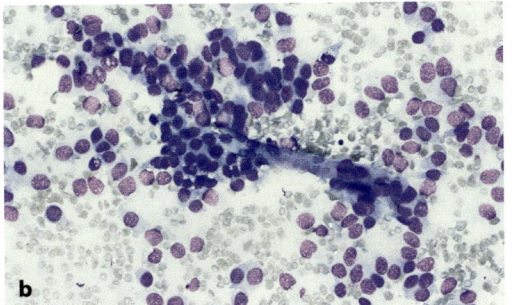

Fig. 9.9
FNAC breast. Stroma and lookalikes. **a** Fibroadenoma with some epithelial discohesion and a very cellular stroma. **b** Ductal carcinoma with marked discohesion and bare nuclei of epithelial cells that may mimic stromal cells. **c** Mucinous carcinoma shows a monotonous population of epithelial cells in a background of mucin, both of which may be mistaken for a fibroadenoma

Cytological diagnosis of PT remains difficult. The presence of large size, low epithelial/stromal ratio, epithelial atypia, columnar stromal cells with visible cytoplasm and stromal giant cells favours a diagnosis of PT over fibroadenoma [25] (Figs. 9.10 and 9.11). Some histologically benign tumors may be misdiagnosed as carcinoma. Possible reasons for overdiagnosis include: high cellularity of the smears, the presence of atypical ductal hyperplasia, paucity of the stromal component in the aspirates and occasional dissociation of epithelial cells [26]. Deen et al. found no differences in the glandular elements, the myoepithelial and single stromal cells, and the type of stromal fragments seen in the three benign groups [27]. The stromal nuclei, the number of leaf-shaped fragments and the numbers of spindle-cell groups present showed a spectrum of changes varying from those of fibroadenomas at one end to those of benign PT at the other. Malignant PT has characteristic features that are quite different from those of the benign lesions [27].

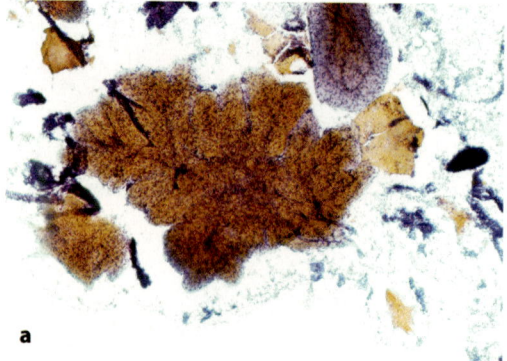

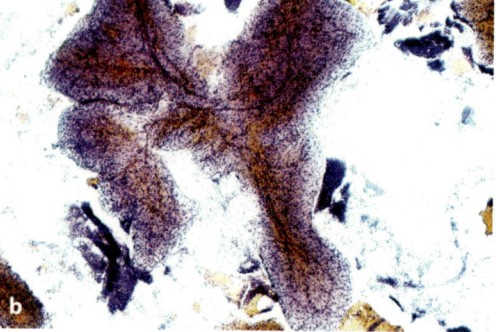

Fig. 9.10
FNAC breast. Fibroadenoma. **a** Large leaf-like stromal fragments suggestive of phyllodes tumour may be seen in a fibroadenoma. **b** Cellular and vascular leaf-like fragments of stroma in an aspirate from a fibroadenoma. The stromal nuclei, the number of leaf-shaped fragments and the numbers of spindle-cell groups present show a spectrum of changes varying from those of fibroadenomas at one end to those of benign phyllodes tumour at the other

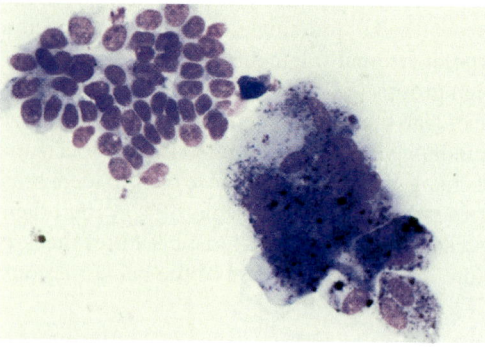

Fig. 9.11
FNAC breast. Fibroadenoma. Multinucleate foreign-body-type giant cells may be seen in fibroadenoma as well as in phyllodes tumour

9.2 Papillary Lesions

Papillary lesions of the breast include a wide spectrum of benign and malignant lesions, all of which may pose diagnostic dilemmas both cytologically and histologically. Cytological features that may be evaluated include cellularity, architecture, apocrine/single/columnar cells, nuclear atypia, intranuclear inclusions, calcifications, background, myoepithelial cells, and bipolar, naked nuclei [28]. Dawson et al. found that the common features of papillary lesions include: increased cellularity, papillary groups and single columnar epithelial cells [29]. Papillary carcinomas are characterised by higher cellularity, more complex papillae with thin disorganised fronds, mild to moderate nuclear atypia, and prominent dissociation with many single papillae and single cells (Fig. 9.12). Fibrovascular cores are more common in papillary carcinoma than intraduct papilloma in which detached fibrous tissue fragments are frequently seen [30]. Apocrine metaplasia is variably present in papilloma, atypical intraduct papilloma and fibroadenoma, but absent in carcinomas (Fig. 9.13). Papillomas may have marked nuclear atypia with background necrosis and inflammation, representing infarcted papillomas, a potential pitfall in the diagnosis of carcinoma. Markedly increased cellularity and numerous single cells favour a diagnosis of papillary carcinoma (Fig. 9.14). More specific diagnostic clues are the FNAC findings of nuclear hyperchromasia, stratification and absence of benign background cells and apocrine metaplasia. In the papilloma there is less material; the papillae have cohesive stalks surrounded by columnar cells in a honeycomb pattern. Apocrine metaplasia and bipolar naked nuclei are also present [31]. Invasive micropapillary carcinoma is a rare variant of infiltrating duct carcinoma. It has a strong tendency for lymphatic spread. Cytological features include: moderate to high cellularity, angulated small groups or clusters of cohesive cells with papillary configurations without fibrovascular cores (morula-like, inside out) and abundant single cells with nuclear atypia and intact cytoplasm in the background (Fig. 9.15) [32]. Neoplastic cells show moderate to high nuclear atypia, irregular nuclear contours and prominent nucleoli. They may cluster in the form of rosette-like microacinar structures without a central space. Psammoma bodies may be present [33].

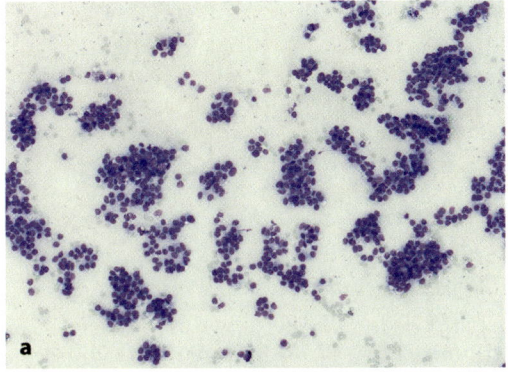

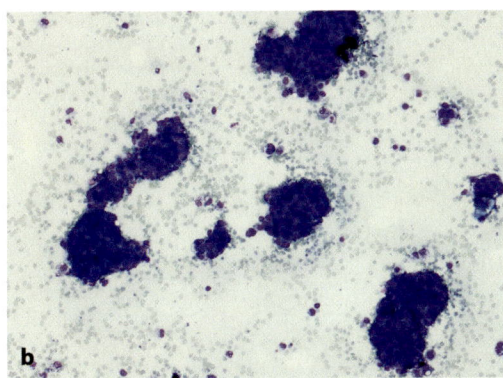

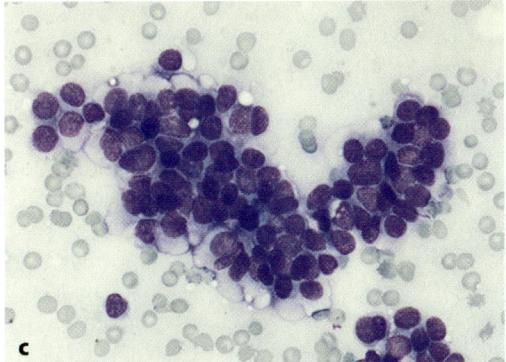

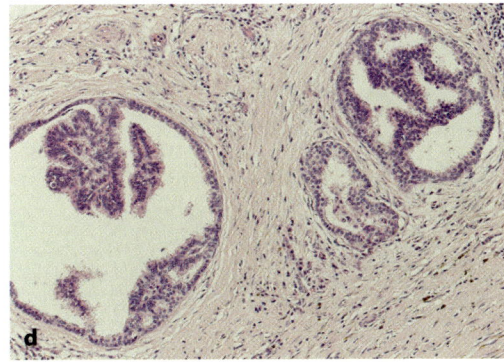

Fig. 9.12
FNAC breast. Papillary lesion. Histology shows papillary carcinoma. **a** Papillary carcinomas are characterised by higher cellularity, more complex papillae with thin disorganised fronds, mild to moderate nuclear atypia and prominent dissociation with many single papillae and single cells. **b** Markedly increased cellularity and numerous single cells favour a diagnosis of papillary carcinoma. **c** Nuclear hyperchromasia, stratification and absence of benign background cells may be helpful in the diagnosis of carcinoma. **d** HLE histology

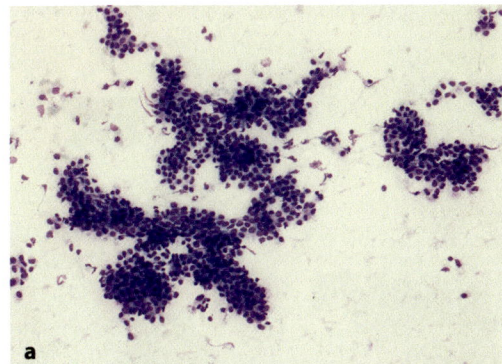

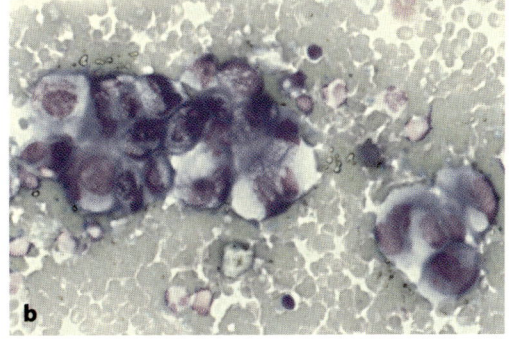

Fig. 9.13
FNAC breast. Papillary lesion. (see next page)

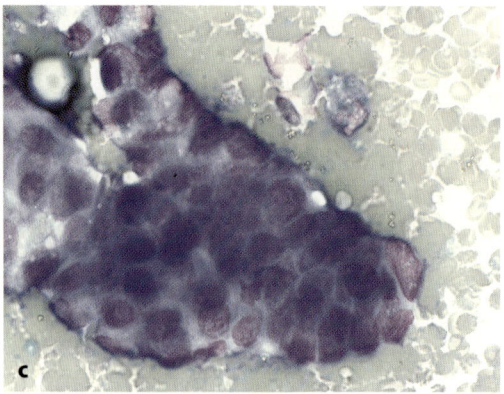

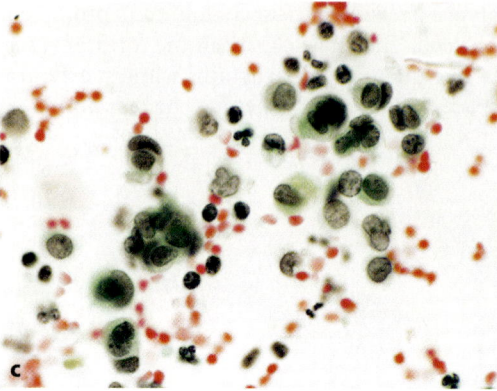

Fig. 9.13
Continued from previous page. FNAC breast. Papillary lesion. **a** Multiple branching clusters in this case of benign papilloma. **b** Apocrine metaplasia is variably present in papilloma, atypical intraduct papilloma and fibroadenoma, but absent in carcinomas. This was a papilloma, reported as suspicious on FNAC. **c** Papillomas may have marked nuclear atypia with background necrosis and inflammation, representing infarcted papillomas, a potential pitfall in the diagnosis of carcinoma.. The papillae have cohesive stalks surrounded by columnar cells in a honeycomb pattern. In this case, histology confirmed a papilloma

Fig. 9.14
FNAC breast. Papillary lesion. **a** Cellular smear with papillary clusters. **b** Some cytological atypia and absence of myoepithelial cells. **c** Inflammatory cells and single epithelial cells in the background. The lesion was reported as a papillary lesion. Histology showed papillary carcinoma. Lesions that fall short of a definitive benign diagnosis should be placed into an indeterminate category. This approach will guide the surgeon to provide better patient management

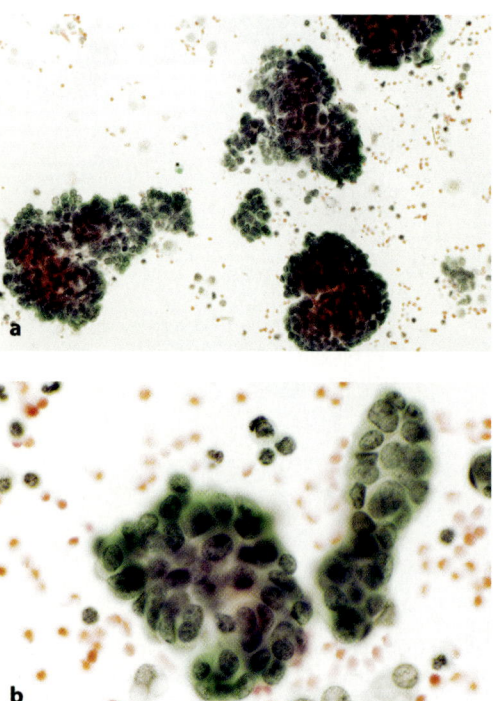

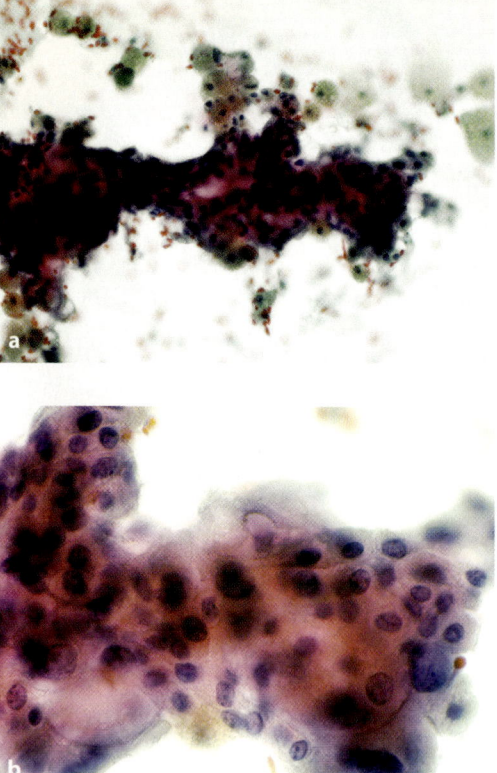

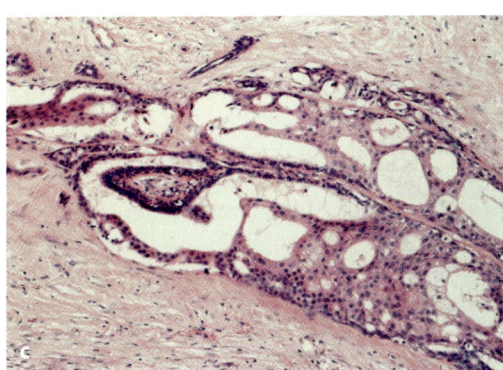

Fig. 9.15
FNAC breast. Papillary lesion. **a** Angulated small groups or clusters of cohesive cells with papillary configurations without fibrovascular cores (morula-like, inside out) and abundant single cells with nuclear atypia and intact cytoplasm in the background. **b** The neoplastic cells show moderate to high nuclear atypia, irregular nuclear contours and prominent nucleoli. They may cluster in the form of rosette-like microacinar structures without a central space. Psammoma bodies may be present.
c Histology of the lesion shows micropapillary ductal carcinoma in situ (DCIS)

A significant portion of lesions displaying a papillary pattern on FNAC are found to be non-papillary on follow-up (Fig. 9.16). They include fibroadenoma (Fig. 9.7b), fibrocystic change, mucinous carcinoma (Fig. 9.5a) and cribriform ductal carcinoma in situ [19, 30](Fig. 9.17). Intraductal papilloma can be distinguished from fibroadenoma by its broad ruffled branches, scalloped borders, and tiny tongue-like projections. True papillae are commonly covered by tall columnar cells. Myoepithelial cells are few in intraduct papilloma but numerous in fibroadenoma. Epithelial fragments in non papillary lesions present as cellular spheres and/or complex sheets with finger-like projections but lack fibrovascular cores and columnar cells [30]. The micropapillary variant of mucinous carcinoma of the breast demonstrates characteristic cytological and histological features that warrant special attention. It may represent the mucinous counterpart of invasive micropapillary carcinoma. FNAC preparations are of moderate cellularity, with cohesive clusters and micropapillae of mildly pleomorphic tumour cells among a mucoid background (Fig. 9.5a). True tumor papillae with fibrovascular cores are absent. Nuclear hobnailing is observed commonly and occasional psammoma bodies may be found. Scanty isolated tumour cells and the pseudoacinar pattern may be appreciated more readily in the cell-block sections [34].

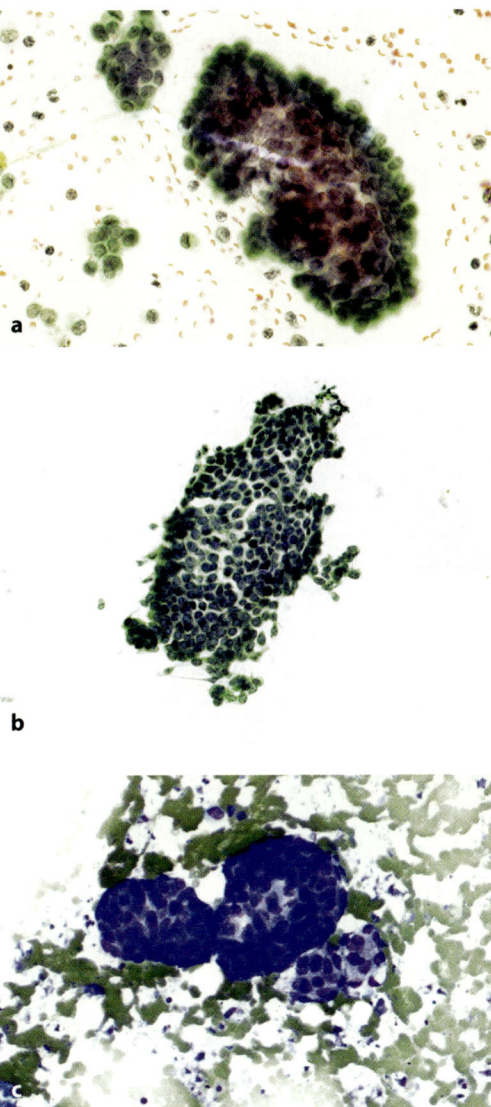

Fig. 9.16
FNAC breast. Papillary lesions. **a** Papilla in papillary carcinoma. **b** The epithelial fragments in non-papillary lesions (here: fibroadenoma) present as cellular spheres and/or complex sheets with finger-like projections, but lack fibrovascular cores and columnar cells. **c** Invasive ductal carcinoma may show micropapillary pattern

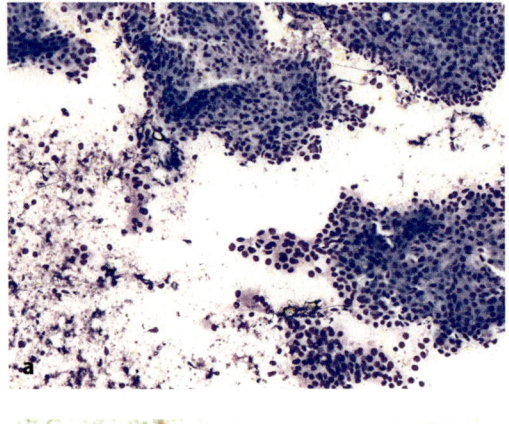

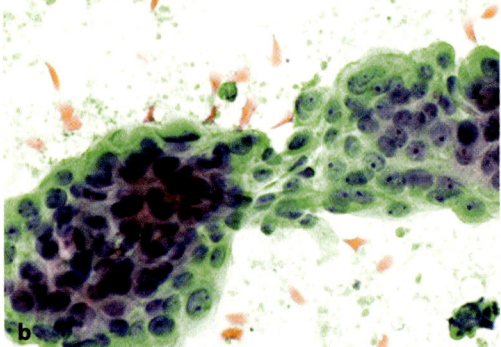

In spite of the overlapping features of true papillary lesions and their cytological look-alikes, the majority can be classified accurately into benign or atypical categories by FNAC. Lesions that fall short of a definitive benign diagnosis should be placed into an indeterminate category. This approach will guide the surgeon to provide better patient management [35]. As to the preference for using core biopsy (CB) in these cases, Masood et al. suggest that both FNAC and CB share similar diagnostic challenges and a follow-up surgical excision is indicated when diagnosis of a papillary lesion is considered by either or both of the procedures [36] (Fig. 9.18).

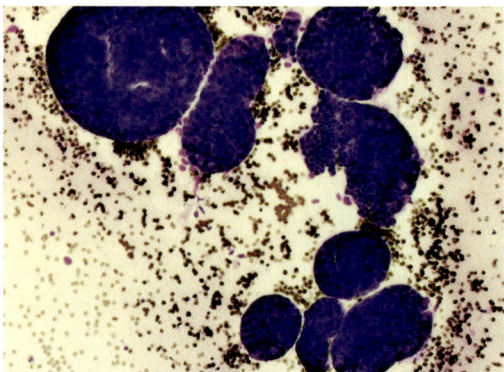

Fig. 9.18
FNAC axillary node. Papillary lesion. Multiple well-outlined three-dimensional clusters of relatively uniform epithelium represent an axillary metastasis of an invasive ductal carcinoma

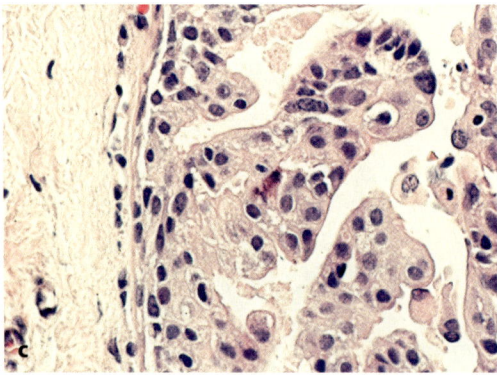

Fig. 9.17
FNAC breast. Cribriform DCIS mimicking papillary lesion. **a** Low-power view showing epithelial aggregates with pseudopapillary projections. **b** Higher-power view showing relatively monotonous epithelium with prominent nucleoli and absent myoepithelial cells. **c** Histology shows cribriform DCIS

Case history 9.1: Patient with a long-term history of bloodstained nipple discharge and a previous biopsy of a benign papillary lesion underwent FNAC for a radiologically suspicious lesion. Magnetic resonance imaging showed an 11-mm mass. CBs, attempted earlier, were negative. Cytology was reported as highly suggestive of papillary carcinoma. At surgery, the surgeon could not find any tumour mass and took multiple biopsy samples (Fig. 9.19).

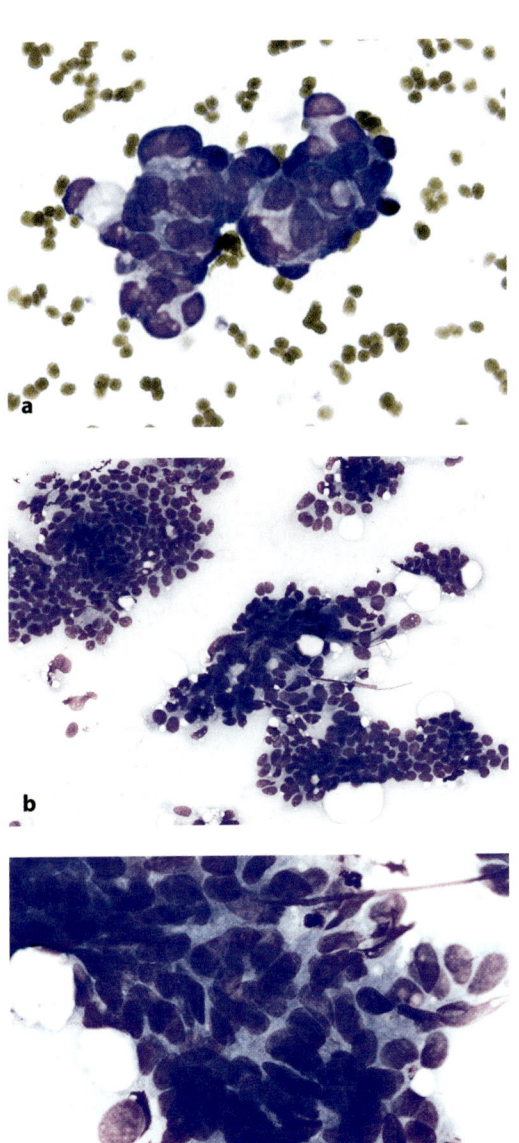

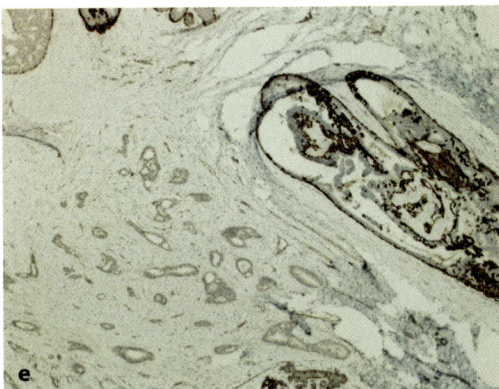

Fig. 9.19
Nipple discharge and FNAC breast. Papillary lesion.
a Papillary cluster of ductal cells in the nipple discharge.
b FNAC: Multiple papillary clusters of duct epithelium, some showing marked overlapping and crowding of the epithelial cells. **c** Higher power view of another cluster with marked cytological atypia suggestive of malignancy. **d** Histology shows papilloma and a tubular carcinoma adjacent to it. **e** CK 5 staining highlights myoepithelial cells present within the papilloma and absent in the adjacent tubular carcinoma

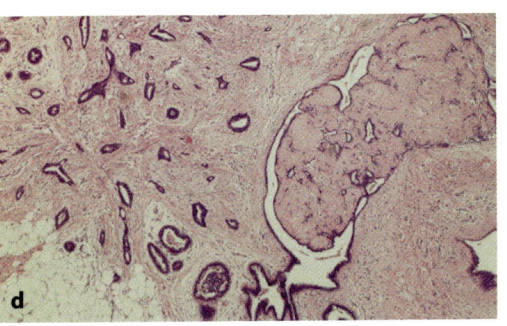

9.3 Apocrine Changes

Apocrine changes are seen in a wide spectrum of breast lesions, ranging from microscopic cysts to invasive carcinoma (Fig. 9.20). Although apocrine change in many cases do not present any diagnostic difficulty, apocrine proliferations demonstrating cytological atypia may be challenging [37]. In particular, distinguishing a low-grade apocrine carcinoma from atypical apocrine metaplasia may be difficult [38] (Fig. 9.21). Clinically, in apocrine carcinoma, the average age of patients (65 years) is more than 20 years older than the average age for apocrine metaplasia. In apocrine carcinoma, FNAC is highly cellular, with apocrine cells occurring singly or in syncytial aggregates. The background contains numerous degenerated apocrine cells and characteristic cell debris. The cells have marked nuclear abnormalities, including hyperchromasia and irregular nuclear shape, frequently with irregular nucleoli; more nuclei measure ≥12 μm in diameter than in atypical apocrine metaplasia

[39]. Histiocytoid carcinoma cells also exhibit apocrine differentiation, as demonstrated by immunocytochemical and in situ hybridisation studies. These tumours can be easily misinterpreted as either fibrohistiocytic or myoblastomatoid (granular cell) tumours [40] (Fig. 9.22).

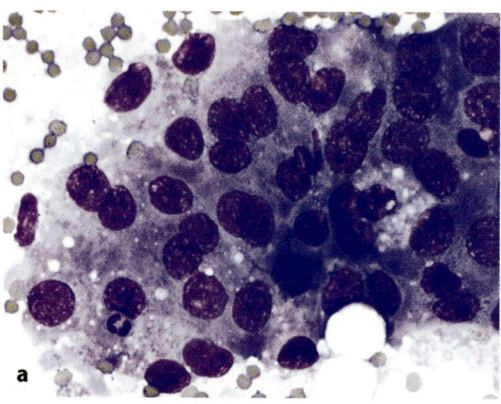

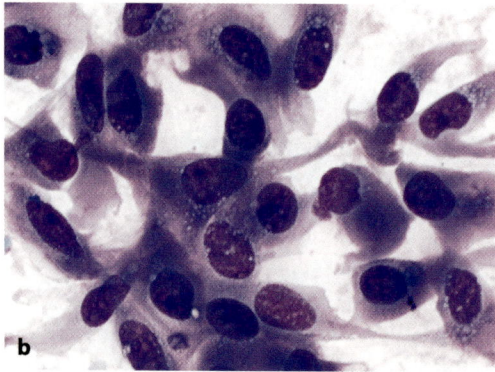

Fig. 9.20
FNAC breast. Apocrine change. **a** High-power view of apocrine change in a benign papilloma. **b** Spindle cell shape of apocrine cells in a benign breast change. Although apocrine change in many cases does not present any diagnostic difficulty, apocrine proliferations demonstrating cytological atypia may be challenging

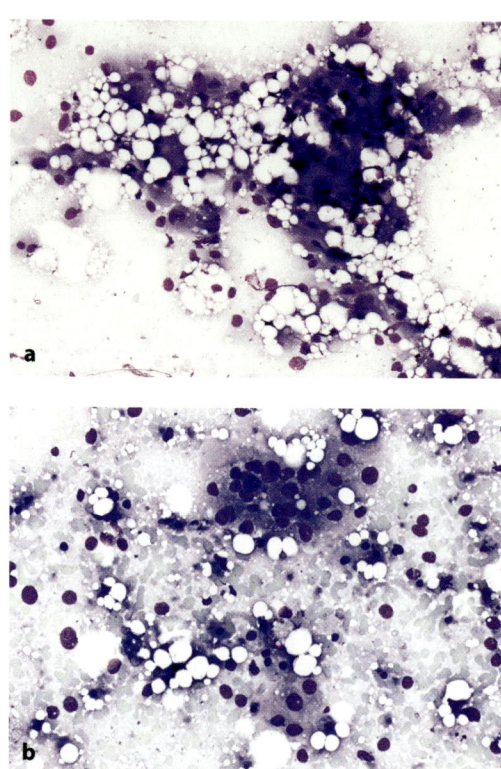

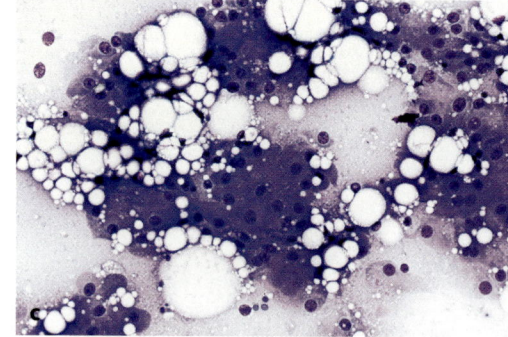

Fig. 9.21
FNAC breast. Apocrine differentiation. **a** Low-grade apocrine carcinoma. FNAC is highly cellular with apocrine cells occurring singly or in syncytial aggregates. The background contains numerous degenerated apocrine cells and characteristic cell debris. The cells have marked nuclear abnormalities, including hyperchromasia and an irregular nuclear shape, frequently with irregular nucleoli; more nuclei measure ≥12 μm in diameter than in atypical apocrine metaplasia. **b** Apocrine carcinoma, different case. **c** Benign apocrine metaplasia in a patient with a history of breast carcinoma in the contralateral breast

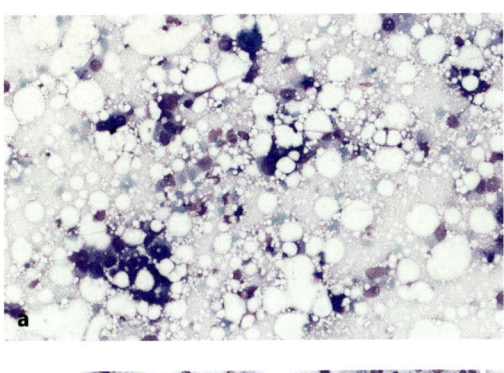
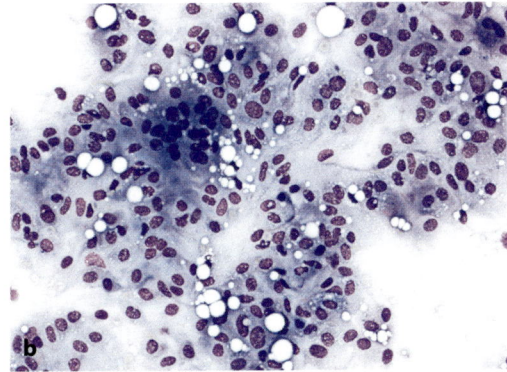

Fig. 9.22
FNAC breast. Histiocytoid appearance. **a** Histiocytoid carcinoma cells also exhibit apocrine differentiation, as demonstrated by immunocytochemical and in situ hybridisation studies. These tumours can be easily misinterpreted as either fibrohistiocytic or myoblastomatoid (granular cell) tumours. **b** Different case. Macrophages and giant cells from fat necrosis

9.4 Mucinous Lesions

Mammary mucinous lesions include mucocoele-like lesions and mucinous carcinoma. In the case of mucocoele-like lesions, patients present with breast lumps and are much younger (mean age 34.8 years) than for mucinous carcinoma (67.9 years) [41]. Radiologically, mucocoele-like lesions have a non-specific mammographic appearance and show a cystic lesion on sonography. However, the mammographic image may sometimes mimic that of ductal carcinoma in situ [42]. Mucinous carcinoma appears as a solid mass on sonography and as a distinct, smoothly outlined nodule or a lobulated mass with only slight irregularities on mammography. Clinically, it may be missed in up to 25% of cases [29]. Histologically, mucocoele-like lesion is characterised by mucinous cysts that may rupture and discharge their contents into the surrounding tissue. The lining epithelium is bland and epithelial cells are rare in the mucin pool. In contrast, mucinous carcinoma is formed by large mucin pools that are devoid of lining epithelium and contain numerous tumour cells. FNAC sampling yields grossly visible jelly-like mucous substance for both benign and malignant lesions. Cytologically, all smears show abundant mucus in the background. Simple mucocoele-like lesions and mucocoele-like with ductal hyperplasia show scant cellularity, no or rare intact single ductal cells, monolayered arrangement and absence of nuclear atypia. In contrast, most mucinous carcinomas show higher cellularity, more single ductal cells, three-dimensional clusters and minimal nuclear atypia (Fig. 9.23) [29, 43]. Marked nuclear atypia is confined predominantly to cases with mixed mucinous and ductal carcinoma [44]. Diffuse cytoplasmic hyalinisation and resulting eospinophila is a peculiar morphologic change that is apparently unique to pure mucinous carcinoma [45]. A distinct feature is also the presence of thin-walled capillaries [44]. Mucocoele-like lesions with atypical ductal hyperplasia may show cytological features overlapping with mucinous carcinoma. The most important features distinguishing benign mucocoele-like lesions from mucinous carcinoma are: scant cellularity, rare intact single ductal cells and ductal cells arranged in cohesive monolayered clusters lacking significant nuclear atypia. Myxoid fibroadenoma is more cellular than benign mucocoele-like lesions and can be distinguished from carcinoma by the absence of dissociation and presence of numerous bare nuclei of bland morphology in the background. The mucoid material of myxoid fibroadenoma stain bright pink rather than magenta as in mucocoele-like tumours using the Diff Quik stain [46].

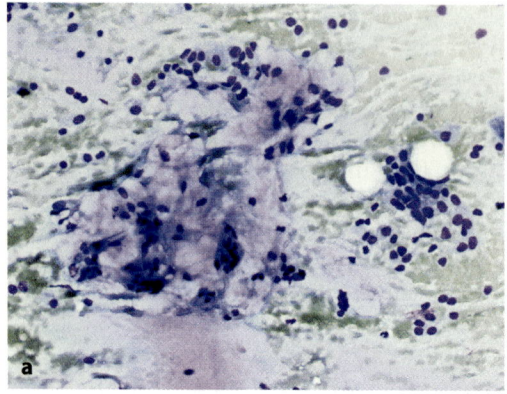

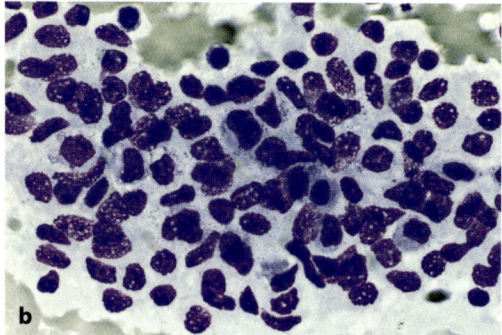

Fig. 9.23
FNAC breast. Mucinous carcinoma. **a** Preparations show pools of mucin and monotonous ductal cells. **b** High-power view revealing nuclear atypia and some overlapping and crowding. Marked nuclear atypia is confined predominantly to cases with mixed mucinous and ductal carcinoma

Based on the combination of FNAC and image findings, benign mucocoele-like lesions can be correctly distinguished from adenocarcinoma before surgery. However, Farshid et al. report 70% of mucocoele-like lesions having been reported as atypical or suspicious on FNAC preceding surgery [42]. Operative therapy can be performed for definite cases of mucinous carcinoma without further biopsy. However, excisional biopsy is advised in mucocoele-like lesions for further separation into benign and malignant categories [47]. CB may not suffice in these cases [48].

9.5 Lobular Carcinoma

FNAC of invasive lobular carcinoma (ILC) is associated with high rates of false-negative and equivocal diagnoses [50]. Smear cellularity, presence of single intact epithelial cells, nuclear size, nuclear atypia, palpability of the tumour and histological type of ICL (classic versus non-classic) are all statistically significant in establishing an unequivocally positive diagnosis [50]. Hwang et al. found that the cytological cellularity of the lesion does not reflect the actual cellularity of the tumour, but instead is an indicator of the architectural arrangement of the neoplastic cells; tumours that form epithelial cell groups, such as in non-classic ILC, tend to yield more cellular aspirates that are diagnostic for carcinoma [51] (Fig. 9.24). In contrast, classic ILC, in which single neoplastic cells are embedded in fibrous stroma, is more likely to yield a paucicellular smear with subtle atypia and rare single intact epithelial cells. As such, an inconclusive diagnosis in a certain percentage of classic ILC cases may be unavoidable. Rajesh et al. found the overall sensitivity in detection of malignancy in ILC cases to be 76%, smears showing moderate (52%) to abundant (32%) cellularity and the cells of ILC arranged both in clusters and in dissociation (72%). Individual cells were monomorphic (40%) to mildly pleomorphic (60%), and the cells were smaller, showed a smooth, regular nuclear margin, bland chromatin and indistinct nucleoli. An Indian-file arrangement was frequently observed (28%). Nuclear moulding (28%) and intranuclear inclusions (16%) were also noted. Intracytoplasmic lumina were seen in occasional cases [51]. Cytological differential diagnosis of ductal versus lobular carcinoma remains difficult [53] (Figs. 9.25 and 9.26). On evaluating MGG-stained FNAC smears, cytoplasmic vacuolation was observed in 70% and positivity with PAS-d staining was observed in 90% of cases of ductal carcinoma [54]. Pleomorphic lobular carcinoma of the breast is a subtype of lobular carcinoma of the breast that is well recognised in the surgical pathology literature. FNAC recognition of this subtype is important because the subtype characteristically pursues an aggressive clinical course as compared to classic lobular carcinoma of the breast [55].

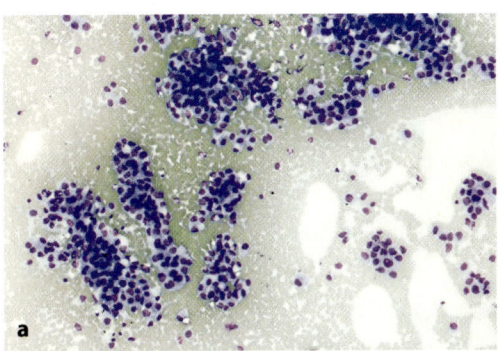

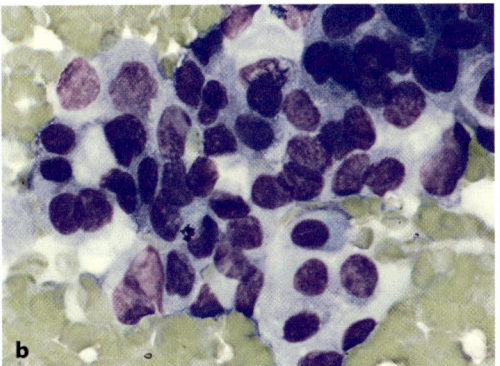

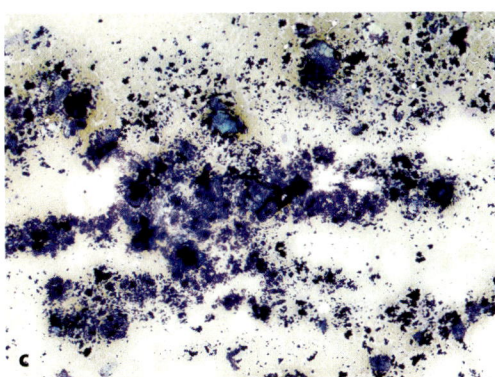

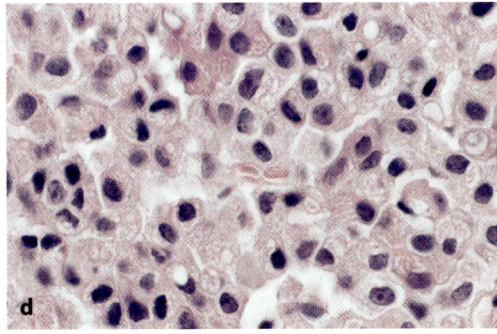

Fig. 9.24
FNAC breast. Lobular carcinoma. **a** The cellularity of the lesion does not reflect the actual cellularity of the tumour, but instead is an indicator of the architectural arrangement of the neoplastic cells; tumours that form epithelial cell groups, as in non-classic invasive lobular carcinoma, tend to yield more cellular aspirates that are diagnostic for carcinoma. **b** High-power view; some carcinoma cells with eccentric nuclei and cytoplasmic vacuole. Cytoplasmic vacuolation is also observed in the majority of ductal carcinomas. **c** Lobular carcinoma may show prominent calcification. **d** Histology shows similar cell features

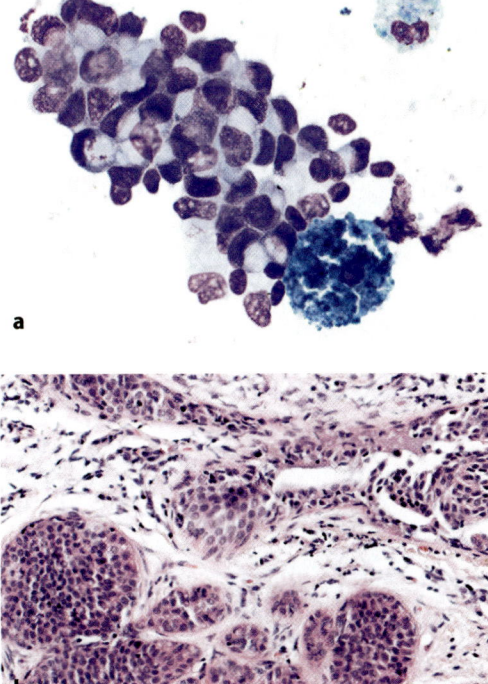

Fig. 9.25
FNAC breast. Lobular carcinoma. (see next page)

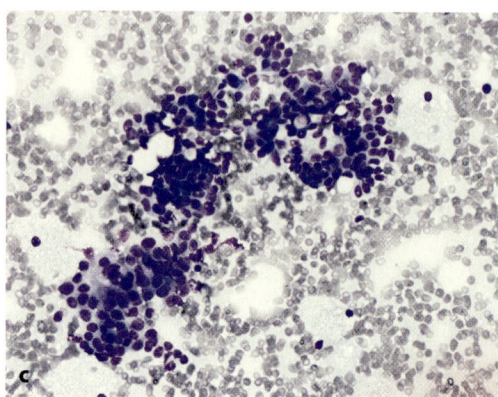

Fig. 9.25
Continued from previous page. FNAC breast. Lobular carcinoma. **a** Cluster of cells showing nuclear moulding, intranuclear inclusions and intracytoplasmic lumina. Macrophage indicates cystic change/necrosis. Differentiation from ductal carcinoma remains difficult.
b Histology shows lobular carcinoma. **c** Different case. Ductal carcinoma may also show both cytoplasmic and nuclear vacuolation

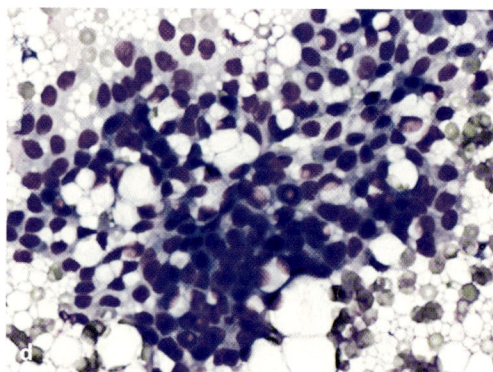

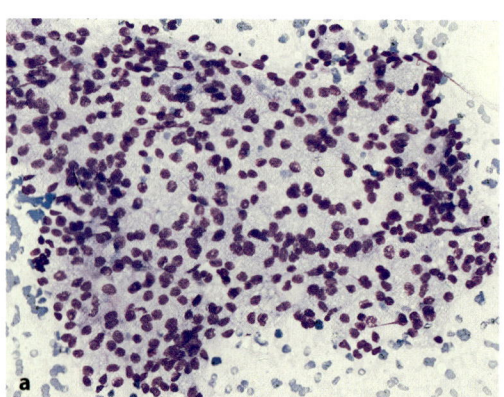

Fig. 9.26
FNAC breast. Lobular carcinoma. **a** Monotonous appearance of lobular epithelium resembling salivary gland acinar epithelium. **b** Aggregates of lobular and ductal epithelium showing no prominent pleomorphism.
c Same case, another area. Very bland nuclear features in this case of in situ and invasive lobular carcinoma. **d** Lactation change in a fibroadenoma may cause cytoplasmic vacuolation, mimicking lobular carcinoma

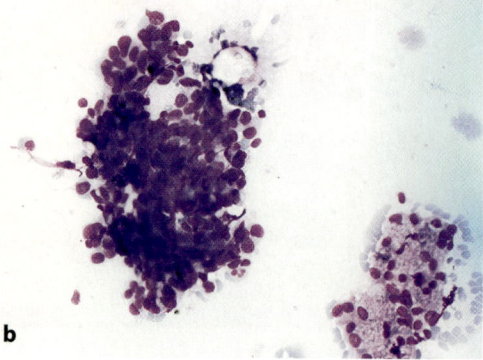

9.6 In Situ or Invasive Carcinoma?

Clinical management of in situ carcinoma of the breast is different from invasive carcinomas. Thus, it is important to find cytomorphological criteria to distinguish between these two entities. Klijanjenko et al. tried to predict the status of stromal invasion by applying strict cytological criteria including cellular clustering, eosinophilic differentiation, necrosis, tubular structures, dirty background, nuclear anisonucleosis, cellular pleomorphism, cribriform pattern and stromal infiltration (Figs. 9.27-9.30). Among the parameters examined, stromal infiltration was the most powerful predictor of status of invasion. Stromal infiltration was significantly higher in invasive (88%) than in situ carcinoma (11%). In contrast, cribriform pattern (16% vs. 36%) and necrosis (19% vs. 59%) were more frequently seen in situ than in invasive carcinomas [56]. The combination of stromal infiltration and cribriform pattern and necrosis in aspirates may provide an opportunity in introducing a predictive index with which to differentiate between an in situ versus an invasive process.

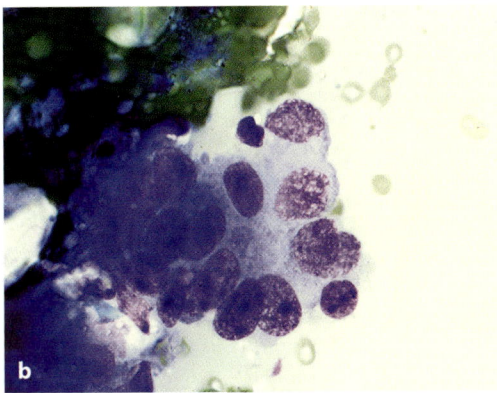

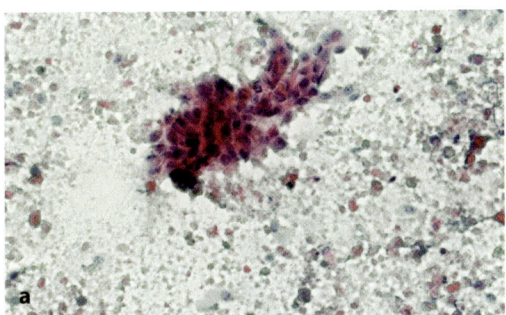

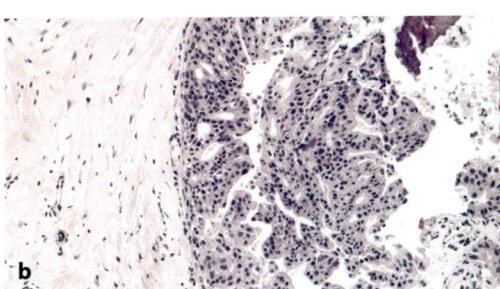

Fig. 9.27
FNAC breast. In situ or invasive? **a** Flat sheets of ductal epithelium against a dirty, necrotic background is frequently seen in DCIS. **b** Histology of the tumour showed cribriform DCIS

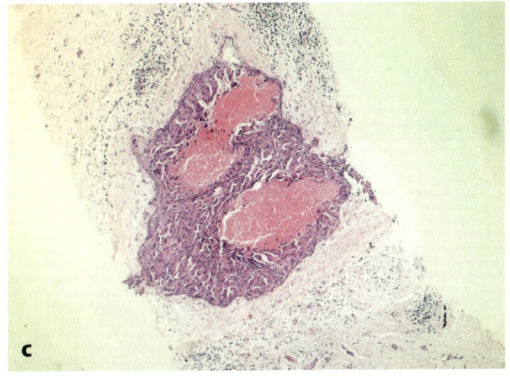

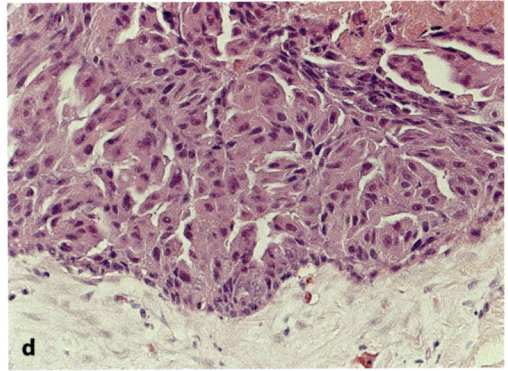

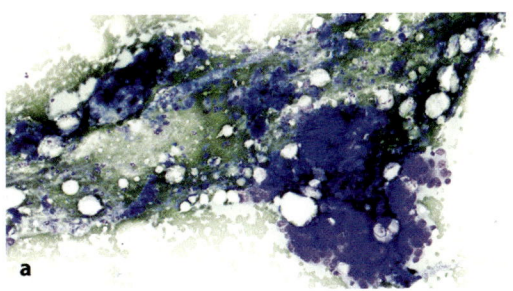

Fig. 9.28
FNAC breast. In situ or invasive? **a** Malignant cells appear to be associated with fatty fragments. In fact the association is due to fibrin from the blood clot.
b High-power view showing a high-nuclear-grade tumour. **c** Histology shows a high-grade DCIS. **d** Higher-power view of histology showing cells similar to those seen in FNAC

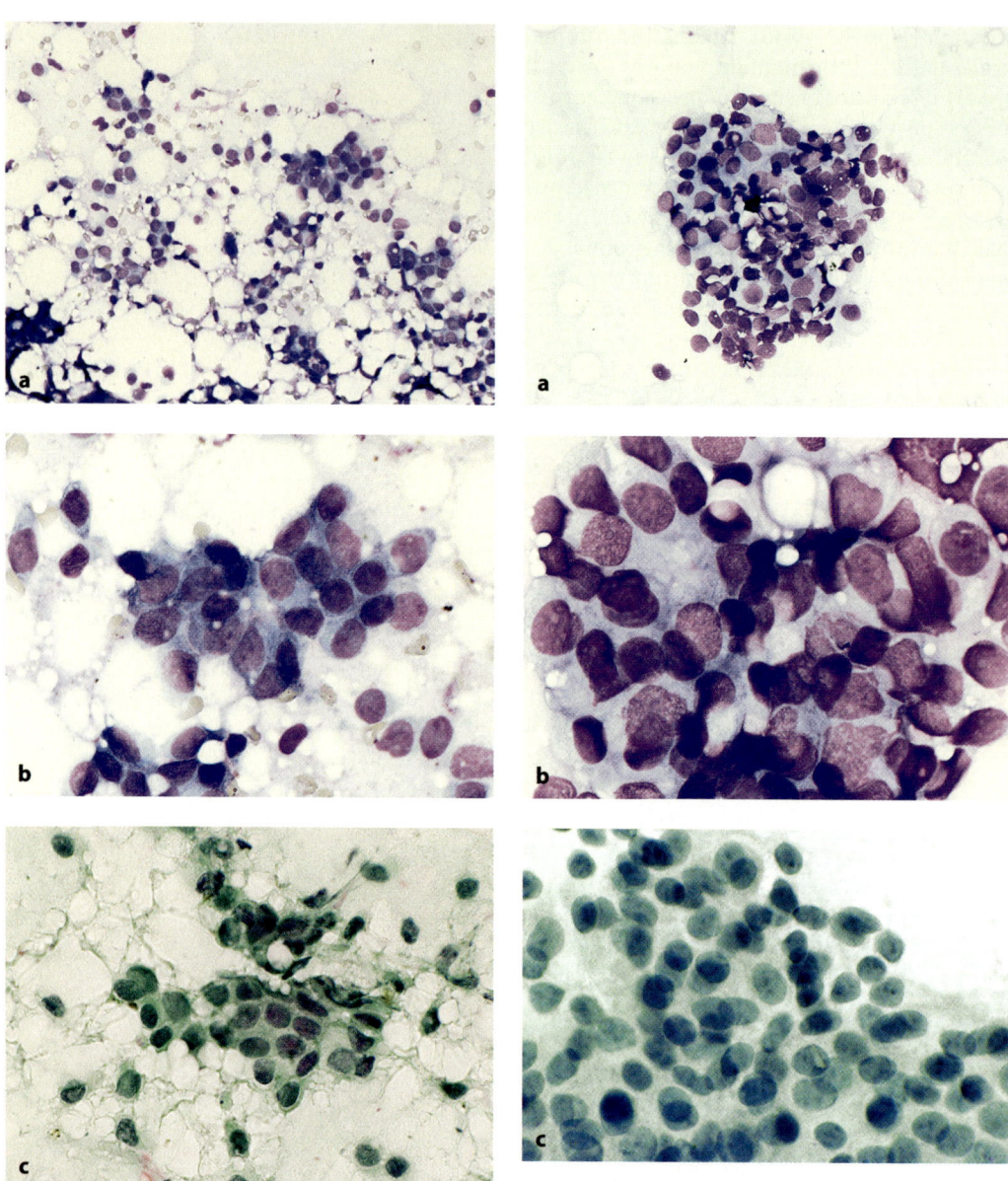

Fig. 9.29
FNAC breast. In situ or invasive of this case of invasive caricoma. **a** Infiltration of fat or stroma by malignant cells was present in 72% of invasive cases, but was not present in any of the in situ cases reported my McKee et al. [57]. **b** Intracytoplasmic vacuoles were seen in 50% of invasive cases and 21% of in situ lesions. **c** Individual cell infiltration of the fat may be difficult to asses on FNAC

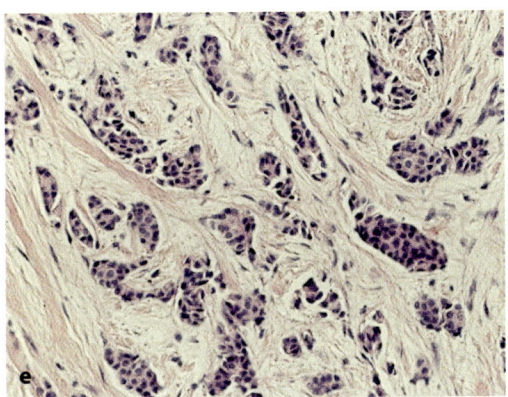

Fig. 9.30
FNAC breast. In situ or invasive? **a** Cytospin preparations of FNAC breast give impression of two cell populations, epithelial and myoepithelial. **b** The presence of myoepithelial cells overlying clusters of tumour cells was seen in 86% of in situ tumours and 7% of invasive cases. **c** Same case, Pap stain. Distinction between the two populations appears to have been blurred, suggesting that the phenomenon shown in a and b may have been apoptosis and air-drying artefact. **d** Different case. Calcification is present in 71% of in situ and 15% of the invasive breast carcinomas. **e** Same case. Histology shows invasive carcinoma

Bondesen and Lindholm analysed 11 features in an attempt to predict invasiveness in malignant breast lesions by FNAC. Four findings appeared to be useful in this context: (1) malignant cell clusters with tubular structure, (2) cytoplasmic lumen formation in malignant cells, (3) fibroblast proliferation and (4) fragments of elastoid stroma. When any combination of two or more of these key features was seen in a smear being diagnostic of malignancy, the positive predictive value regarding invasiveness was 96%. The accuracy of this prediction in terms of sensitivity and specificity was 48% and 96%, respectively [57]. In a similar study, McKee et al. assessed 17 cytological features and found that 6 of them showed a statistically significant difference between the invasive and in situ cases [58]. These were: infiltration of fat or stroma by malignant cells (72% of invasive cases demonstrated this feature, but it was not present in any of the in situ cases, P=0.0002), the presence of myoepithelial cells overlying clusters of tumour cells (seen in 86% of in situ tumours and 7% of invasive cases, P<0.00001), calcification (present in 71% of in situ and 15% of the invasive group, P=0.001), foamy macrophages (noted in 64% of in situ tumors and 16% of invasive carcinomas, P=0.0007), intracytoplasmic vacuoles (seen in 50% of invasive cases and 21% of in situ lesions, P=0.08) and tubules (present in 30% of invasive and 7% of in situ tumours, P=0.10). They demonstrated that invasion could be suggested in the FNAC of carcinomas provided that true infiltration of fibrofatty connective tissue by neoplastic cells is present. (Fig 9.28) In situ disease has characteristic features, but the presence of invasion cannot be excluded, even in the presence of stromal or adipose tissue fragments without tumour infiltration [57].

Sauer et al. claim that they were able to distinguish between invasive and in situ carcinoma in 294 out of 320 directly diagnosed invasive carcinomas (91.8%) [58]. The positive predictive value of a diagnosis of invasive carcinoma in their series was 97%. Their data showed that definitive cytological diagnosis of invasive carcinoma was possible in more than 90% of fully diagnostic smears, allowing definitive primary surgery in these women [58].

Bofin et al. found that nuclear morphology, myoepithelial cells, signs of invasion and degree of cellular dissociation are among the most potent factors discriminating between benign epithelial proliferations, atypical intraductal hyperplasia, ductal carcinoma in situ and invasive carcinoma [59].

In conclusion, studies so far show that using FNAC analysis it is possible to speculate about possible stromal invasion. However, even with the features suggesting an in situ condition, invasion cannot be excluded.

9.7 Rare Lesions

9.7.1 Radial Scar/Complex Sclerosing Lesion

Radial scar/complex sclerosing lesion (RS/CSL) of the breast has become more frequently detected during the mammography performed in breast screening. Clinical examination and mammography often do not show specific features differentiating RS/CSL from carcinoma of the breast. Cytology of RS/CSL without associated malignant changes shows bland epithelial clusters and bipolar naked nuclei. Apocrine cells, papillary clusters, foam cells and fibrillary elastoid material are also frequently seen [60]. Cases of radial scar with apocrine adenosis, showing atypical cells may be misleading and diagnosed as suspicious. Deb et al. found that radial scars constituted 6.2% of C3 and 10.4% of C4 FNAC diagnoses [6]. RS/CSL may be associated with carcinomas that are characterised by the presence of single atypical cells or a few tubular clusters without myoepithelial cells (in case of a tubular carcinoma; Fig. 9.31). Although the cytology of RS/CSL without associated carcinoma does not seem characteristic, in most cases a diagnosis of a benign condition can be made accurately. Some authors advocate CB as the preferred method for preoperative diagnosis when sampling FNAC provides scarce material and suspicion of a fibrotic and collagenous lesion such as lobular carcinoma and radial scar [61]. There are few reports of these fibrosclerotic lesions associated with metaplastic tumours [62].

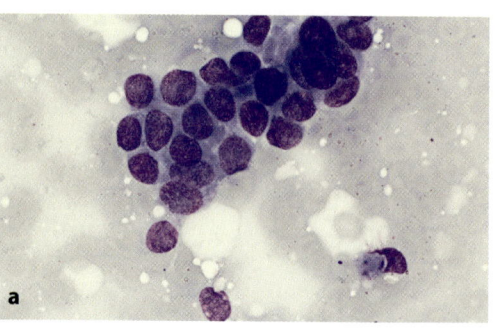

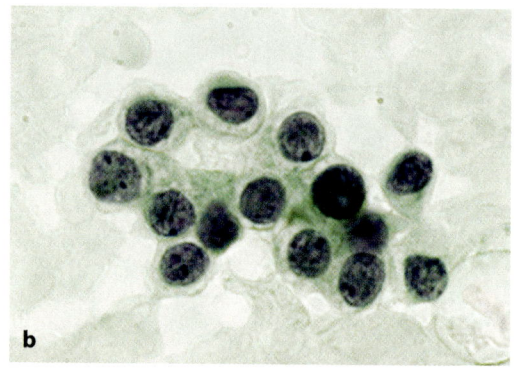

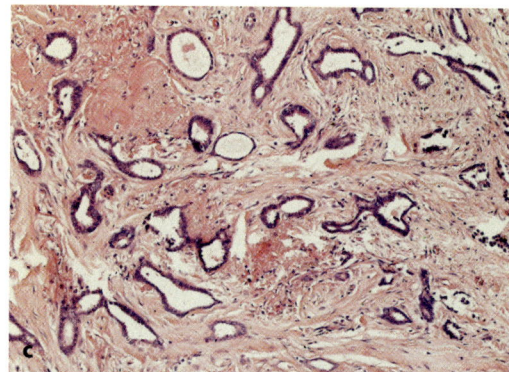

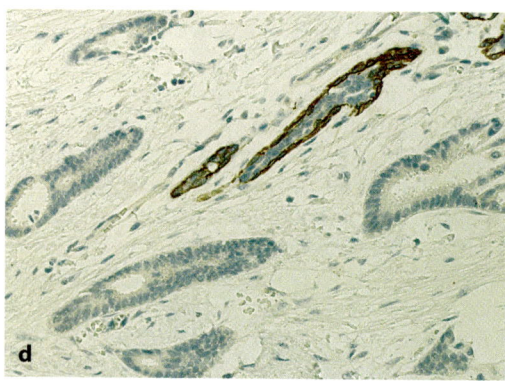

Fig. 9.31
FNAC breast. Tubular carcinoma. **a** Radial scar/central sclerosing lesion (RS/CSL) may be associated with carcinoma characterised by the presence of single atypical cells or a few tubular clusters without myoepithelial cells in case of a tubular carcinoma. **b** Pap appearances are similarly bland, cells are in a tubular arrangement and lack myoepithelial cells. **c** Histology of tubular carcinoma may also be difficult to distinguish from RS/CSL. **d** CK14 immunoperoxidase stain shows the presence of myoepithelium in the benign duct and absence thereof in the tubular carcinoma

9.7.2 Collagenous Spherulosis

Collagenous spherulosis is a rare incidental finding seen in association with benign breast lesions. The presence of pink hyaline globules surrounded by benign myoepithelial cells in MGG-stained smears is a diagnostic feature (Fig. 9.32). Associated lesions were atypical papillary hyperplasia and fibroadenoma. Adenoid cystic carcinoma was the close differential diagnosis on cytology [63, 64]. Awareness of this entity is important to avoid a false-positive diagnosis of malignancy.

9.7.2 Ductal Adenoma

Ductal adenoma is an uncommon breast lesion that can histologically and clinically mimic carcinoma [65]. Cytologically, the lesion has features overlapping with those of mucinous carcinoma, mucocoele-like lesion, lactating adenoma and intraductal papilloma. The smears are highly cellular and contain numerous monolayered sheets of ductal cells with prominent punched-out, small vacuoles distending the cytoplasm. The nuclei are mostly round to oval and contain bland chromatin. Occasionally cells with enlarged nuclei and conspicuous nucleoli are present. The background shows large mucin pools, scattered single cells with mild nuclear atypia, some with apocrine metaplasia, rare stripped nuclei and a fibrovascular stromal component. Calcifications may be present. Ductal adenoma may represent a diagnostic pitfall on FNAC. Increased awareness of its cytological appearances may help prevent a misdiagnosis.

9.7.3 Gynaecomastia

Gynaecomastia may have some common cytological findings, such as apocrine metaplasia, cellular atypia and foamy macrophages, that can be misinterpreted as evidence of malignancy [66]. Duct ectasia may occasionally present diagnostic dilemma on FNAC, particularly if there are associated degenerative changes (Fig. 9.33).

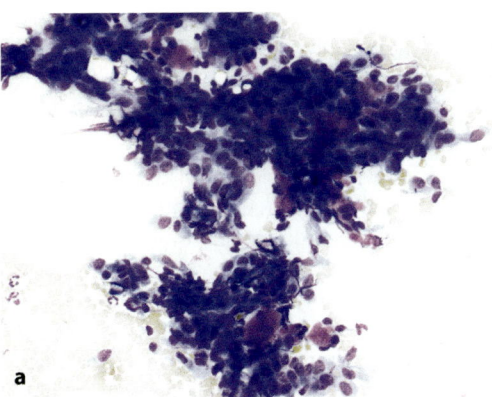

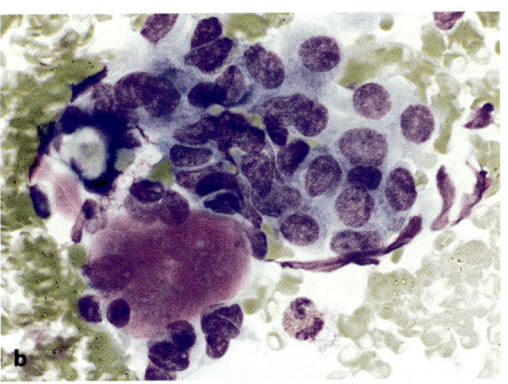

Fig. 9.32
FNAC breast. Collagenous spherulosis. **a** The presence of pink hyaline globules surrounded by benign myoepithelial cells in MGG-stained smears is a diagnostic feature. Associated lesions were atypical papillary hyperplasia and fibroadenoma. **b** Same lesion, high-power view of the collagen globule

9.7.5 Spindle-Cell and Mesenchymal Lesions of the Breast

Spindle cell and mesenchymal lesions of the breast include a variety of benign and malignant conditions and may be a cause of potential diagnostic pitfalls [67]. Chhieng et al. found that 0.87% of the 5306 breast FNAC in their series contained a significant spindle-cell or mesenchymal component [68]. They can be classified into four categories: (1) reactive conditions, including diabetic mastopathies, granulation tissue specimens and granulomatous lesions, (2) benign neoplastic conditions, including mammary hamartoma [69, 70], dermatofibroma, fibromatosis [71, 72], granular cell tumour [73, 74], angiolipoma, cellular fibroadenoma, neurilemmoma [75, 76], spindle-cell lipoma [77], myofibroblastoma [78, 79] and low-grade malignant neoplastic lesions, including low grade PTs and (4) high-grade malignant neoplastic lesions, including metaplastic carcinoma with chondroid stroma, pleomorphic liposarcoma, osteosarcoma, leiomyosarcoma, angiosarcoma [80, 81] and metastatic tumours [82, 83]. A specific diagnosis may be given in 82.6% of cases [68]. Angiosarcoma may be cytologically mistaken for granulation tissue. Review of the cytological features revealed findings that should suggest angiosarcoma [84], especially when correlated with the clinical history (see Fig. 8.4)(see 8.8.2). Atypical haemangioma should therefore be included in the differential diagnosis of angiosarcoma and other benign and malignant spindle-cell lesions of the breast encountered on cytological samples [85]. Breast lesions with a significant spindle-cell or mesenchymal component are rarely encountered in FNAC and constitute a heterogeneous group that may pose a diagnostic dilemma. FNAC should be the initial diagnostic procedure for investigating these lesions [81]. (see chapter 8)

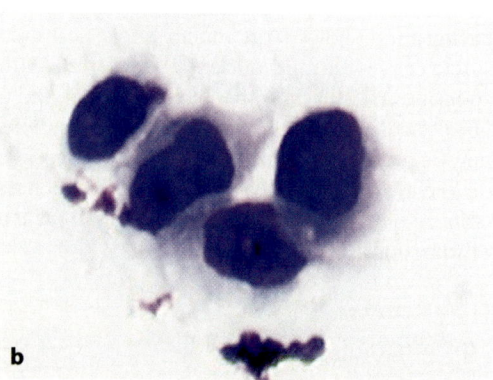

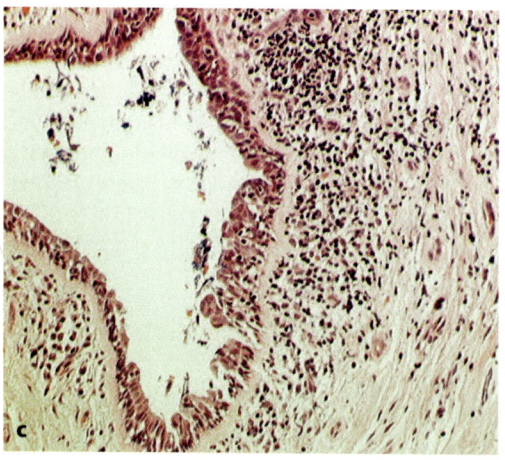

Fig. 9.33
FNAC breast. Duct ectasia. **a** FNAC may contain atypical epithelial cells, which may raise the suspicion of malignancy. **b** Same case, higher-power view of the epithelium. **c** Histology shows atypia of the epithelium lining the ectatic duct with the associated inflammation in the wall

9.7.6 Pseudoangiomatous Stromal Hyperplasia

Pseudoangiomatous stromal hyperplasia of the breast occurs in patients within the age range 34–56 years, some may be males with gynaecomastia [86]. FNAC of pseudoangiomatous stromal hyperplasia closely resembles that of fibroadenoma. FNAC often does not yield a satisfactory cellular yield for diagnosis. In diagnostic cases, FNAC shows a moderate cellularity with cohesive clusters of bland-looking ductal cells in a background of single, naked nuclei and some spindle cells containing fine chromatin and a discernible amount of cytoplasm. Occasional ductal cell clusters assuming a „staghorn" pattern, a feature commonly seen in fibroadenoma, are also present. In addition, scantly, loose and hypocellular stromal tissue fragments containing spindle cells and occasional paired, elongated nuclei embedded in a fibrillary matrix are seen. Histology shows many slit-like spaces rimmed by CD34-positive myofibroblasts/fibroblasts in a focally hyalinised stroma. Sometimes, ill-formed, fusiform aggregates of fibroblasts are also observed. A definitive diagnosis is unlikely on the basis of the cytological examination alone. Pseudoangiomatous stromal hyperplasia needs to be distinguished from borderline lesions, such as PT, and more sinister conditions, which sometimes have a similar cytological appearance [86].

9.7.7 Metaplastic Tumours

Metaplastic tumours show a dominant spindle-cell component with various degrees of atypia, ranging from fibromatosis-like to a low-grade, intermediate-grade and high-grade fibrosarcoma phenotype. Squamous metaplasia may be present as well as low-grade glandular elements. Some tumours have a low-grade adenosquamous growth pattern. The low-grade tumours are histologically similar to limited areas of stromal reaction and myofibroblastic proliferation, seen in partially sclerotic micropapillomas/papillomas and complex sclerosing lesions, but usually more cellular. Cytokeratin positivity supports the metaplastic nature of the more plump spindled cells. The spindle cells are also positive for vimentin and smooth-muscle and muscle-specific actins. Spindle-cell metaplastic tumours, from fibromatosis-like to fibrosarcoma, may arise within a variety of fibrosclerotic breast lesions [62]. The cytological findings suggesting a diagnosis of metaplastic carcinoma include a liquid aspirate, a proteinaceous or chondromyxoid background and a poorly differentiated tumour with multinucleated giant cells, neoplastic or histiocytic. A definite diagnosis requires the presence of both carcinomatous and metaplastic (squamous/mesenchymal) components [87].

9.7.8 Secretory Carcinoma

Secretory carcinoma of the breast is a rare variant of breast malignancy and its cytological features in FNAC include cellular material with malignant cells exhibiting diffuse, prominent, intracytoplasmic vacuoles and secretion as well as occasional signet-ring like forms [88–90]. Cytochemical stains show diffuse positivity for mucin by alcian blue stain in the vacuolated cells, which is PAS positive and resistant to diastase digestion (PAS-d). Oil-red O staining is negative. Immunopositivity to CEA, cytokeratin (CAM 5.2), B72.3 and epithelial membrane antigen (EMA) is found in malignant cells. Lipid-secreting carcinoma is a rare type of invasive carcinoma of the breast that was first described by Aboumrad et al. in 1963; it is a specific type of breast carcinoma that can be differentiated from invasive lobular carcinoma [91].

9.7.9 Tumoral Calcinosis

Tumoral calcinosis relates to calcific deposits in soft tissue that may clinically resemble a tumour. Extensive accumulation of acellular calcific material in the breast may be diagnosed by FNAC [92]. In these cases a routine mammogram shows a partially cystic opacity. All other investigations are normal and no significant family or medical history is usually found. Cytology shows abundant acellular calcium. The patients have no further treatment and on follow-up are clinically well with no changes.

9.7.10 Clear-Cell Hidradenoma

Clear-cell hidradenoma, a benign tumor of sweat gland, may present as a breast lump with ulceration of overlying skin. Failure to identify its cytological features on FNAC may lead to a wrong diagnosis of breast carcinoma. Cytology shows the presence of many clear cells amidst polygonal tumour cells, but no tubular lumina are seen. Accurate diagnosis remains a problem [93]. Other benign skin appendage tumours (e.g. pilomatrixoma) may pose a diagnostic pitfall in FNAC diagnosis [94].

9.7.11 Tubular Adenoma

Tubular adenoma shows cells arranged as small, three-dimensional balls or clusters, tubules of different shapes and less frequently as closely approximated acini [95]. Cells are uniform, with pale cytoplasm, which may exhibit magenta granules in MGG-stained smears. The tubules in tubular adenomas always show myoepithelial cells along with sheets of ductal cells and bipolar naked nuclei, and are more open than the angulated tubules of tubular carcinoma. Stroma is conspicuously scanty or absent. Confusion with fibroadenoma may occur due to the presence of a „staghorn" pattern of ductal cells. However, straight tubules closely approximated acini and intracytoplasmic granules are not seen in aspirates from fibroadenomas [96].

9.7.12 Adenomyoepithelioma

Adenomyoepithelioma shows cytologically a biphasic cell population composed of clusters and sheets of benign apocrine cells admixed with clumps of bland-looking oval- to spindle-shaped cells. The apocrine cells contain larger, round nuclei, prominent solitary nucleoli, and ample eosinophilic, granular cytoplasm. In contrast, the spindle cells have oval nuclei, fine chromatin, inconspicuous nucleoli and scanty amphophilic cytoplasm. A small number of nuclei and foamy macrophages may be noted in the background. The characteristic stromal elements usually seen in fibroepithelial tumour of the breast are not found. The myoepithelial nature of the spindle cells may be confirmed by immunohistochemical and ultrastructural studies. Recognition of the peculiar combination of benign apocrine cells and clumps of nondescript spindle cells should alert the cytologist to this rare but distinct entity, which carries a propensity for malignant transformation [97].

9.7.13 Squamous Cells

Squamous cells may be present in a variety of breast conditions, for example metaplastic carcinoma, fibroepithelial tumour, duct ectasia, subareolar abscess, intraduct papilloma and benign breast cyst [98]. Subareolar breast abscess shows a spectrum of cytological findings including diagnostic anucleated squames associated with numerous neutrophils, keratinous debris, cholesterol crystals, parakeratosis and strips of squamous epithelium. A foreign-body reaction, with sheets of histiocytes and multinucleated foreign-body-type giant cells is noted in some of the cases. Potential pitfalls for a false-positive diagnosis of malignancy include the presence of groups of atypical ductal cells, squamous atypia and fragments of exuberant granulation tissue [99]. The pathogenesis of the lesions is shown in dilated lactiferous ducts undergoing squamous metaplasia with rupture and surrounding extensive acute and chronic inflammation with foreign-body reaction.

Lymphoproliferative diseases of the breast include lymphocytic mastopathy, primary and secondary NHL, Hodgkin's lymphoma and leukaemic deposits [100] (see chapter 5.2.4). The tumours manifest mostly as a unilateral mass but may present as bilateral breast lumps. The regional lymph nodes may be involved [101].

9.7.14 Inflammatory Myofibroblastic Tumour

Inflammatory myofibroblastic tumour of the breast is a very rare tumour-like lesion. FNAC shows an unusual inflammatory lesion with occasional aggregates of cellular connective tissue fragments, sheets of uniform ductal epithelial cells with myoepithelial cells, spindle cells, lymphocytes and histiocyte-like cells. Many new lesions may appear in both breasts and may result in a bilateral mastectomy procedure. Although inflammatory myofibroblastic tumour of the breast has benign cytology and histology, clinically and on imaging, it resembles a carcinoma. Awareness of the condition may help prevent a false-diagnosis of carcinoma [102].

9.8 FNAC or core biopsy?

Core biopsy (CB) has gained remarkable popularity since the 1980s, and in many institutions it has replaced FNAC. However, similar to FNAC, its limitation lies in the ability of this procedure to reliably diagnose a small, but prognostically significant, number of breast lesions. These include entities such as atypical ductal hyperplasia, fibroepithelial tumours, radial scar, papillary lesions and lobular neoplasia [36]. Masood et al. analysed the diagnostic accuracy of CB vs. FNAC in the same breast lesions and reviewed the cases of papillary lesions of the breast. Their study suggests that both FNAC and CB share similar diagnostic challenges, and a follow-up surgical excision is indicated when diagnosis of a papillary lesion is entertained by both procedures [36]. Berner et al. analysed cases with both FNAC and CB using the methodology detailed in the NHS-BSP guidelines [1, 61]. High specificity and sensitivity, as calculated for satisfactory specimens, were achieved with the use of both FNAC and CB. False-positive and false-negative diagnoses were seen in 7/404 (1.7%) and 45/635 (7.1%) of biopsy-proven specimens sampled by FNAC, respectively. The corresponding values for CB were 0% and 5.7%, respectively. Inadequate sampling (15.1%) with use of FNAC was seen particularly in collagenous lesions and in submitted specimens sampled by physicians lacking experience with the FNAC procedure. The authors conclude that FNAC is a valuable method, although moderately less sensitive than CB. CB is the preferred method for preoperative diagnosis when sampling FNAC provides scarce material and suspicion of a fibrotic and collagenous lesion such as lobular carcinoma and radial scar arises. FNAC is most accurate when experienced cytologists are available and when immediate assessment by professionals is performed for the evaluation of material adequacy, so that additional aspirations can be done when needed.

9.9 Radiation Changes

The range of radiation-induced changes in FNAC of the breast may show three patterns of non-neoplastic lesions: epithelial atypia, fat necrosis and poorly cellular smears without epithelial atypia or fat necrosis. It is important to be familiar with the patterns of radiation-induced epithelial atypia, since such atypia may lead to a misdiagnosis of recurrent carcinoma. These atypical cells may show impressive anisocytosis and anisonucleosis; however, the N/C ratio remains normal and an admixture of bipolar cells is present. Cell dissociation and necrotic cell debris, as often seen in breast cancer smears, were never encountered in FNAC smears from irradiated non-neoplastic breasts [103].

References

1. NHSBSP. Guidelines to Cytology Procedures and Reporting in Breast Cancer Screening. NHSBSP Publication 1993;No. 22,:18-19.

2. The uniform approach to breast fine-needle aspiration biopsy. National Cancer Institute Fine-Needle Aspiration of Breast Workshop Subcommittees. Diagn Cytopathol 1997;16(4):295-311.
3. Boerner S, Fornage BD, Singletary E, Sneige N. Ultrasound-guided fine-needle aspiration (FNA) of nonpalpable breast lesions: a review of 1885 FNA cases using the National Cancer Institute-supported recommendations on the uniform approach to breast FNA. Cancer 1999;87(1):19-24.
4. Lim JC, Al-Masri H, Salhadar A, Xie HB, Gabram S, Wojcik EM. The significance of the diagnosis of atypia in breast fine-needle aspiration. Diagn Cytopathol 2004;31(5):285-8.
5. al-Kaisi N. The spectrum of the „gray zone" in breast cytology. A review of 186 cases of atypical and suspicious cytology. Acta Cytol 1994;38(6):898-908.
6. Deb RA, Matthews P, Elston CW, Ellis IO, Pinder SE. An audit of „equivocal" (C3) and „suspicious" (C4) categories in fine needle aspiration cytology of the breast. Cytopathology 2001;12(4):219-26.
7. Moyes C, Dunne B. Predictive power of cytomorphological features in equivocal (C3, C4) breast FNAC. Cytopathology 2004;15(6):305-10.
8. Mander BJ, Beresford PA, Tildsley G, Qureshi T, Wishart GC. Management of patients with intermediate (C3) cytology and a solitary breast lump. Breast 2001;10(2):163-5.
9. Osin P. Abolish C3. Cytopathology 2004;15(1):64.
10. Arif S, Singh N. Abolish C3. Cytopathology 2004;15(1):63-4.
11. Trott PA. Why abolish C3? Cytopathology 2003;14(6):352.
12. Kanhoush R, Jorda M, Gomez-Fernandez C, Wang H, Mirzabeigi M, Ghorab Z, et al. ‚Atypical' and ‚suspicious' diagnoses in breast aspiration cytology. Cancer 2004;102(3):164-7.
13. Mottahedeh M, Rashid MH, Gateley CA. Final diagnoses following C3 (atypical, probably benign) breast cytology. Breast 2003;12(4):276-9.
14. Al-Adnani M, Etessami N, Freeman A, Falzon M. Why abolish C3? Cytopathology 2003;14(5):302-303.
15. Purnell D, Walker RA. Analysis of C3 and C4 breast cytology: can unnecessary cytospins be avoided? Cytopathology 2004;15(6):337-8.
16. Troxel DB. Diagnostic Pitfalls in Surgical Pathology- Uncovered by a Review of Malpractice Claims: Part II. Breast Fine Needle Aspirations. Int J Surg Pathol 2000;8(3):229-231.
17. Stanley MW, Tani EM, Skoog L. Fine-needle aspiration of fibroadenomas of the breast with atypia: a spectrum including cases that cytologically mimic carcinoma. Diagn Cytopathol 1990;6(6) 1990;6(6):375-82.
18. Benoit JL, Kara R, McGregor SE, Duggan MA. Fibroadenoma of the breast: diagnostic pitfalls of fine-needle aspiration. Diagn Cytopathol 1992;8(6):643-7; discussion 647-8.
19. Myers T, Wang HH. Fibroadenoma mimicking papillary carcinoma on ThinPrep of fine-needle aspiration of the breast. Arch Pathol Lab Med 2000;124(11):1667-9.
20. Simsir A, Waisman J, Cangiarella J. Fibroadenomas with atypia: causes of under- and overdiagnosis by aspiration biopsy. Diagn Cytopathol 2001;25(5):278-84.
21. Sturgis CD, Sethi S, Cajulis RS, Hidvegi DF, Yu GH. Diagnostic significance of ‚benign pairs' and signet ring cells in fine needle aspirates (FNAs) of the breast. Cytopathology 1998;9(5):308-19.
22. Veneti S, Manek S. Benign phyllodes tumour vs fibroadenoma: FNA cytological differentiation. Cytopathology 2001;12(5):321-8.
23. Krishnamurthy S, Ashfaq R, Shin HJ, Sneige N. Distinction of phyllodes tumor from fibroadenoma: a reappraisal of an old problem. Cancer 2000;90(6):342-9.
24. Scolyer RA, McKenzie PR, Achmed D, Lee CS. Can phyllodes tumours of the breast be distinguished from fibroadenomas using fine needle aspiration cytology? Pathology 2001;33(4):437-43.
25. Tse GM, Ma TK, Pang LM, Cheung H. Fine needle aspiration cytologic features of mammary phyllodes tumors. Acta Cytol 2002;46(5):855-63.
26. Dusenbery D, Frable WJ. Fine needle aspiration cytology of phyllodes tumor. Potential diagnostic pitfalls. Acta Cytol 1992;36(2):215-21.
27. Deen SA, McKee GT, Kissin MW. Differential cytologic features of fibroepithelial lesions of the breast. Diagn Cytopathol 1999;20(2):53-6.
28. Nayar R, De Frias DV, Bourtsos EP, Sutton V, Bedrossian C. Cytologic differential diagnosis of papillary pattern in breast aspirates: correlation with histology. Ann Diagn Pathol 2001;5(1):34-42.
29. Dawson AE, Mulford DK. Fine needle aspiration of mucinous (colloid) breast carcinoma. Nuclear grading and mammographic and cytologic findings. Acta Cytol 1998;42(3):668-72.
30. Michael CW, Buschmann B. Can true papillary neoplasms of breast and their mimickers be accurately classified by cytology? Cancer 2002;96(2):92-100.
31. Gomez-Aracil V, Mayayo E, Azua J, Arraiza A. Papillary neoplasms of the breast: clues in fine needle aspiration cytology. Cytopathology 2002;13(1):22-30.
32. Wong SI CH, Tse GM. Fine needle aspiration cytology of invasive micropapillary carcinoma of the breast. A case report. Acta Cytol 2000;44(6):1085-9.
33. Onguru O, Deveci S, Gunhan O. Cytological findings of invasive micropapillary carcinoma of the breast: a report of two cases. Cytopathology 2002;13(3):160-3.
34. Ng WK. Fine-needle aspiration cytology findings of an uncommon micropapillary variant of pure mucinous carcinoma of the breast: review of patients over an 8-year period. Cancer 2002;96(5):280-8.

35. Simsir A, Waisman J, Thorner K, Cangiarella J. Mammary lesions diagnosed as „papillary" by aspiration biopsy: 70 cases with follow-up. Cancer 2003;99(3):156-65.
36. Masood S, Loya A, Khalbuss W. Is core needle biopsy superior to fine-needle aspiration biopsy in the diagnosis of papillary breast lesions? Diagn Cytopathol 2003;28(6):329-34.
37. O'Malley FP BA. The spectrum of apocrine lesions of the breast. Adv Anat Pathol 2004;11(1):1-9.
38. Ng WK, Kong JH, Wong WW. Atypical apocrine metaplasia: a diagnostic pitfall in fine needle aspiration cytology of the breast. Acta Cytol 2003;47(4):698-701.
39. Yoshida K, Inoue M, Furuta S, Sakai R, Imai R, Hayakawa S, et al. Apocrine carcinoma vs. apocrine metaplasia with atypia of the breast. Use of aspiration biopsy cytology. Acta Cytol 1996;40(2):247-51.
40. Eusebi V, Foschini MP, Bussolati G, Rosen PP. Myoblastomatoid (histiocytoid) carcinoma of the breast. A type of apocrine carcinoma. Am J Surg Pathol 1995;19(5):553-62.
41. Wong NL, Wan SK. Mucocele-like lesion of the breast-histopathology and fine needle aspiration cytology changes. Zhonghua Bing Li Xue Za Zhi 1999;28(5):327-30.
42. Farshid G PS, King JM, Robinson J. Mucocele-like lesions of the breast: a benign cause for indeterminate or suspicious mammographic microcalcifications. Breast J 2005;11(1):15-22.
43. Cheng L, Lee WY, Chang TW. Benign mucocele-like lesion of the breast: how to differentiate from mucinous carcinoma before surgery. Cytopathology 2004;15(2):104-8.
44. Ventura K CJ, Lee I, Moreira A, Weisman J, Simsir A. Aspiration biopsy of mammary lesions with abundant mucinous material. Review of 43 cases with surgical follow up. Am J Clin Pathol 2003;120(2):194-202.
45. Ng WK. Mammary mucinous carcinoma with marked cytoplasmic hyalinization. A report of 2 cases with emphasis on fine needle aspiration cytologic findings. Acta Cytol 2003;47(6):1045-9.
46. Yeoh GP, Cheung PS, Chan KW. Fine-needle aspiration cytology of mucocelelike tumors of the breast. Am J Surg Pathol 1999;23(5):552-9.
47. Wong NL, Wan SK. Comparative cytology of mucocelelike lesion and mucinous carcinoma of the breast in fine needle aspiration. Acta Cytol 2000;44(5):765-70.
48. Carder PJ MC, Liston JC. Surgiccal excision warranted following a core biopsy diagnosis of mucocoele like lesion of the breast. Histopathology 2004;45(2):148-54.
49. Lerma E FV, Carreras A, Esteva E, Prat J. Undetected invasive lobular carcinoma of the breast: review of false -negative smears. Diagn Cytopathol 2000;23(5):303-7.
50. Hwang S, Ioffe O, Lee I, Waisman J, Cangiarella J, Simsir A. Cytologic diagnosis of invasive lobular carcinoma: factors associated with negative and equivocal diagnoses. Diagn Cytopathol 2004;31(2):87-93.
51. Rajesh L, Dey P, Joshi K. Fine needle aspiration cytology of lobular breast carcinoma. Comparison with other breast lesions. Acta Cytol 2003;47(2):177-82.
52. de las Morenas A CP, Moroz K, Donelly MM. Cytologic diagnosis of ductal versus lobular carcinoma of the breast. Acta Cytol 1995;39(5):865-9.
53. Nijhawan R, Rajwanshi A, Gautam U, Gupta SK. Cytoplasmic vacuolation, intracytoplasmic lumina, and DPAS staining in ductal carcinoma of the breast. Diagn Cytopathol 2003;28(6):291-4.
54. Dabbs DJ, Grenko RT, Silverman JF. Fine needle aspiration cytology of pleomorphic lobular carcinoma of the breast. Duct carcinoma as a diagnostic pitfall. Acta Cytol 1994;38(6):923-6.
55. Klijanienko J, Katsahian S, Vielh P, Masood S. Stromal infiltration as a predictor of tumor invasion in breast fine-needle aspiration biopsy. Diagn Cytopathol 2004;30(3):182-6.
56. Bondeson L, Lindholm K. Prediction of invasiveness by aspiration cytology applied to nonpalpable breast carcinoma and tested in 300 cases. Diagn Cytopathol 1997;17(5):315-20.
57. McKee GT, Tambouret RH, Finkelstein D. Fine-needle aspiration cytology of the breast: Invasive vs. in situ carcinoma. Diagn Cytopathol 2001;25(1):73-7.
58. Sauer T, Young K, Thoresen SO. Fine needle aspiration cytology in the work-up of mammographic and ultrasonographic findings in breast cancer screening: an attempt at differentiating in situ and invasive carcinoma. Cytopathology 2002;13(2):101-10.
59. Bofin AM, Lydersen S, Hagmar BM. Cytological criteria for the diagnosis of intraductal hyperplasia, ductal carcinoma in situ, and invasive carcinoma of the breast. Diagn Cytopathol 2004;31(4):207-15.
60. Bonzanini M, Gilioli E, Brancato B, Pellegrini M, Mauri MF, Dalla Palma P. Cytologic features of 22 radial scar/complex sclerosing lesions of the breast, three of which associated with carcinoma: clinical, mammographic, and histologic correlation. Diagn Cytopathol 1997;17(5):353-62.
61. Berner A, Davidson B, Sigstad E, Risberg B. Fine-needle aspiration cytology vs. core biopsy in the diagnosis of breast lesions. Diagn Cytopathol 2003;29(6):344-8.
62. Gobbi H, Simpson JF, Jensen RA, Olson SJ, Page DL. Metaplastic spindle cell breast tumors arising within papillomas, complex sclerosing lesions, and nipple adenomas. Mod Pathol 2003;16(9):893-901.
63. Jain S, Kumar N, Sodhani P, Gupta S. Cytology of collagenous spherulosis of the breast: a diagnostic dilemma--report of three cases. Cytopathology 2002;13(2):116-20.

64. Saqi A, Mercado CL, Hamele-Bena D. Adenoid cystic carcinoma of the breast diagnosed by fine-needle aspiration. Diagn Cytopathol 2004;30(4):271-4.
65. Mesonero CE, Tabbara S. Fine-needle aspiration cytology of ductal adenoma: report of a case associated with a mucocele-like lesion. Diagn Cytopathol 1995;13(3):252-6.
66. Amrikachi M, Green LK, Rone R, Ramzy I. Gynecomastia: cytologic features and diagnostic pitfalls in fine needle aspirates. Acta Cytol 2001;45(6):948-52.
67. Silverman JF, Geisinger KR, Frable WJ. Fine-needle aspiration cytology of mesenchymal tumors of the breast. Diagn Cytopathol 1988;4(1):50-8.
68. Chhieng DC, Cangiarella JF, Waisman J, Fernandez G, Cohen JM. Fine-needle aspiration cytology of spindle cell lesions of the breast. Cancer 1999;87(6):359-71.
69. Gomez-Aracil V, Mayayo E, Azua J, Mayayo R, Azua-Romeo J, Arraiza A. Fine needle aspiration cytology of mammary hamartoma: a review of nine cases with histological correlation. Cytopathology 2003;14(4):195-200.
70. Herbert M, Schvimer M, Zehavi S, Mendlovic S, Karni T, Pappo I, et al. Breast hamartoma: fine-needle aspiration cytologic finding. Cancer 2003;99(4):255-8.
71. Chhieng DC, Cohen JM. Fine needle aspiration (FNA) cytology of mammary fibromatosis: a case report and review of literature. Cytopathology 1999;10(5):354-9.
72. Pereira S, Tani E, Skoog L. Diagnosis of fibromatosis colli by fine needle aspiration (FNA) cytology. Cytopathology 1999;10(1):25-9.
73. Pieterse AS, Mahar A, Orell S. Granular cell tumour: a pitfall in FNA cytology of breast lesions. Pathology 2004;36(1):58-62.
74. Salto-Tellez M, Saunders C, Kocjan G. Diagnosis of multiple granular cell tumours by fine needle aspiration cytology. Cytopathology 2000;11(3):191-3.
75. Fisher PE, Estabrook A, Cohen MB. Fine needle aspiration biopsy of intramammary neurilemoma. Acta Cytol 1990;34(1):35-7.
76. Staklenac B, Pauzar B, Pajtler M, Loncar B, Dmitrovic B. An unusual tumour of the breast: cytological findings. Cytopathology 2004;15(3):160-2.
77. Lew WY. Spindle cell lipoma of the breast: a case report and literature review. Diagn Cytopathol 1993;9(4):434-7.
78. Lopez-Rios F, Burgos F, Madero S, Ballestin C, Martinez-Gonzalez MA, de Agustin P. Fine needle aspiration of breast myofibroblastoma. A case report. Acta Cytol 2001;45(3):381-4.
79. Powari M, Srinivasan R, Radotra BD. Myofibroblastoma of the male breast: a diagnostic problem on fine-needle aspiration cytology. Diagn Cytopathol 2002;26(5):290-3.
80. Munitiz V, Rios A, Canovas J, Ferri B, Sola J, Canovas P, et al. Primitive leiomyosarcoma of the breast: case report and review of the literature. Breast 2004;13(1):72-6.
81. Jun Wei X, Hiotis K, Garcia R, Hummel Levine P. Leiomyosarcoma of the breast: a difficult diagnosis on fine-needle aspiration biopsy. Diagn Cytopathol 2003;29(3):172-8.
82. Choi HJ, Park IA. Fine needle aspiration cytology of metastatic choriocarcinoma presenting as a breast lump. A case report. Acta Cytol 2004;48(1):91-4.
83. Hejmadi RK, Day LJ, Young JA. Extramammary metastatic neoplasms in the breast: a cytomorphological study of 11 cases. Cytopathology 2003;14(4):191-4.
84. Carson KF, Hirschowitz SL, Nieberg RK, Sadeghi S. Pitfalls in the cytologic diagnosis of angiosarcoma of the breast by fine-needle aspiration: a case report. Diagn Cytopathol 1994;11(3):297-9; discussion 299-300.
85. Galindo LM, Shienbaum AJ, Dwyer-Joyce L, Garcia FU. Atypical hemangioma of the breast: a diagnostic pitfall in breast fine-needle aspiration. Diagn Cytopathol 2001;24(3):215-8.
86. Ng WK, Chiu CS, Han KC, Chow JC. Mammary pseudoangiomatous stromal hyperplasia. A reappraisal of the fine needle aspiration cytology findings. Acta Cytol 2003;47(3):373-80.
87. Nogueira M, Andre S, Mendonca E. Metaplastic carcinomas of the breast--fine needle aspiration (FNA) cytology findings. Cytopathology 1998;9(5):291-300.
88. Gupta RK, Kenwright D, Naran S, Lallu S, Fauck R. Fine needle aspiration cytodiagnosis of secretory carcinoma of the breast. Cytopathology 2000;11(6):496-502.
89. Jayaram G, Looi LM, Yip CH. Fine needle aspiration cytology of secretory carcinoma of breast: a case report. Malays J Pathol 1997;19(1):69-73.
90. Pohar-Marinsek Z, Golouh R. Secretory breast carcinoma in a man diagnosed by fine needle aspiration biopsy. A case report. Acta Cytol 1994;38(3):446-50.
91. Insabato L, Russo R, Cascone AM, Angrisani P. Fine needle aspiration cytology of lipid-secreting breast carcinoma. A case report. Acta Cytol 1993;37(5):752-5.
92. Gupta RK, Lallu S, Naran S, Fauck R, Gaskell D. Aspiration cytodiagnosis of the breast with abundant acellular calcific material indicative of soft tissue calcinosis (a study of 3 cases). Cytopathology 2002;13(2):111-5.
93. Kumar N, Verma K. Clear cell hidradenoma simulating breast carcinoma: a diagnostic pitfall in fine-needle aspiration of breast. Diagn Cytopathol 1996;15(1):70-2.
94. Pascual A, Casado I, Colmenero I, Pelayo A, Asenjo JA. Fine needle aspiration cytology of pilomatrixoma of the breast. Acta Cytol 2000;44(2):274-6.

95. Shet TM, Rege JD. Aspiration cytology of tubular adenomas of the breast. An analysis of eight cases. Acta Cytol 1998;42(3):657-62.
96. Kumar N, Kapila K, Verma K. Characterization of tubular adenoma of breast--diagnostic problem in fine needle aspirates (FNAs). Cytopathology 1998;9(5):301-7.
97. Ng WK. Adenomyoepithelioma of the breast. A review of three cases with reappraisal of the fine needle aspiration biopsy findings. Acta Cytol 2002;46(2):317-24.
98. Ng WK, Kong JH. Significance of squamous cells in fine needle aspiration cytology of the breast. A review of cases in a seven-year period. Acta Cytol 2003;47(1):27-35.
99. Silverman JF, Lannin DR, Unverferth M, Norris HT. Fine needle aspiration cytology of subareolar abscess of the breast. Spectrum of cytomorphologic findings and potential diagnostic pitfalls. Acta Cytol 1986;30(4):413-9.
100. Salto-Tellez M, Kocjan G. Lymphocytic mastopathy in a patient with previous breast cancer diagnosed by fine-needle aspirate. Diagn Cytopathol 2000;23(2):141-2.
101. Singh NG, Kapila K, Dawar R, Verma K. Fine needle aspiration cytology diagnosis of lymphoproliferative disease of the breast. Acta Cytol 2003;47(5):739-43.
102. Zardawi IM, Clark D, Williamsz G. Inflammatory myofibroblastic tumor of the breast. A case report. Acta Cytol 2003;47(6):1077-81.
103. Markovic-Glamocak M, Sucic M, Krizanac S, Ries S, Gjadrov-Kuvezdic K, Boban D. Cytodiagnosis in irradiated breast cells--its value and pitfalls. Lijec Vjesn 2003;125(7-8):180-3.

Chapter 10

Principles of Safe Practice: the Role of FNAC in Clinical Management

Contents

10.1   FNAC Breast Lesions 214

10.2   FNAC Thyroid 215

10.3   FNAC Head and Neck Conditions 216

10.4   FNAC Lymph Nodes 216

10.5   FNAC Adrenal and Kidney 217

10.6   FNAC Gastrointestinal Tract 217

10.7   FNAC Soft Tissue 218

10.8   FNAC Bone 218

10.9   FNAC in Children 218

10.10 FNAC for HIV-Related Lesions 219

10.11 Transrectal Digitally Guided FNAC 219

10.12 FNAC in Gynaecology 219

10.13 Diagnostic Accuracy and
        Cost-Effectiveness of FNAC 219

References 220

FNAC has been widely used as a diagnostic tool for the past 50 years. Differing from large-bore cutting needle biopsy sampling, FNAC utilises 22- to 27-gauge needles. The cell samples aspirated from a lesion are characteristically smeared onto glass slides for immediate microscopic evaluation. An adequacy report and a preliminary diagnostic impression can be given within approximately 10–15 min. A final report is generally available within 24 h [1]. This method has been used as one of the most cost-effective, complication-free and rapid techniques for preoperative investigation of tumours and tumour-like conditions. Its usefulness in the diagnosis and management of patients is emphasised in this chapter.

Successful FNAC requires a specimen with adequate cellularity, a high-quality preparation, an experienced aspirator and a cytopathologist [2]. Up to 32% of FNAC procedures in various organs (e.g. thyroid, breast, lung) may be non-diagnostic due to scant cellularity and poor preparation [3]. On-site immediate evaluation of FNAC specimens can be beneficial in the determination of adequacy, triage for ancillary studies and in providing a preliminary diagnosis of the specimen, which often facilitates rapid clinical decisions [3]. Including the number of relevant cells/cell clusters, as a parameter of adequacy, could reduce the rate of false-negative FNAC diagnoses. However, the presence or even abundance of diagnostic cells does not eliminate the potential for a false-negative cytological diagnosis. This must be correlated with clinical and imaging findings, where available.

The last 7 years has seen a dramatic increase in the use of core biopsy (CB) over that of FNAC in the diagnosis of breast cancer [4]. In the UK, in 1997, 17% of all screen-detected breast carcinomas were diagnosed by CB, compared with 73% in 2003 [5]. By contrast, 19% of preoperative tissue diagnoses were made solely by FNAC in 2001, this figure falling to 10% in 2003. Although the use of FNAC alone for the diagnosis of breast carcinoma has undoubtedly fallen, there is still a need for rapid diagnosis using a robust, simple and cost-effective method. The majority of women attending breast clinics with palpable or screen-detected lesions will have a benign disease, and for many, the reassurance that a patient may get from being told she has a benign condition in either a rapid-access or one-stop clinic setting cannot be underestimated [6, 7].

10.1 FNAC Breast Lesions

The role of FNAC in the management of breast lesions has been clearly defined by the National Health Service Breast Screening Programme (NHSBSP) [8]. According to these recommendations, FNAC of the breast is reported using the C1–C5 scale where C1 is unsatisfactory, C2 negative, C3 atypical, probably benign, C4 suspicious, probably malignant and C5 malignant. The triple assessment rule requires complete agreement between the cytologist, radiologist and surgeon, if definitive management is to be based on a cytology report without the tissue biopsy. The National Cancer Institute (NCI) uses a similar system, FNAC is classified as benign, indeterminate/atypical, suspicious/probably malignant or malignant [9]. The application of the NCI-supported diagnostic categories to FNAC of breast lesions is useful in stratifying aspirates based on the likelihood of underlying malignancy. The subcategories of FNAC diagnosed as atypical or suspicious require tissue biopsy to exclude carcinoma. Benign and inadequate FNAC diagnoses must be correlated with the clinical and imaging findings, and in non-correlative cases the patient should undergo a biopsy procedure [10, 11]. Supported by appropriately trained on-site cytopathologists and in conjunction with follow-up mammography, ultrasound-guided FNAC appears to be efficient in the management of patients with abnormal radiological findings [12].

FNAC has also proved to be a useful and reliable tool in the evaluation and management of masses involving the adolescent breast. The majority of breast masses in adolescents are benign, and lesions can be managed conservatively in this age group. The use of non-invasive diagnostic procedures such as FNAC and ultrasound can reduce the need for open surgery during breast development [13]. Ultrasound-guided FNAC for non-palpable breast lesions is highly accurate, and helps direct patient management [14]. Cytological specimens of breast lesions are also used in the evaluation of individual prognostic and predictive factors as well as for genomic and proteomic studies [15]. Such investigative studies are under way and offer great potential for revolutionising the prediction of patient outcomes and disease response to therapy, as well as assessment of the risk of developing breast cancer [16].

There is a well-recognised incidence of false-positive and -negative diagnoses for FNAC due both to sampling and interpretive errors [4, 8]. The latter range from common look-alikes such as fibroadenomas with loss of cellular cohesion mimicking carcinoma and the under-calling of ILC due to the low cell numbers of lesional cells to more esoteric diagnoses only achieved retrospectively after examining the histological resection specimen (see Chap 9). However, CB is not a perfect vehicle for interpretation, as caveats also exist with this modality. Up to 24% of patients diagnosed on preoperative CB with in situ carcinoma will have invasive disease at surgery, presumably reflecting a sampling error [5]. Furthermore, a 4% false-negative rate for breast malignancy on core biopsy was recorded in a multi-institutional study [17]. This was due to missed sampling of the lesion, benign calcification adjacent to a mammographically undetected carcinoma and microscopic interpretative errors by the reporting pathologist.

Intraoperative imprint cytology of axillary lymph nodes in the assessment of axillary node metastases has been used more recently. It is an accurate and relatively simple method and can be a useful intraoperative tool [18, 19]. FNAC of the breast has improved decision-making and the selection of patients for biopsy and has contributed to saving time in the clinical management of breast lumps. It is an indispensable diagnostic tool in the management of breast lesions [20].

10.2 FNAC Thyroid

FNAC of the thyroid is a reliable, safe, cost-effective, and widely used test. Its introduction and application have had a significant impact in the management of nodular thyroid diseases in adults [21]. In non-iodine-deficient areas, 4–7% of the population is reported to have thyroid abnormalities. Prophylactic operations of these nodules in the thyroid are not indicated and not cost effective, as at least four out of five nodules are colloid goitre and only a few are malignant [22]. FNAC of the thyroid can be used as a diagnostic test or a triage tool. As a diagnostic test, it can diagnose papillary carcinoma, poorly differentiated carcinoma, medullary carcinoma, anaplastic carcinoma, metastatic malignancy, thyroiditis, and most benign nodular goitres and cysts [23]. However, follicular adenoma, well-differentiated carcinoma and some hypercellular goitres are indistinguishable in FNAC preparations. As a triage tool, FNAC can be used to distinguish thyroid nodules that might have a higher risk of malignancy (i.e. neoplasms), and would thus require surgical excision, from nodular goitres or thyroiditis, which can be managed medically. Although FNAC can reduce the number of diagnostic thyroidectomies by identifying benign lesions that need not be removed, it does not and cannot eliminate all diagnostic operations. Some patients with thyroid nodules who are referred for operation after FNAC are actually found to have benign disease because of our inability to distinguish accurately between follicular adenoma, well-differentiated carcinoma and some cellular goitres on FNAC. The commonest thyroid lesions in one particular district general hospital were nodular goitre (52.4%), followed by thyroiditis (17.6%) and neoplasia (13.9%) [24]. When compared with clinical diagnoses based on non-invasive diagnostic investigations, FNAC has an essential role in the diagnosis and management of 23% of our own patients, a confirmatory role in 61% of patients, a non-contributory role in 13% when specimens were inadequate and was misleading in 3% where results were false negative. The positive identification of thyroiditis and neoplasia stands on its own as a justification for FNAC of the thyroid [25]. Non-diagnostic FNAC may be associated with a high probability of thyroid malignancy. They should not be considered benign. In these cases a re-aspiration followed by selective surgical treatment is recommended [26]. Repeated FNAC in the follow-up of patients with benign nodular thyroid disease with or without any clinical changes is of limited use [27]. As the consequence of the decreasing incidence of follicular thyroid carcinoma, one wonders whether cytopathologists should stop reporting follicular neoplasms to minimise unnecessary thyroidectomies if the follicular variant of papillary carcinoma (FVPC) has been excluded. Yang et al. showed that FVPC cannot be excluded completely from follicular neoplasms by FNAC because of the patchy distribution of papillary carcinoma nuclei in the encapsulated variant. [28]. Given the difference in surgical management between follicular neoplasms and PTC, the sensitivity of FNAC and intraoperative frozen section in establishing a diagnosis of FVPC were compared and how these techniques impact on operative management [29]. The sensitivity of FNAC for diagnosis of FVPC was 9% versus 42% for intraoperative frozen section. Kesmodel et al. recommend that although the sensitivity of FNAC in establishing a diagnosis of FVPC is low, FNAC identifies patients with suspicious lesions in whom intraoperative frozen section is important in guiding operative management [29]. As regards the use of intraoperative frozen section of the thyroid, as compared with preoperative FNAC, Duek et al. showed that the sensitivity and specificity of FNAC were 78.1% and 96.5%, respectively, demonstrating an overall accuracy of 91.3%. The sensitivity, specificity and accuracy rates for frozen section were 83.3%, 95.2% and 91.7%, respectively [30]. Wong et al. recommend that when the FNAC result is malignant, an intraoperative frozen section is unnecessary and contributes little to the management. A frozen section, however, is considered to be of value when the FNAC result is reported as benign, suspicious or inadequate

[31]. Taking into account all of the above caveats, FNAC is the most reliable and cost-effective method of distinguishing benign from suspicious or malignant thyroid nodules [32].

10.3 FNAC Head and Neck Conditions

FNAC is a well-established tool for investigating many head and neck conditions. Its application in parotid tumours is still controversial amongst some head and neck surgeons. Cytological examination aims to determine if a process is inflammatory and/or reactive, benign or malignant neoplasm and if possible gives a specific diagnosis. It has been argued that in the area of salivary gland tumours, surgical management relies less heavily on a specific preoperative diagnosis, because almost all neoplastic salivary gland lesions will undergo surgical excision. However, knowing beforehand if a lesion is malignant or benign will aid in planning surgery and may prompt or postpone decisions for surgical intervention [33]. Wong et al. aimed at defining the exact role of FNAC in the diagnostic workup of patients and found that the methodological interpretation of FNAC results provides useful preoperative information, enables more reliable patient counselling and reduces pathological surprises [34]. Its enhancement of the preoperative recognition of malignant parotid tumours may bring about a more stringent attention to the operative margin and hence better tumour clearance [34]. Errors of cytodiagnosis are due to the morphological variability of salivary gland tumours, which makes the interpretation highly dependent upon adequate sampling [35].

Reactive intraparotid lymph nodes and lymphomas present as parotid enlargements that are indistinguishable from pleomorphic adenomas. FNAC is the only method of accurately establishing a preoperative diagnosis in these patients [36, 37]. It is a valuable tool in the primary diagnosis and management of cystic parotid gland lesions. The diagnostic accuracy of this procedure can be significantly improved by acquiring a detailed clinical history, obtaining an adequate cellular specimen and having knowledge of the variety and frequencies of possible diagnostic entities that may present as cystic parotid-gland lesions. By using FNAC, an operation was avoided in 70% and 79% of patients with a non-neoplastic lesion and a metastasis, respectively [36]. Although the definitive subclassification of some lesion types was poor, FNAC was useful in patient triage [38]. FNAC is a safe, accurate means of diagnosing carotid body paragangliomas. It can provide essential information for treatment planning and patient management [39]. EUS-FNAC provides a viable approach to the diagnosis and staging of tumours in the head and neck region when there is a suggestion of oesophageal invasion on CT or magnetic resonance imaging, or enlarged mediastinal lymph nodes. EUS-FNAC may avoid the need for mediastinoscopy or other more invasive techniques for staging of these neoplasms [40].

10.4 FNAC Lymph Nodes

FNAC is a first level diagnostic technique in the screening of lymphadenopathies. The most common cytological diagnosis from lymph node FNAC is metastatic carcinoma, followed by reactive lymphadenopathy and lymphoma. Patients with a history of malignancy are more than twice as likely to show malignancy on lymph node FNAC compared to those without such a history (87% versus 41%) [41]. FNAC offers a rapid and accurate approach for the diagnosis of recurrent Hodgkin's disease and its initial recognition [42]. FNAC of enlarged palpable nodules in nodal basins in patients with melanoma is accurate, rapid and cost-efficient and forms part of an algorithm for the management of patients with melanoma who have palpable nodes [43]. Although surgical biopsy examination is considered the gold standard for lymphoma diagnostics, FNAC offers several advantages in that it is quick, inexpensive and the aspiration procedure has very few complications. The diagnosis is accurate if corroborated by immunophenotyping and/or molecular techniques [44];, however, an increasing use of FNAC for primary diagnosis and classification of lymphomas may result in a loss of archival tissue for complementary analyses, reclassification and research purposes. In addition, some of the lymphoma entities are impossible to diagnose using the FNAC technique [45]. FNAC of tuberculous lymphadenopathy provides a high level of diagnostic accuracy, as shown by a 1.7% false-negative and a zero false-positive rate, acting as an initial evaluating procedure for diagnosis and making it suitable for wider application in developing countries with scant resources [46]. All lymphadenopathies showing acute suppuration without granulomas or AFB on the first FNAC should be re-evaluated by follow-up FNAC and staining for AFB. This will enhance the diagnostic yield of TB in developing countries, where molecular diagnostics are either too costly or unavailable [47].

10.5 FNAC Adrenal and Kidney

FNAC of adrenal masses using a simple diagnostic tree allows the correct classification of the majority of specimens as benign or malignant (accuracy 97.6%), differentiation of primary tumours from metastatic depositions remaining the most difficult task [48]. The indications for renal FNAC are changing as radiological imaging allows better assessment of cystic lesions and incidentally identifies an increasing percentage of renal lesions. Cytological criteria and pitfalls for the diagnosis of a wide variety of benign and malignant lesions have been delineated and refined [49]. The increasing use of partial rather than radical nephrectomy for some renal lesions suggests that accurate distinction between these lesions may have important therapeutic implications. FNAC does not contribute to the diagnosis of malignancy in large (>5 cm) masses, as good radiological imaging is nearly always diagnostic. For smaller (<5 cm) masses and complex cysts, FNAC can occasionally confirm malignancy, but lack of diagnostic yield and low sensitivity means that FNAC is unreliable as a diagnostic tool and will rarely help in the routine management of these patients [50].

10.6 FNAC Gastrointestinal Tract

The role of EUS-FNAC has come out as an important modality for the diagnosis and staging of benign and malignant lesions of the gut wall and surrounding structures of the mediastinum, abdomen and pelvis. It is also used as a diagnostic tool for the evaluation of submucosal masses of the upper gastrointestinal tract and the rectosigmoid, for locating pancreatic endocrine tumours and for the assessment of vascular disease. EUS-FNAC is used for obtaining cell samples, for pseudocyst drainage, and for delivery of local therapy. The widest application of EUS is, however, in the diagnosis and staging of oesophageal, gastric, rectal and pancreaticobiliary carcinoma. EUS-FNAC has been shown to change the approach to clinical management in a significant proportion of patients to a less costly, risky or invasive strategy [51]. It is a highly sensitive method for the detection of pancreatic masses. The indications for pancreatic EUS-FNAC comprise the definite diagnosis of malignancy and pathological confirmation of adenocarcinoma before surgical resection, chemo/radiotherapy, or coeliac plexus neurolysis [52]. Whilst EUS-FNAC of the pancreas achieves high diagnostic accuracy in the diagnosis of malignancy, it is not able to provide conclusive results of benign conditions. Difficulties may be encountered in diagnosing well-differentiated carcinoma and neuroendocrine tumours and distinguishing them from reactive epithelium and islet cell hyperplasia [53]. Cystic lesions of the pancreas are increasingly recognised and usually represent pseudocysts or cystic pancreatic tumours, but also include congenital cysts, acquired cysts, extrapancreatic cysts or cystic degeneration of solid tumours (see chapter 4.2). It is important to distinguish these lesions given their varied prognosis and therapy. Mucinous varieties (mucinous cystic neoplasms and intraductal papillary mucinous tumours) are pre-malignant or malignant, and surgical resection is generally recommended in good operative candidates [54]. In contrast, non-mucinous cystic pancreatic lesions include serous cystadenomas with a very low malignant potential, or pseudocysts, which are always benign. As a result, non-mucinous cystic pancreatic tumours are generally resected only when inducing symptoms or complications. As a minimally invasive procedure, EUS and EUS-FNAC avoid the risk of cutaneous or peritoneal contamination that may occur with CT or ultrasound-guided investigations and is less invasive than surgical interventions. As a result, EUS-FNAC of pancreatic masses is becoming the standard for obtaining cytological diagnosis [55]. The relatively limited accuracy of FNAC and other diagnostic modalities requires consideration of the combined results when making management decisions [54].

EUS-FNAC is a safe and sensitive, minimally invasive method for evaluating patients with a solid lesion of the mediastinum suspected by CT scanning. The most common indication for EUS-FNAC of the mediastinum is non-diagnostic transbronchial FNAC. EUS-FNAC is a valuable diagnostic method for sampling mediastinal lymph nodes and affecting management. False-negative results do not appear to delay appropriate treatment or adversely affect clinical outcome [56]. EUS-FNAC should be considered for diagnosing the spread of cancer to the mediastinum in patients with lung cancer considered for surgery (staging), as well as for the primary diagnosis of solid lesions located in the mediastinum adjacent to the oesophagus [57].

10.7 FNAC Soft Tissue

FNAC as a diagnostic modality for the evaluation of soft tissue neoplasms and non-neoplastic soft tissue mass lesions is uncommon and controversial. This procedure contrasts with more traditional diagnostic methods such as marginal excision, incisional (open) biopsy, or even CB to obtain tissue from somatic sites [58]. However, using FNAC can be an accurate and minimally invasive method for the initial pathological diagnosis of primary benign and malignant soft tissue masses, for the confirmation of metastatic tumours to soft tissue, and for the documentation of locally recurrent soft-tissue neoplasms. FNAC is capable of specifically subtyping a large percentage of primary and metastatic soft-tissue tumours if cellular material, either in the form of a cell block or flow cytometry, is obtained in addition to cell smears [58]. (see chapter 8)

10.8 FNAC Bone

FNAC of bone lesions is a reliable and easily performed diagnostic test for metastatic and primary bone tumours. False-positive results have major therapeutic implications; hence a conservative diagnostic approach is recommended. Areas of difficulty are due to inadequate sampling or misclassification with regard to the exact type of malignancy. The simplicity and accuracy of this procedure, which does not require any surgical incisions (open biopsy or manipulation), supports its important role in triaging and managing bone lesions with minimum risk or morbidity [59, 60]. FNAC is also a good technique for studying bone-graft responses without interfering with graft uptake. It is helpful in the early detection of subclinical infection or any other pathology at the graft site [61].

10.9 FNAC in Children

FNAC is of proven benefit in the paediatric population. For the procedure to be of maximum benefit, several aspects unique to children and paediatric lesions must be considered [62]. FNAC is a valuable diagnostic tool in the management of children with the clinical presentation of a suspicious neck mass. The technique reduces the need for more invasive and costly procedures. Early surgical biopsy should be considered in rapidly enlarging masses, in the presence of persistent systemic symptoms and when repeated FNAC is non-diagnostic [63]. The use of FNAC in thyroid masses prevents unnecessary surgery in 60% and improves surgical selection of children with thyroid malignancy. It is recommended as the first diagnostic test for paediatric patients with nodular thyroid lesions [21, 64].

10.10 FNAC for HIV-Related Lesions

FNAC is a very useful simple and cost-effective procedure for the diagnosis of HIV-related lesions and in the management of these patients [65–67]. Material can be taken for mycobacterial culture at the same time [68]. With the advent of antiretroviral therapy, patients live longer and, given the increased incidence of malignancy in this population, can be diagnosed by FNAC.

10.11 Transrectal Digitally Guided FNAC

Transrectal digitally guided FNAC taken through intact mucosa or from intraluminal rectal tumours achieves a sensitivity of 88% versus 68% for CB [69]. The simple and cost-effective digitally guided transrectal FNAC may be adequate for an early morphological diagnosis, avoiding the more expensive CT or ultrasonically guided biopsies. It is safe and easy to perform and the complication rate is low. Surgical treatment for locally recurrent rectal cancer is justified. In combination with radiation therapy, it offers pain relief and improves quality of life. Survival is prolonged and cure can be achieved in up to one-third of patients [69]. FNAC is a minimally invasive method of obtaining testicular cells for diagnostic purposes. It can evaluate accurately all classically defined histological types, and may have the potential to replace testis biopsy in the assessment of spermatogenesis [70]. FNAC of penile tumours is a successful, well-tolerated procedure capable of providing a cytological diagnosis and useful information for patient management [71].

10.12 FNAC in Gynaecology

In gynaecology, FNAC achieves an overall accuracy of 94.5% in the differentiation between benign and malignant tumours [72]. Despite many controversial views regarding its safety, FNAC has been accepted as an innocuous procedure that can be accomplished with minimal discomfort or complications and, in association with laparoscopy, assist in the management of ovarian cysts and masses [72]. Although FNAC cannot be considered the first-hand diagnostic procedure for ovarian cancer in postmenopausal patients, it may be extremely helpful in young women, even during pregnancy, to safely differentiate functional and other benign ovarian cysts from malignant ones [72]. In postmenopausal women, especially those in the high-risk group for surgical procedures and those undergoing a second-look intervention following radiation or chemotherapy, FNAC may provide sufficient information to warrant abandoning unnecessary surgery [72]. During laparotomy for suspected unilateral disease, FNAC may provide sufficient data about the opposite ovary to allow that organ to remain in place, thus preserving its function in a young patient [72].

FNAC has a role in the clinical management of solid-organ transplant population [73]. Over 50% of the aspirates are benign, justifying a conservative approach in the clinical management of these patients with an overall specificity of 100% and a sensitivity of 97% [73].

10.13 Diagnostic Accuracy and Cost-Effectiveness of FNAC

The establishment of FNAC clinics, with a pathologist as the aspirator, has improved specimen adequacy and therefore diagnostic accuracy of FNAC [74–78]. The advantages of having a pathologist as the aspirator are that a rapid evaluation can be made regarding specimen adequacy and the need for repeating the procedure established immediately. In addition, pathologists can direct the distribution of aspirated material for other tests such as culture study, flow cytometry and electron microscopy, as indicated by preliminary evaluation of the smears. (see chapter 2.8) These factors significantly lower the proportions of unsatisfactory specimens and improve the diagnostic accuracy of the FNAC procedure [79]. The introduction of such a service in our own institution, where aspirates are taken by the cytopathologist, reduced the number of inadequate specimens within 12 months from 43% to 9%. The establishment of the clinic resulted in a threefold reduction in the cost of diagnosing breast lesions alone [80, 81]. At the same time, the rates of cancer following inadequate FNAC fell from 15.7% to 4.2% [11]. FNAC of solid palpable breast lesions should be the diagnostic procedure of choice for those patients classified clinically as probably benign or clinically as highly suspicious for cancer.

FNAC is a cost-effective method of obtaining a pathological diagnosis, which is usually required to determine definitive management for a palpable lesion. In this era of cost control, FNAC provides a low-cost alternative to open excisional biopsy. Rimm et al. aimed to quantify the savings resulting from the use of FNAC on superficial palpable lesions to obtain a diagnosis. FNAC provided a sufficient pathological diagnosis to avoid open surgical biopsy in 63–85% of the cases [82]. Estimation of cost savings on the basis of the distribution of cases and indications for surgery suggest a savings of $250,000–750,000 per 1000 FNAC procedures performed [82]. This and other studies have proven the use of FNAC instead of an open biopsy to represent substantial cost savings [83–89]. Cost analysis revealed that elimination of an open biopsy in cases of benign and clinically suspicious breast lumps would save $1,100 per patient [84]. Traditional open biopsy in an outpatient setting for these tumours is twice as costly as FNAC [83].

On-site FNAC interpretation is cost effective [90]. If patients would undergo a repeat FNAC for each non-diagnostic specimen, the estimated additional cost in direct institutional charges, without on-site evaluation, would outweigh the otherwise higher cost of on-site evaluation [3]. In one study it was shown that total resource savings when using the FNAC clinic setting (£135,544) exceeded the expenses of the FNAC clinic (£27,290) [91]. Potential cost savings per case are greatest for thyroid aspirates. The FNAC clinic where the pathologist takes, stains and reports optimally prepared specimens, provides a high quality and accurate service upon which clinicians can confidently base clinical management decisions. FNAC of the thyroid has improved selectivity for surgery in patients with nodular thyroid disease and has reduced the number of patients who undergo thyroidectomy for benign disease. The result is an increasing yield of malignant lesions found at surgical intervention. FNAC has had a substantial cost-saving effect on thyroid practice [92].

References

1. Wu M, Burstein DE. Fine needle aspiration. Cancer Invest 2004;22(4):620-8.
2. Kocjan G. Fine needle aspiration cytology. Cytopathology 2003;14(6):307-8.
3. Nasuti JF, Gupta PK, Baloch ZW. Diagnostic value and cost-effectiveness of on-site evaluation of fine-needle aspiration specimens: review of 5,688 cases. Diagn Cytopathol 2002;27(1):1-4.
4. Levine T. Breast cytology--is there still a role? Cytopathology 2004;15(6):293-6.
5. NBSPaA, BASO BSa. An Audit of Screen Detected Breast Cancers for the Year of Screening April 2002 March 2003. http//www.cancerscreening.nhs.uk/breastscreen/publications.
6. Dey P BN, Gibbs A et al. Costs and benefits of a one stop clinic compared with a dedicated breast clinic: randomised controlled trial. BMJ 2002;324:507-9.
7. Kocjan G. Is £35.00 too high a price for instant peace of mind. BMJ 2002;324:electronic response to Dey et al 324:507-9.
8. NHSBSP. Breast Screening Programme: Guidelines for Non-operative Diagnostic Procedures and Reporting in Breast Cancer Screening. NHS BSP Publication No 50 June 2001.
9. Institute. NC. The uniform approach to breast fine-needle aspiration biopsy. Diagnostic Cytopathology 1997;16:295-311.
10. Boerner S, Fornage BD, Singletary E, Sneige N. Ultrasound-guided fine-needle aspiration (FNA) of nonpalpable breast lesions: a review of 1885 FNA cases using the National Cancer Institute-supported recommendations on the uniform approach to breast FNA. Cancer 1999;87(1):19-24.
11. Lazda EJ, Kocjan G, Sams VR, Wotherspoon AC, Taylor I. Fine needle aspiration (FNA) cytology of the breast: the influence of unsatisfactory samples on patient management. Cytopathology 1996;7(4):262-7.
12. Buchbinder SS, Gurell DS, Tarlow MM, Salvatore M, Suhrland MJ, Kader K. Role of US-guided fine-needle aspiration with on-site cytopathologic evaluation in management of nonpalpable breast lesions. Acad Radiol 2001;8(4):322-7.

13. Pacinda SJ, Ramzy I. Fine-needle aspiration of breast masses. A review of its role in diagnosis and management in adolescent patients. J Adolesc Health 1998;23(1):3-6.
14. Liao J, Davey DD, Warren G, Davis J, Moore AR, Samayoa LM. Ultrasound-guided fine-needle aspiration biopsy remains a valid approach in the evaluation of nonpalpable breast lesions. Diagn Cytopathol 2004;30(5):325-31.
15. Nizzoli R, Guazzi A, Naldi N, Fraciosi V, Bozzetti C. HER-2/neu evaluation by fluorescence in situ hybridization on destained cytologic smears from primary and metastatic breast cancer. Acta Cytol 2005;49(1):27-30.
16. Sneige N. Utility of cytologic specimens in the evaluation of prognostic and predictive factors of breast cancer: current issues and future directions. Diagn Cytopathol 2004;30(3):158-65.
17. Verkooijen HM, Hoorntje LE, Peeters PH. False-negative core needle biopsies of the breast: an analysis of clinical, radiologic, and pathologic findings in 27 consecutive cases of missed breast cancer. Cancer 2004;100(5):1104-5; author reply 1105-6.
18. Ravichandran D, Kocjan G, Falzon M, Ball RY, Ralphs DN. Imprint cytology of the sentinel lymph node in the assessment of axillary node status in breast carcinoma. Eur J Surg Oncol 2004;30(3):238-42.
19. Pogacnik A, Klopcic U, Grazio-Frkovic S, Zgajnar J, Hocevar M, Vidergar-Kralj B. The reliability and accuracy of intraoperative imprint cytology of sentinel lymph nodes in breast cancer. Cytopathology 2005;16(2):71-6.
20. Feichter GE, Haberthur F, Gobat S, Dalquen P. Breast cytology. Statistical analysis and cytohistologic correlations. Acta Cytol 1997;41(2):327-32.
21. Gharib MH, Zimmerman MD, Goellner MJ, Bridley RS, LeBlanc RS. Fine-needle aspiration biopsy: use in diagnosis and management of pediatric thyroid diseases. Endocr Pract 1995;1(1):9-13.
22. Werga P, Wallin G, Skoog L, Hamberger B. Expanding role of fine-needle aspiration cytology in thyroid diagnosis and management. World J Surg 2000;24(8):907-12.
23. Suen KC. Fine-needle aspiration biopsy of the thyroid. CMAJ 2002;167(5):491-5.
24. El Hag IA, Kollur SM, Chiedozi LC. The role of FNA in the initial management of thyroid lesions: 7-year experience in a district general hospital. Cytopathology 2003;14(3):126-30.
25. Godinho-Matos L, Kocjan G, Kurtz A. Contribution of fine needle aspiration cytology to diagnosis and management of thyroid disease. J Clin Pathol 1992;45(5):391-5.
26. Chow LS, Gharib H, Goellner JR, van Heerden JA. Nondiagnostic thyroid fine-needle aspiration cytology: management dilemmas. Thyroid 2001;11(12):1147-51.
27. Merchant SH, Izquierdo R, Khurana KK. Is repeated fine-needle aspiration cytology useful in the management of patients with benign nodular thyroid disease? Thyroid 2000;10(6):489-92.
28. Yang GC, Liebeskind D, Messina AV. Should cytopathologists stop reporting follicular neoplasms on fine-needle aspiration of the thyroid? Cancer 2003;99(2):69-74.
29. Kesmodel SB, Terhune KP, Canter RJ, Mandel SJ, LiVolsi VA, Baloch ZW, et al. The diagnostic dilemma of follicular variant of papillary thyroid carcinoma. Surgery 2003;134(6):1005-12; discussion 1012.
30. Duek SD, Goldenberg D, Linn S, Krausz MM, Hershko DD. The role of fine-needle aspiration and intraoperative frozen section in the surgical management of solitary thyroid nodules.857-61.
31. Wong CK, Wheeler MH. Thyroid nodules: rational management. World J Surg 2000;24(8):934-41.
32. Castro MR, Gharib H. Thyroid fine-needle aspiration biopsy: progress, practice, and pitfalls. Endocr Pract 2003;9(2):128-36.
33. Schindler S, Nayar R, Dutra J, Bedrossian CW. Diagnostic challenges in aspiration cytology of the salivary glands. Semin Diagn Pathol 2001;18(2):124-46.
34. Wong DS, Li GK. The role of fine-needle aspiration cytology in the management of parotid tumors: a critical clinical appraisal. Head Neck 2000;22(5):469-73.
35. Kocjan G, Nayagam M, Harris M. Fine needle aspiration cytology of salivary gland lesions: advantages and pitfalls. Cytopathology 1990;1(5):269-75.
36. MacCallum PL, Lampe HB, Cramer H, Matthews TW. Fine-needle aspiration cytology of lymphoid lesions of the salivary gland: a review of 35 cases. J Otolaryngol 1996;25(5):300-4.
37. Chhieng DC, Cangiarella JF, Cohen JM. Fine-needle aspiration cytology of lymphoproliferative lesions involving the major salivary glands. Am J Clin Pathol 2000;113(4):563-71.
38. Raab SS, Sigman JD, Hoffman HT. The utility of parotid gland and level I and II neck fine-needle aspiration. Arch Pathol Lab Med 1998;122(9):823-7.
39. Fleming MV, Oertel YC, Rodriguez ER, Fidler WJ. Fine-needle aspiration of six carotid body paragangliomas. Diagn Cytopathol 1993;9(5):510-5.
40. Wildi SM, Fickling WE, Day TA, Cunningham CD, 3rd, Schmulewitz N, Varadarajulu S, et al. Endoscopic ultrasonography in the diagnosis and staging of neoplasms of the head and neck. Endoscopy 2004;36(7):624-30.
41. Schafernak KT, Kluskens LF, Ariga R, Reddy VB, Gattuso P. Fine-needle aspiration of superficial and deeply seated lymph nodes on patients with and without a history of malignancy: review of 439 cases. Diagn Cytopathol 2003;29(6):315-9.

42. Jimenez-Heffernan JA, Vicandi B, Lopez-Ferrer P, Hardisson D, Viguer JM. Value of fine needle aspiration cytology in the initial diagnosis of Hodgkin's disease. Analysis of 188 cases with an emphasis on diagnostic pitfalls. Acta Cytol 2001;45(3):300-6.
43. Basler GC, Fader DJ, Yahanda A, Sondak VK, Johnson TM. The utility of fine needle aspiration in the diagnosis of melanoma metastatic to lymph nodes. J Am Acad Dermatol 1997;36(3 Pt 1):403-8.
44. Ribeiro A, Vazquez-Sequeiros E, Wiersema LM, Wang KK, Clain JE, Wiersema MJ. EUS-guided fine-needle aspiration combined with flow cytometry and immunocytochemistry in the diagnosis of lymphoma. Gastrointest Endosc 2001;53(4):485-91.
45. Landgren O, Porwit MacDonald A, Tani E, Czader M, Grimfors G, Skoog L, et al. A prospective comparison of fine-needle aspiration cytology and histopathology in the diagnosis and classification of lymphomas. Hematol J 2004;5(1):69-76.
46. Handa U, Palta A, Mohan H, Punia RP. Fine needle aspiration diagnosis of tuberculous lymphadenitis. Trop Doct 2002;32(3):147-9.
47. Kumar N, Jain S, Murthy NS. Utility of repeat fine needle aspiration in acute suppurative lesions. Follow-up of 263 cases. Acta Cytol 2004;48(3):337-40.
48. Fassina AS, Borsato S, Fedeli U. Fine needle aspiration cytology (FNAC) of adrenal masses. Cytopathology 2000;11(5):302-11.
49. Renshaw AA, Granter SR, Cibas ES. Fine-needle aspiration of the adult kidney. Cancer 1997;81(2):71-88.
50. Brierly RD, Thomas PJ, Harrison NW, Fletcher MS, Nawrocki JD, Ashton-Key M. Evaluation of fine-needle aspiration cytology for renal masses. BJU Int 2000;85(1):14-8.
51. Opacic M, Rustemovic N. [Endoscopic ultrasonography and diagnostic algorithms in diseases of the gastrointestinal tract]. Lijec Vjesn 2003;125(7-8):192-9.
52. Jinga M, Gheorghe C, Dumitrescu M, Gheorghe L, Nicolaie T. Endoscopic ultrasound guided fine needle aspiration biopsy in the diagnosis of pancreatic masses. Rom J Gastroenterol 2004;13(1):49-54.
53. Kocjan G, Rode J, Lees WR. Percutaneous fine needle aspiration cytology of the pancreas: advantages and pitfalls. J Clin Pathol 1989;42(4):341-7.
54. Levy MJ, Clain JE. Evaluation and management of cystic pancreatic tumors: Emphasis on the role of EUS FNA. Clin Gastroenterol Hepatol 2004;2(8):639-53.
55. Horwhat JD, Gress FG. Defining the diagnostic algorithm in pancreatic cancer. JOP 2004;5(4):289-303.
56. Hernandez LV, Mishra G, George S, Bhutani MS. A descriptive analysis of EUS-FNA for mediastinal lymphadenopathy: an emphasis on clinical impact and false negative results. Am J Gastroenterol 2004;99(2):249-54.
57. Larsen SS, Krasnik M, Vilmann P, Jacobsen GK, Pedersen JH, Faurschou P, et al. Endoscopic ultrasound guided biopsy of mediastinal lesions has a major impact on patient management. Thorax 2002;57(2):98-103.
58. Wakely PE, Jr., Kneisl JS. Soft tissue aspiration cytopathology. Cancer 2000;90(5):292-8.
59. Bommer KK, Ramzy I, Mody D. Fine-needle aspiration biopsy in the diagnosis and management of bone lesions: a study of 450 cases. Cancer 1997;81(3):148-56.
60. Handa U, Bal A, Mohan H, Bhardwaj S. Fine needle aspiration cytology in the diagnosis of bone lesions. Cytopathology 2005;16(2):59-64.
61. Garg M, Dev G, Misra K, Tuli SM. Early biologic behavior of bone grafts. A fine needle aspiration cytology study. Acta Cytol 1997;41(3):765-70.
62. Buchino JJ, Lee HK. Specimen collection and preparation in fine-needle aspirations in children. Am J Clin Pathol 1998;109(4 Suppl 1):S4-8.
63. Liu ES, Bernstein JM, Sculerati N, Wu HC. Fine needle aspiration biopsy of pediatric head and neck masses. Int J Pediatr Otorhinolaryngol 2001;60(2):135-40.
64. Lugo-Vicente H, Ortiz VN, Irizarry H, Camps JI, Pagan V. Pediatric thyroid nodules: management in the era of fine needle aspiration. J Pediatr Surg 1998;33(8):1302-5.
65. Grossl NA, Mosunjac MI, Wallace TM. Utility of fine needle aspiration in HIV-positive patients with corresponding CD4 counts. Four years' experience in a large inner city hospital. Acta Cytol 1997;41(3):811-6.
66. Kocjan G, Miller R. The cytology of HIV-induced immunosuppression. Changing pattern of disease in the era of highly active antiretroviral therapy. Cytopathology 2001;12(5):281-96.
67. Reid AJ, Miller RF, Kocjan GI. Diagnostic utility of fine needle aspiration (FNA) cytology in HIV-infected patients with lymphadenopathy. Cytopathology 1998;9(4):230-9.
68. Harrison AC, Jayasundera T. Mycobacterial cervical adenitis in Auckland: diagnosis by fine needle aspirate. N Z Med J 1999;112(1080):7-9.
69. Larsen SG, Wiiu JN, Giercksky KE, Berner A. [Transrectal specimens in recurrent rectal cancer]. Tidsskr Nor Laegeforen 1999;119(28):4170-2.
70. Meng MV, Cha I, Ljung BM, Turek PJ. Testicular fine-needle aspiration in infertile men: correlation of cytologic pattern with biopsy histology. Am J Surg Pathol 2001;25(1):71-9.
71. Skoog L, Collins BT, Tani E, Ramos RR. Fine needle aspiration cytology of penile tumors. Acta Cytol 1998;42(6):1336-40.
72. Ganjei P. Fine-needle aspiration cytology of the ovary. Clin Lab Med 1995;15(3):705-26.

73. Gattuso P, Reddy VB, Kizilbash N, Kluskens L, Selvaggi SM. Role of fine-needle aspiration in the clinical management of solid organ transplant recipients: a review. Cancer 1999;87(5):286-94.
74. Mayall F, Denford A, Chang B, Darlington A. Improved FNA cytology results with a near patient diagnosis service for non-breast lesions. J Clin Pathol 1998;51(7):541-4.
75. Padel AF, Coghill SB, Powis SJ. Evidence that the sensitivity is increased and the inadequacy rate decreased when pathologists take aspirates for cytodiagnosis. Cytopathology 1993;4(3):161-5.
76. Rubenchik I, Sneige N, Edeiken B, Samuels B, Fornage B. In search of specimen adequacy in fine-needle aspirates of nonpalpable breast lesions. Am J Clin Pathol 1997;108(1):13-8.
77. Saxe A, Phillips E, Orfanou P, Husain M. Role of sample adequacy in fine needle aspiration biopsy of palpable breast lesions. Am J Surg 2001;182(4):369-71.
78. Vural G, Hagmar B, Lilleng R. A one-year audit of fine needle aspiration cytology of breast lesions. Factors affecting adequacy and a review of delayed carcinoma diagnoses. Acta Cytol 1995;39(6):1233-6.
79. Al-Marzooq YM, Chopra R, Al-Bahrani AT, Younis M, Al-Mulhim AS, Al-Mommatten MI. Comparison of specimen adequacy in fine-needle aspiration biopsies performed by surgeons and pathologists. Ann Saudi Med 2004;24(2):124-6.
80. Kocjan G. Evaluation of the cost effectiveness of establishing a fine needle aspiration cytology clinic in a hospital out-patient department. Cytopathology 1991;2(1):13-8.
81. Hamill J, Campbell ID, Mayall F, Bartlett AS, Darlington A. Improved breast cytology results with near patient FNA diagnosis. Acta Cytol 2002;46(1):19-24.
82. Rimm DL, Stastny JF, Rimm EB, Ayer S, Frable WJ. Comparison of the costs of fine-needle aspiration and open surgical biopsy as methods for obtaining a pathologic diagnosis. Cancer 1997;81(1):51-6.
83. Smith TJ, Safaii H, Foster EA, Reinhold RB. Accuracy and cost-effectiveness of fine needle aspiration biopsy. Am J Surg 1985;149(4):540-5.
84. Rubin M, Horiuchi K, Joy N, Haun W, Read R, Ratzer E, et al. Use of fine needle aspiration for solid breast lesions is accurate and cost-effective. Am J Surg 1997;174(6):694-6; discussion 697-8.
85. Lifrange E, Kridelka F, Colin C. Stereotaxic needle-core biopsy and fine-needle aspiration biopsy in the diagnosis of nonpalpable breast lesions: controversies and future prospects. Eur J Radiol 1997;24(1):39-47.
86. Logan-Young W, Dawson AE, Wilbur DC, Avila EE, Tomkiewicz ZM, Sheils LA, et al. The cost-effectiveness of fine-needle aspiration cytology and 14-gauge core needle biopsy compared with open surgical biopsy in the diagnosis of breast carcinoma. Cancer 1998;82(10):1867-73.
87. Sheikh FA, Tinkoff GH, Kline TS, Neal HS. Final diagnosis by fine-needle aspiration biopsy for definitive operation in breast cancer. Am J Surg 1987;154(5):470-4.
88. Peterson IM, Brink WJ. Fine-needle aspiration biopsy. When is it most beneficial? Postgrad Med 1990;88(3):119-22, 124, 126.
89. Skrzynski MC, Biermann JS, Montag A, Simon MA. Diagnostic accuracy and charge-savings of outpatient core needle biopsy compared with open biopsy of musculoskeletal tumors. J Bone Joint Surg Am 1996;78(5):644-9.
90. Dray M, Mayall F, Darlington A. Improved fine needle aspiration (FNA) cytology results with a near patient diagnosis service for breast lesions. Cytopathology 2000;11(1):32-7.
91. Brown LA, Coghill SB. Cost effectiveness of a fine needle aspiration clinic. Cytopathology 1992;3(5):275-80.
92. Hadi MM, Gharib MFH, Goellner MJ, Heerden MJ. Has fine-needle aspiration biopsy changed thyroid practice? Endocr Pract 1997;3(1):9-13.

Chapter 11

Principles of Safe FNAC Practice: FNAC versus Core Biopsy

Contents

11.1 Breast Lesions 225

11.2 Lung Lesions 227

11.3 Hepatic Lesions 227

11.4 Abdominal Lesions 227

11.5 Prostate Cancer 228

11.6 Thyroid Lesions 228

11.7 Gynaecological Lesions 228

11.8 Soft-Tissue Lesions 228

11.9 Skeletal Lesions 228

11.10 Summary 229

References 229

There appears to be a growing movement in favour of the use of core biopsy (CB) over FNAC in making a tissue diagnosis. The new technology available enables both surgeons and radiologists to take tissue samples by CB. This apparently requires less technical skill and the sample is easier to transport to the laboratory; a piece of tissue is simply dropped into formalin rather than having to prepare multiple glass slides, label, dry and fix them and, despite this, frequently failing to produce adequate samples. On the other hand, most pathologists welcome the situation where material is sent in the format suitable for tissue processing with all the advantages that is carries: the preparation and staining is standardised and not dependent on the operator, material can be cut into multiple levels and special stains can be applied in case of need. The morphology is familiar and the clinicians trust the tissue diagnosis implicitly, because they can understand the concept of the architecture of the lesion easily. Patients, having discovered a lump, find themselves overwhelmed by the new situation and their level of anxiety is raised. They often leave it to the surgeon to choose the optimal method of investigation. Which will he/she choose? This chapter discusses some of the arguments for and against the use of FNAC or CB in a variety of clinical settings.

11.1 Breast Lesions

FNAC of the breast has long been recognised as a useful diagnostic tool and has been used in many institutions because it provides a rapid, accurate and cost-effective evaluation (see chapter 9) [1]. However, the use of CB is increasing and vacuum-assisted biopsy devices have been developed to produce larger specimens for analysis. CB is useful because the frequency of inadequate specimens is lower than in FNAC, and it requires a less invasive procedure than open biopsy [1]. CB is also more widely used than FNAC because it can provide a more definitive diagnosis of borderline lesions and can be used to distinguish between invasive ductal and invasive lobular carcinoma. Therefore, the use of CB with mammographic or ultrasonographic guidance is especially high for non-palpable tumours [1]. FNAC of palpable breast lesions is the more sensitive method for the detection of carcinoma regardless of tumour type, size or differentiation. Contrary to other reports, Ballo and Sneige found that not only was FNAC alone more sensitive than CB alone, the addition of CB to an already negative FNAC failed to increase sensitivity in the detection of carcinoma [2]. However, CB did contribute to a more definitive diagnosis in some cases. These authors also found FNAC to be more cost-effective than CB for palpable breast lesions when time and effort are taken into consideration. CB may be an alternative method for preoperative diagnosis when experienced cytopathologists are not available. CB is superior to FNAC in fibrotic and collagenous lesions such as lobular carcinoma and radial scar because of low cellularity [3]. Patients with a discrete breast lump and unclear cytology results require CB [4]. FNAC is the more accurate method when an immediate assessment by a cytopathologist is performed for the evaluation of adequate material so that additional aspirations can be done if needed. When comparing stereotactic FNAC with stereotactic CB in the evaluation of radiographically clustered mammary microcalcification, FNAC was superior to CB for the confirmation of clustered mammary microcalcification (99% versus 94%) and in the identification of cancer associated with microcalcification (false-negative rate of 4% versus 8%) [5]. Foster et al. found that 17% of patients with lobular carcinoma in situ or atypical lobular hyperplasia diagnosed on CB were upgraded to invasive cancer or ductal carcinoma in situ after excision biopsy [6]. Excisional biopsy is supported when lobular carcinoma in situ, atypical lobular hyperplasia, or atypical ductal hyperplasia is diagnosed at CB [6]. Cheung et al. have carried out a statistical comparison showing that there was no significant difference between FNAC and CB [7]. Masood et al. analysed the relative merits of FNAC and CB in the diagnosis of papillary lesions and found that both FNAC and CB share similar diagnostic challenges and recommended a follow-up surgical excision when diagnosis of a papillary lesion is entertained by both procedures [8, 9]. The combined result of both FNAC and CB was superior to clinical examination when non-diagnostic samples were excluded [7]. With the routine use of both techniques, frozen section was avoided in 73% of all cancers and unnecessary operations were avoided in 33.5% of patients, including those with breast cysts, benign mammary dysplasia and inflammatory lesions [7]. Where there is access to skilled cytopathologists, FNAC can provide a highly accurate, rapid and cost-effective means of triage of patients who would benefit most from the more expensive CB [10]. Stereotactic CB was more accurate than stereotactic FNAC in the diagnosis of non-palpable breast cancer [11]. Florentine et al. found that the addition of CB is especially useful for: (1) providing a definitive diagnosis of infiltrating carcinoma in those cases in which the FNAC diagnosis was reported as suspicious, (2) providing ample tissue for ancillary studies, and (3) differentiating a PT from a fibroadenoma. A false-negative diagnosis of breast carcinoma was found to be more common in CB performed without image guidance, but occurred to a lesser degree in image-guided biopsies [12, 13]. A pathologist performing FNAC is the physician best qualified to perform the combined FNAC/CB procedure should he/she deem it necessary [14]. A combination of CB and FNAC can markedly improve the preoperative diagnosis of breast cancer [15], particularly where there is no access to skilled cytopathologists or where the inadequate rate of FNAC is exceptionally high [16, 17].

FNAC is a rapid and non-invasive procedure that is useful for mass lesions. The accuracy of FNAC for non-palpable lesions is relatively low and depends upon the skill of the aspirators, cytoscreeners and cytopathologists involved in the procedure. However, FNAC for palpable masses, together with a physical and mammographic examination (the triple test) is highly accurate for a diagnosis of breast cancer when all three modalities indicate malignancy, and for a benign lesion when all three are negative [1].

11.2 Lung Lesions

FNAC versus CB of the lung achieves diagnostic accuracy of 94% for FNAC and 59% for CB (P<0.01) [18]. The addition of CB significantly increases the diagnostic accuracy only for the subset of benign lesions that are not acute infections [18, 19]. Some authors use cytological imprints of the CB. Using both CB imprints and FNAC smears in the immediate assessment of lung biopsy specimens, Chandan et al. could assign a specific malignant histological cell type in 92%, compared to FNAC smears alone of only 64% [20]. CB offers no substantial advantage over FNAC in the evaluation of peripheral malignant lung lesions. Greif et al. recommend the use of FNAC as the initial diagnostic procedure in all cases of suspected malignancy [21]. The use of the CB technique is recommended when the diagnosis of malignancy by FNAC is uncertain or when a more detailed characterisation of the lesion is required [21].

11.3 Hepatic Lesions

CB is the established procedure for histopathological diagnosis of hepatic lesions. In recent years FNAC has emerged as a minimally invasive, relatively inexpensive and rapid method of pathologic evaluation of primary or metastatic hepatic masses. It can be performed percutaneously or, nowadays more frequently, under endoscopic ultrasound guidance (EUS-FNAC). The specificity and the positive predictive value of FNAC are very high. However, the sensitivity of the procedure ranges between 67% and 93% [22]. The two major areas of diagnostic difficulties are differentiation of benign and non-neoplastic hepatic nodules from a well-differentiated hepatocellular carcinoma and identification of obviously malignant cells as hepatocellular carcinoma, cholangiocarcinoma or metastasis. Preparation of cell blocks, immunohistochemical stains and application of other ancillary techniques is often helpful in difficult cases. In the presence of characteristic features, a diagnosis of hepatocellular carcinoma can be established on FNAC; a negative result does not, however, exclude malignancy. The role of pathological diagnosis in the assessment of large hepatic masses is well established, although its role in the evaluation of small hepatic nodules (<3 cm) detected during surveillance of high risk patients is still evolving [22]. Considering the overall advantages and cost-analysis, FNAC can be suggested as the initial method of choice for evaluation of hepatic masses in most clinical settings. The final choice of the diagnostic procedure should be decided on the basis of a working clinical diagnosis and the institutional experience [22]. FNAC and CB have the same diagnostic accuracy (78%) when considered separately and 88% when considered in combination [23]. Franca et al. also found sensitivity, specificity and positive predictive value to be similar for both techniques [23]. EUS-FNAC of liver tumours is a powerful, reliable and safe procedure for the diagnosis of malignant liver lesions. Optimal diagnostic results are achieved by combining cytological with histological assessment. Hence, EUS-FNAC is an alternative to percutaneous biopsy, particularly in patients at risk of bleeding or with small lesions of the liver [24].

11.4 Abdominal Lesions

FNAC is more sensitive and accurate than NCB in the diagnosis of abdominal lesions, and also offers more rapid diagnosis [25]. However, the combination of these sampling techniques increases the diagnostic sensitivity and occasionally provides more accurate classification of tumours and benign lesions. The techniques should be considered complementary in the investigation of abdominal lesions [25]. The accuracy of EUS-FNAC depends on immediate specimen review by a cytopathologist. Stromal tumours, lymphoma and well-differentiated pancreatic cancer are difficult to diagnose on the basis of cytology alone. To overcome these limitations, a 19-gauge Trucut needle has been developed to obtain histological samples at EUS. The diagnostic accuracy of the new EUS-Trucut needle biopsy is comparable to that of EUS-FNAC. However, in the experience of some authors, the overall efficacy and safety profile of the CB appears modest [26].

11.5 Prostate Cancer

The sensitivity of FNAC for detection of prostate cancer is 81%, and both specificity and positive predictive value are 98% [27]. FNAC is easily performed, has negligible morbidity and offers prompt results. The data suggest that FNAC is a reasonable initial diagnostic procedure for the detection of prostate cancer [27]. CB may be reserved for patients with negative cytology who are clinically suspected of having prostate cancer. In selected patients, FNAC may be used as an alternative to CB for diagnosis, treatment planning and follow-up [27].

11.6 Thyroid Lesions

Karstup et al. demonstrated that neither ultrasound-guided CB nor the combination of ultrasound-guided FNAC and CB were superior to ultrasound-guided FNAC of the thyroid [28]. Ultrasound-guided CB is only recommended in a few selected patients [28]. Quinn et al. reported sonographically guided CB of the thyroid to be safe and effective [29]. Their results using CB were better than those obtained using FNAC, but the best results were obtained when both needles were used in the same patient [29]. The complication rate of this approach was 0.98% [29].

11.7 Gynaecological Lesions

FNAC in combination with CB in gynaecological lesions is a simple and safe operation that requires the use of needle guides. In comparison with FNAC, the sensitivity for CB is lower but the specificity is higher [30]. No significant differences were found in accuracy between the two methods. CB should be considered in the subset of patients where additional information about the tumour is desired for planning the treatment of recurrent disease [30]. (see chapter 10.12)

11.8 Soft-Tissue Lesions

Analysis of the role of FNAC versus CB in the diagnosis of soft-tissue lesions found that there was a 100% correlation between FNAC and CB when sarcoma was diagnosed [31]. CB may have the advantage of subtyping selected sarcomas diagnosed by FNAC. Unsatisfactory FNAC should be evaluated further by a repeat aspirate or CB. Performance of FNAC by cytopathologists can reduce the number of unsatisfactory specimens and allow repeat FNAC procedures. Most of the unsatisfactory FNACs are from retroperitoneal and pelvic lesions, performed under radiographic guidance. Many of these lesions, however, may be as readily accessible via CB as they are via FNAC. (see chapter 8)

11.9 Skeletal Lesions

Koscick et al. compared the diagnostic sensitivity and specificity of FNAC and CB in the diagnosis of skeletal lesions in order to determine if a complementary role exists for the two modalities [32]. They evaluated FNAC and CB over a 21-year period and found that FNAC and CB concurred in 73% of diagnostic cases [32]. The two modalities agreed in 78% of cases diagnosed as metastatic carcinoma and in 59% of primary malignant tumours of bone excluding Ewing's sarcoma. FNAC alone was diagnostic in 8% of cases, including metastatic carcinomas, chondrosarcomas, Ewing's sarcoma and osteomyelitis. CB alone was diagnostic in 19% of cases. Given these findings, CB is more specific in the evaluation, grading and typing of skeletal lesions, in particular malignant primary bone tumours. Overall, there is excellent agreement between FNAC and CB, especially in the evaluation of benign primary bone tumours. Most importantly, FNAC improved the diagnostic yield in 24% of cases when CB was normal or unsatisfactory, obviating the need for a repeat biopsy. FNAC should be performed concurrently with CB in the evaluation of skeletal lesions since the two modalities are complementary [32].

11.10 Summary

There are multiple published papers comparing the relative merits of FNAC and CB, used separately and together. Their results vary depending on the perspective that they are written from. FNAC still has an important part to play, although this is very much dependent upon local circumstances. If taken by a skilled aspirator, it remains a method of choice as a first-line investigation of any mass in the body. The majority of lesions turn out to be benign. Many unnecessary biopsy procedures can be avoided by prudent use of FNAC. However, FNAC does require a dedicated aspirator and a dedicated interpreter. (see chapter 2.3) In the absence of either of these, a CB is a second-best option for the patient in the first instance [33]. Utilisation of each of these modalities and of their full benefits ultimately depends on the proper clinical setting and the experience of the clinician and pathologist. Decisions about the relative values of FNAC and CB should be taken by a multi-disciplinary team within the context of its own results and practice, but in order for the use of FNAC to continue, the maintenance of the relevant expertise is of major importance [34].

References

1. Oyama T, Koibuchi Y, McKee G. Core Needle Biopsy (CNB) as a Diagnostic Method for Breast Lesions: Comparison with Fine Needle Aspiration Cytology (FNA). Breast Cancer 2004;11(4):339-42.
2. Ballo MS, Sneige N. Can core needle biopsy replace fine-needle aspiration cytology in the diagnosis of palpable breast carcinoma. A comparative study of 124 women. Cancer 1996;78(4):773-7.
3. Berner A, Sigstad E, Reed W, Risberg B. [Fine-needle aspiration cytology or core biopsy when diagnosing tumours of the breast]. Tidsskr Nor Laegeforen 2003;123(12):1677-9.
4. Carty NJ, Ravichandran D, Carter C, Mudan S, Royle GT, Taylor I. Randomized comparison of fine-needle aspiration cytology and Biopsy-Cut needle biopsy after unsatisfactory initial cytology of discrete breast lesions. Br J Surg 1994;81(9):1313-4.
5. Cangiarella JF, Waisman J, Weg N, Tata M, Gross J, Symmans WF. The Use of Stereotaxic Core Biopsy and Stereotaxic Aspiration Biopsy as Diagnostic Tools in the Evaluation of Mammary Calcification. Breast J 2000;6(6):366-372.
6. Foster MC, Helvie MA, Gregory NE, Rebner M, Nees AV, Paramagul C. Lobular carcinoma in situ or atypical lobular hyperplasia at core-needle biopsy: is excisional biopsy necessary? Radiology 2004;231(3):813-9.
7. Cheung PS, Yan KW, Alagaratnam TT. The complementary role of fine needle aspiration cytology and Tru-cut needle biopsy in the management of breast masses. Aust N Z J Surg 1987;57(9):615-20.
8. Masood S, Loya A, Khalbuss W. Is core needle biopsy superior to fine-needle aspiration biopsy in the diagnosis of papillary breast lesions? Diagn Cytopathol 2003;28(6):329-34.
9. Mottahedeh M, Rashid MH, Gateley CA. Final diagnoses following C3 (atypical, probably benign) breast cytology. Breast 2003;12(4):276-9.
10. Farshid G, Rush G. The use of fine-needle aspiration cytology and core biopsy in the assessment of highly suspicious mammographic microcalcifications: analysis of outcome for 182 lesions detected in the setting of a population-based breast cancer screening program. Cancer 2003;99(6):357-64.
11. Leifland K, Lagerstedt U, Svane G. Comparison of stereotactic fine needle aspiration cytology and core needle biopsy in 522 non-palpable breast lesions. Acta Radiol 2003;44(4):387-91.
12. Shah VI, Raju U, Chitale D, Deshpande V, Gregory N, Strand V. False-negative core needle biopsies of the breast: an analysis of clinical, radiologic, and pathologic findings in 27 consecutive cases of missed breast cancer. Cancer 2003;97(8):1824-31.
13. Verkooijen HM, Hoorntje LE, Peeters PH. False-negative core needle biopsies of the breast: an analysis

of clinical, radiologic, and pathologic findings in 27 consecutive cases of missed breast cancer. Cancer 2004;100(5):1104-5; author reply 1105-6.
14. Florentine BD, Cobb CJ, Frankel K, Greaves T, Martin SE. Core needle biopsy. A useful adjunct to fine-needle aspiration in select patients with palpable breast lesions. Cancer 1997;81(1):33-9.
15. Hatada T, Ishii H, Ichii S, Okada K, Fujiwara Y, Yamamura T. Diagnostic value of ultrasound-guided fine-needle aspiration biopsy, core-needle biopsy, and evaluation of combined use in the diagnosis of breast lesions. J Am Coll Surg 2000;190(3):299-303.
16. Ibrahim AE, Bateman AC, Theaker JM, Low JL, Addis B, Tidbury P, et al. The role and histological classification of needle core biopsy in comparison with fine needle aspiration cytology in the preoperative assessment of impalpable breast lesions. J Clin Pathol 2001;54(2):121-5.
17. Westenend PJ, Sever AR, Beekman-De Volder HJ, Liem SJ. A comparison of aspiration cytology and core needle biopsy in the evaluation of breast lesions. Cancer 2001;93(2):146-50.
18. Boiselle PM, Shepard JA, Mark EJ, Szyfelbein WM, Fan CM, Slanetz PJ, et al. Routine addition of an automated biopsy device to fine-needle aspiration of the lung: a prospective assessment. AJR Am J Roentgenol 1997;169(3):661-6.
19. Greif J, Marmor S, Schwarz Y, Staroselsky AN. Percutaneous core needle biopsy vs. fine needle aspiration in diagnosing benign lung lesions. Acta Cytol 1999;43(5):756-60.
20. Chandan VS, Zimmerman K, Baker P, Scalzetti E, Khurana KK. Usefulness of core roll preparations in immediate assessment of neoplastic lung lesions: comparison to conventional CT scan-guided lung fine-needle aspiration cytology. Chest 2004;126(3):739-43.
21. Greif J, Marmor S, Schwarz Y, Man A, Staroselsky AN. Percutaneous core cutting needle biopsy compared with fine-needle aspiration in the diagnosis of peripheral lung malignant lesions: results in 156 patients. Cancer 1998;84(3):144-7.
22. Jain D. Diagnosis of hepatocellular carcinoma: fine needle aspiration cytology or needle core biopsy. J Clin Gastroenterol 2002;35(5 Suppl 2):S101-8.
23. Franca AV, Valerio HM, Trevisan M, Escanhoela C, Seva-Pereira T, Zucoloto S, et al. Fine needle aspiration biopsy for improving the diagnostic accuracy of cut needle biopsy of focal liver lesions. Acta Cytol 2003;47(3):332-6.
24. Hollerbach S, Willert J, Topalidis T, Reiser M, Schmiegel W. Endoscopic ultrasound-guided fine-needle aspiration biopsy of liver lesions: histological and cytological assessment. Endoscopy 2003;35(9):743-9.
25. Stewart CJ, Coldewey J, Stewart IS. Comparison of fine needle aspiration cytology and needle core biopsy in the diagnosis of radiologically detected abdominal lesions. J Clin Pathol 2002;55(2):93-7.
26. Varadarajulu S, Fraig M, Schmulewitz N, Roberts S, Wildi S, Hawes RH, et al. Comparison of EUS-guided 19-gauge Trucut needle biopsy with EUS-guided fine-needle aspiration. Endoscopy 2004;36(5):397-401.
27. Engelstein D, Mukamel E, Cytron S, Konichezky M, Slutzki S, Servadio C. A comparison between digitally-guided fine needle aspiration and ultrasound-guided transperineal core needle biopsy of the prostate for the detection of prostate cancer. Br J Urol 1994;74(2):210-3.
28. Karstrup S, Balslev E, Juul N, Eskildsen PC, Baumbach L. US-guided fine needle aspiration versus coarse needle biopsy of thyroid nodules. Eur J Ultrasound 2001;13(1):1-5.
29. Quinn SF, Nelson HA, Demlow TA. Thyroid biopsies: fine-needle aspiration biopsy versus spring-activated core biopsy needle in 102 patients. J Vasc Interv Radiol 1994;5(4):619-23.
30. Malmstrom H. Fine-needle aspiration cytology versus core biopsies in the evaluation of recurrent gynecologic malignancies. Gynecol Oncol 1997;65(1):69-73.
31. Bennert KW, Abdul-Karim FW. Fine needle aspiration cytology vs. needle core biopsy of soft tissue tumors. A comparison. Acta Cytol 1994;38(3):381-4.
32. Koscick RL, Petersilge CA, Makley JT, Abdul-Karim FW. CT-guided fine needle aspiration and needle core biopsy of skeletal lesions. Complementary diagnostic techniques. Acta Cytol 1998;42(3):697-702.
33. Clarke D, Sudhakaran N, Gateley CA. Replace fine needle aspiration cytology with automated core biopsy in the triple assessment of breast cancer. Ann R Coll Surg Engl 2001;83(2):110-2.
34. Litherland J. The role of needle biopsy in the diagnosis of breast lesions. Breast 2001;10(5):383-7.

Chapter 12

Principles of Safe FNAC Practice: Medicolegal Issues

More than ever, malpractice is one of the biggest concerns in the medical community. High insurance premiums have caused providers to reduce services and even close services in some areas or specialties, where premiums have increased by 100–200% [1]. Since 1989, in the USA, the claims frequency for pathology (number of claims per 100 insured physicians per year) has increased from 8.8 % to 10%, whereas for all physicians the claims frequency has decreased from 18% to 17.2% [2]. Cytopathologists need to critically evaluate their practices and practice settings to ensure that what they do and how they document what they do will withstand both regulatory and legal scrutiny [3]. Any individual involved in cytology is a potential target of cytology malpractice litigation. Any such individual must participate in a risk management process [3]. In the practice of diagnostic cytopathology, the standard of care must be met in all instances if the possibility of legal action is to be avoided [4]. Constant vigilance, following appropriate guidelines and well-designed quality assurance programs are all important in reducing the possibility of litigation. During most and, intraoperative consultations in particular, direct communication with the surgeon is essential. If an adequate legal defence is to be mounted, documentation of the precautions taken in each individual case is necessary. Outside consultants should be chosen carefully based on their expertise in the area of concern. Trainee pathologists should be given graduated responsibility, but their work should be supervised by a senior pathologist. Trainee physicians in a paediatric teaching hospital were named in 26% of malpractice cases [5]. Risk-management training of trainees may reduce their involvement, and by extension the teaching institution's involvement, in malpractice litigation [5]. As an expert witness, it is important that one's evidence is objective and impartial. One should not attempt to answer questions outside one's area of expertise.

In the majority of litigation cases, there is either a settlement or jury verdict for the plaintiff based largely on the testimony of expert witnesses. Cases are judged on an individual basis without significant consideration of the general performance of the laboratories operating in compliance with national regulations and with documented and comprehensive quality-control practices in place [6]. It is acknowledged that there are problem laboratories and cytology practitioners. There is an emerging issue of automated preparation and screening devices and issues of informed patient consent. The information to the patient should include statements on the use of alternative technology. The profession should develop process guidelines for review of smears in the context of possible litigation, including standardised methods for blind slide review that reduces or eliminates the possibility of litigation [6]. The concept of second opinion in surgical pathology is well established. Multiple studies have demonstrated discrepancy rates between the original and the review histopathological diagnoses of up to 30%, with a mean of approximately 10% [7]. In developing countries, where few laboratories are equipped to function as modern cytopathology units, the second opinion in difficult cases is very important [8]. Ayata et al. applied a probability approach for reporting breast FNAC and assessed its dependence on the cytopathologist's level of experience. They found that the probability approach with defined diagnostic criteria (e.g. categories C1–C5) is an accurate method and can be consistently applied in reporting breast FNAC. Although use of indeterminate (suspicious and atypical) categories is variable, a definite and considerable difference in the probability of carcinoma between these two categories was observed for all pathologists [9].

Professional cytopathology and pathology societies should formulate acceptable guidelines for expert witnesses. The standards should be applicable to both defendant and plaintiff experts. All materials, including consultant opinions, should be available for peer review. Professional cytopathology and pathology societies should monitor expert evidence for objectivity and scientific accuracy. Review of cytological material is often a key component of civil litigation in cases of alleged negligence or medical malpractice. While the outcome of such cases may hinge on the evidence of expert witnesses, determining who is qualified to serve as an expert in such cases is generally left to the parties involved [10].

Laboratories and individuals can reduce the risk of malpractice liability by proactive quality control and quality assurance methods. Consumer education about the benefits and limitations of the test is another key to limiting malpractice claims. Guidelines such as those for uniform reporting terminology and clinical management, form the basis of cytology practice standards upon which legal standards of practice can be based [11]. Clinical pathways, or practice guidelines, have been gaining wider acceptance from physicians and hospitals seeking to constrain increasing operating costs for inpatient care. Properly developed and agreed upon guidelines can be used as appropriate standards of care in determining if medical malpractice has occurred. Adherence to the guidelines could then be asserted by defendants as an affirmative defence in a medical malpractice suit [12]. The consensus-based process of creating clinical standards and guidelines specifically for controlling professional liability losses is itself a powerful and emerging standard for health-care risk-management programmes [13]. If the vague, „reasonable man" standard of care, in negligence law can be supplanted by a scientifically developed, particularised medical practice standard, it is anticipated that spurious claims and defensive medical practice will be discouraged, quality improved and iatrogenic injury and malpractice litigation diminished [14]. Written protocols and standards of practice can, however, create a potential malpractice problem. Lawyers who bring malpractice cases on behalf of patients will use these protocols and standards to measure the practitioner's care [15]. The practice standards are often too high to be reasonably met by practitioners at all times and in all settings. As a result, the practitioner's care may breach those standards [15, 16]. Consensus conference reports, clinical management trials and scientifically valid studies of false-negative rates that analyse the type, frequency and cause of missed cases represent sounder methods of establishing defensible cases.

Breast FNAC accounted for 6% of surgical pathology and FNAC claims reviewed between 1995 and 1997 [17]. The majority of these claims were for false-negative breast FNAC resulting from sampling error in women with a palpable breast mass [17]. Most malpractice complaints related to carcinoma of the breast are instituted by women under the age of 50 years who identified the breast mass by themselves and were assumed by their physicians to have fibrocystic disease of the breast [18]. Complaints can be expected to increase regarding failure to order further diagnostic tests, such as ultrasound or FNAC, despite a negative mammogram. Obstetricians and gynaecologists have been involved in the greatest number of such malpractice cases, followed by family practitioners and internists, general surgeons and radiologists. Although this particular study does not mention pathologists, medicolegal issues affecting breast FNAC are important. Emphasis on early diagnosis has led to the perception that purported delay in diagnosis, however short, even in the presence of a palpable mass, changes the chances of survival [19].

DeMay's advice "what you can do to decrease your risk of being sued" includes laboratory practices, patient contact, informed consent, documentation, record keeping, interpretive problems, triple test, diligence, reporting results and what to do if sued [20].

Controversies concerning the definition of specimen adequacy for breast FNAC form a central part of most breast FNAC litigation claims [17]. Claims for false-positive breast FNAC usually result from interpretive error [17]. Although cytopathologists agree that several parameters relate to the adequacy of an FNAC specimen, there is no unanimity on the role of epithelial cell quantitation in the determination of an adequate FNAC. Including the number of epithelial cell clusters as a parameter of adequacy could reduce the rate of false-negative FNAC diagnoses of palpable breast masses by approximately 50% [21]. However, quantitative parameters alone are insufficient measures for determining specimen adequacy in FNAC of palpable breast lesions. Rather, adequacy remains based upon factors such as confidence of needle placement, cell preservation and correlation with clinical and mammographic findings [22]. The presence or even abundance of epithelial clusters does not eliminate the potential for a false-negative cytological diagnosis. Cytological diagnoses must be correlated with clinical and imaging findings (the triple test) to reduce the rate of false-negative cases, but benign triple-test results do not entirely exclude the possibility of carcinoma, and such cases require periodic follow-up [21]. The cytological diagnosis of breast lesions such as fibroadenoma, fibromatosis, complex sclerosing lesions, papillary lesions, angiosarcoma, low-nuclear-grade in situ and invasive carcinomas, ductal hyperplasia, adenosis tumours, mucocoele-like lesions, nipple adenoma, apocrine cyst with atypia and sclerosing adenosis with radial scar can be the cause of false-positive and false-negative diagnoses (see chapter 9)[23, 24]. Benign and inadequate FNAC diagnoses must be correlated with the clinical and imaging findings and in non-correlative cases the patient should undergo a biopsy procedure. Ultrasound-guided FNAC is a sensitive and specific means with which to diagnose non-palpable breast lesions [25]. In the majority of cases of lobular carcinoma, the cellular yield of FNAC is disproportionately lower than expected when compared with the corresponding histological material. Awareness of modest cellularity and subtle cytological features will minimise false-negative diagnoses [26]. Hypocellularity and relative nuclear monomorphism are the reasons for failure to diagnose malignant breast lesions [27].

Pneumothorax is a rare but recognised complication of FNAC breast and, as such, has been reported as a cause of litigation for alleged negligence [28]. The reported incidence of pneumothorax after diagnostic aspiration of the breast varies between 3 in 100 (3%) and 1 in 10,000 (0.01%), but the weight of evidence tends towards the latter rate [28]. This complication is more common in the hands of trainees [28]. It is not always possible to maintain the aspirating needle parallel or tangential to the chest wall. Pleural puncture may be more common than is apparent, and is most common in the tail of the breast in a thin woman. It is important that breast clinicians are aware of the risk of pneumothorax but, provided appropriate care has been taken, this complication is not the result of a negligent act [28].

There is currently no evidence that the new monolayer technology for processing FNAC breast is better than conventional smears. Biscotti et al. found that although Thin Prep slides (Cytic Corp, USA) had greater cellularity and better nuclear detail than conventional smears, they were just as sensitive in identifying the carcinomas. The difference in specificity between the two techniques was not statistically significant (P=0.065) [29].

The main recommendations for preventing and reducing the number of difficult diagnoses in cytopathology are: (1) development of quality assurance programmes with use of written protocols in each pathology laboratory, (2) knowledge of clinical history to help explain the cytopathology results and (3) availability of complementary patient information (e.g. radiological data) to help explain the cytopathology results [30]. The main recommendation for detecting lesions associated with difficult diagnosis in cytopathology is that tumour types known as potential difficult diagnosis in surgical pathology or cytopathology should be reviewed by a second pathologist (e.g. sarcoma, lymphoma) [30]. The main recommendations for solving a difficult diagnosis in cytopathology are: (1) use of special techniques (immunocyto/histochemistry and molecular biology), additional data from clinicians, a second opinion from a local pathologist, or new specimen can be required to establish the diagnosis, and (2) an outside second opinion by an expert pathologist should be considered if the other steps did not establish a cytopathology diagnosis [31].

What should a pathologist do from the time of an initial threat of a lawsuit to the initial lawsuit, and through to the initial physician/lawyer meeting? [31]. Epstein advises how to avoid judicial process and defines malpractice in pathology: duty, breach of standard of care, proximal cause and damage [31]. The quality of medical care (negligence) is an extremely important determinant of a defendant's medical malpractice liability. In general, plaintiffs are poorly informed about whether there has been negligence, they then file law suits to gather information and either drop the case if they find that negligence was unlikely or settle for a positive payoff if they find that negligence was likely [32]. The cases are resolved earlier in the litigation process when the parties are more certain, one way or the other, about the likelihood of negligence [32]. When evaluating as to how courts used guidelines and how state legislatures link guideline compliance with malpractice defences, Hyams et al. found that although the guidelines are being used for both inculpatory and exculpatory purposes in common-law litigation (a two-way street), legislatures are interested in applying them only for exculpatory purposes (a one-way street) [33].

The mandatory disclosure of medical errors has been advocated to improve patient safety [34]. Many resist mandatory disclosure policies because of concerns about increasing malpractice exposure. It has been countered that malpractice liability actually decreases when there is full disclosure of medical errors [34]. Despite extensive literature on the impact of disclosure on malpractice liability, few well-designed studies have focussed on the real-world impact on the volume and cost of suits following implementation of a full disclosure policy. Many articles examine why patients sue their doctors, suggesting that some lawsuits may be averted by disclosure, but the articles do not allow us to estimate the additional suits that would be created by disclosure [34].

The delayed diagnosis of cancer leading to negligence litigation is associated with significant indemnity payments, often involves patients far younger than the expected age in the general cancer population and is defensible only in the minority after 6 months of diagnostic delay [35].

For the laboratory as a corporate entity, business and technical practices, including quality control and quality assurance procedures, must be contemporary, legitimate and justifiable [3]. Sound scientific evidence and well-subscribed standards of practice supporting an individual's or laboratory's conduct are the best defences to malpractice claims. For the near future, litigation will continue to focus on false-negative smears on a case-by-case basis. Laboratories and individuals can reduce the risk of malpractice liability by directing their attention to proactive quality control and quality assurance methods. Consumer education about the benefits and limitations of FNAC is a key to limiting malpractice claims. The merits of communicating diagnostic error rates to the clinician/patient cannot be overestimated. In the areas of breast FNAC and cervical smears, dissemination of diagnostic error rates in the cytology report is recommended. This would help safeguard against malpractice liability being imposed without showing a deviation by the cytopathologist from reasonable practice standards [36].

A lot of attention and energy has been spent over the past several years on reducing the amount of settlements and awards in malpractice cases. Although these are important issues, the best situation for physicians is not to be sued at all [37]. Therefore, the medical community needs to start focussing on ways to prevent lawsuits from being filed in the first place. Recent studies and publications indicate that physicians may have more control over the lawsuit lottery than they realise. An article appeared on the front page of the May 18, 2004 edition of the Wall Street Journal (Doctors' new tool to fight lawsuits: saying ‚I'm sorry') supports the proposition that the best tool to minimise the possibility of being sued may be as simple as expressing condolence and empathy when there is a bad outcome [38, 39].

References

1. Reiboldt JP. Seven steps to reduce your malpractice risk. J Med Pract Manage 2004;19(6):324-8.
2. Troxel DB, Sabella JD. Problem areas in pathology practice. Uncovered by a review of malpractice claims. Am J Surg Pathol 1994;18(8):821-31.
3. Greening SE. Errors in cervical smears: minimizing the risk of medicolegal consequences. 16-39.
4. Roth LM. Medicolegal issues. An anatomic pathologist's perspective. Am J Clin Pathol 1996;106(4 Suppl 1):S18-24.
5. Grupp-Phelan J, Reynolds S, Lingl LL. Professional liability of residents in a children's hospital. Arch Pediatr Adolesc Med 1996;150(1):87-90.
6. Frable WJ, Austin RM, Greening SE, Collins RJ, Hillman RL, Kobler TP, et al. Medicolegal affairs. International Academy of Cytology Task Force summary. Diagnostic Cytology Towards the 21st Century: An International Expert Conference and Tutorial. Acta Cytol 1998;42(1):76-119; discussion 120-32.
7. Gupta D, Layfield LJ. Prevalence of inter-institutional anatomic pathology slide review: a survey of current practice. Am J Surg Pathol 2000;24(2):280-4.
8. Ahmed Z, Yaqoob N, Muzaffar S, Kayani N, Pervez S, Hasan SH. Diagnostic surgical pathology: the importance of second opinion in a developing country. J Pak Med Assoc 2004;54(6):306-11.
9. Ayata G, Abu-Jawdeh GM, Fraser JL, Garcia LW, Upton MP, Wang HH. Accuracy and consistency in application of a probabilistic approach to reporting breast fine needle aspiration. Acta Cytol 2003;47(6):973-8.
10. Fitzgibbons PL, Austin RM. Expert review of histologic slides and Papanicolaou tests in the context of litigation or potential litigation. Surgical Pathology Committee and Cytopathology Committee of the College of American Pathologists. Arch Pathol Lab Med 2000;124(11):1717-9.
11. Skoumal SM. Establishing standards of care. Diagn Cytopathol 1996;14(3):284-5.
12. Costello MM, Murphy KM. Clinical guidelines: a defense in medical malpractice suits. Physician Exec 1995;21(8):10-2.
13. Holzer JF. The advent of clinical standards for professional liability. QRB Qual Rev Bull 1990;16(2):71-9.
14. King JY. Practice guidelines & medical malpractice litigation. Med Law 1997;16(1):29-39.
15. Moniz DM. The legal danger of written protocols and standards of practice. Nurse Pract 1992;17(9):58-60.
16. O'Connell J, Bryan PB. More Hippocrates, less hypocrisy: „early offers" as a means of implementing the Institute of Medicine's recommendations on malpractice law. J Law Health 2000-2001;15(1):23-51.
17. Troxel DB. Diagnostic Pitfalls in Surgical Pathology- Uncovered by a Review of Malpractice Claims: Part II. Breast Fine Needle Aspirations. Int J Surg Pathol 2000;8(3):229-231.
18. Mitnick JS, Vazquez MF, Kronovet SZ, Roses DF. Malpractice litigation involving patients with carcinoma of the breast. J Am Coll Surg 1995;181(4):315-21.
19. Mitnick JS, Vazquez MF, Plesser KP, Roses DF. Breast cancer malpractice litigation in New York State. Radiology 1993;189(3):673-6.
20. DeMay RM. Medicolegal issues and fine needle aspiration of the breast. What you can do to decrease your risk of being sued. Clin Lab Med 1998;18(3):599-605, vii.
21. Boerner S, Sneige N. Specimen adequacy and false-negative diagnosis rate in fine-needle aspirates of palpable breast masses. Cancer 1998;84(6):344-8.
22. Eckert R, Howell LP. Number, size, and composition of cell clusters as related to breast FNA adequacy. Diagn Cytopathol 1999;21(2):105-11.
23. Sneige N. Fine-needle aspiration of the breast: a review of 1,995 cases with emphasis on diagnostic pitfalls. 106-12.
24. Kumarasinghe MP, Constantine SR. Non-diagnostic smears in aspiration cytology of palpable breast lumps. Ann Acad Med Singapore 1998;27(2):161-7.
25. Boerner S, Fornage BD, Singletary E, Sneige N. Ultrasound-guided fine-needle aspiration (FNA) of nonpalpable breast lesions: a review of 1885 FNA cases using the National Cancer Institute-supported recommendations on the uniform approach to breast FNA. Cancer 1999;87(1):19-24.
26. Abdulla M, Hombal S, al-Juwaiser A, Stankovich D, Ahmed M, Ajrawi T. Cellularity of lobular carcinoma and its relationship to false negative fine needle aspiration results. Acta Cytol 2000;44(4):625-32.
27. Jamal AA, Mansoor I. Analysis of false positive and false negative cytological diagnosis of breast lesions. Saudi Med J 2001;22(1):67-71.
28. Bates T, Davidson T, Mansel RE. Litigation for pneumothorax as a complication of fine-needle aspiration of the breast. Br J Surg 2002;89(2):134-137.
29. Biscotti CV, Shorie JH, Gramlich TL, Easley KA. ThinPrep vs. conventional smear cytologic preparations in analyzing fine-needle aspiration specimens from palpable breast masses. Diagn Cytopathol 1999;21(2):137-41.
30. Coindre JM, Blanc-Vincent MP, Collin F, Mac Grogan G, Balaton A, Voigt JJ, et al. [Standards, options and recommendations: practice guidelines for difficult diagnosis in surgical pathology or cytopathology in cancer patients]. Bull Cancer 2001;88(8):765-73.
31. Epstein JI. Pathologists and the judicial process: how to avoid it. Am J Surg Pathol 2001;25(4):527-37.
32. Farber HS, White MJ. Medical malpractice: an empirical examination of the litigation process. Rand J Econ 1991;22(2):199-217.

33. Hyams AL, Shapiro DW, Brennan TA. Medical practice guidelines in malpractice litigation: an early retrospective. J Health Polit Policy Law 1996;21(2):289-313.
34. Kachalia A, Shojania KG, Hofer TP, Piotrowski M, Saint S. Does full disclosure of medical errors affect malpractice liability? The jury is still out. Jt Comm J Qual Saf 2003;29(10):503-11.
35. Kern KA. Medicolegal analysis of the delayed diagnosis of cancer in 338 cases in the United States. Arch Surg 1994;129(4):397-403; discussion 403-4.
36. Skoumal SM, Florell SR, Bydalek MK, Hunter WJ, 3rd. Malpractice protection: communication of diagnostic uncertainty. Diagn Cytopathol 1996;14(4):385-9.
37. Zimmerman R. Doctors' new tool to fight lawsuits: saying ‚I'm sorry. ‚ Malpractice insurers find owning up to errors soothes patient anger. ‚The risks are extraordinary'. J Okla State Med Assoc 2004;97(6):245-7.
38. Zimmerman R. Doctors' New Tool To Fight Lawsuits: Saying ‚I'm Sorry'. Malpractice Insurers Find Owning Up to Errors Soothes Patient Anger. ‚The Risks Are Extraordinary'. THE WALL STREET JOURNAL 2004;May 18:A1.
39. Woods M. Healing Words: The Power of Apology in Medicine. http://www.sorryworks.net/article5.phtml 2004.

Subject Index

Italic entries refer to images.

A

abdomen 73, 160
accuracy 13, 152, 207, 218, 226, 227, 228
adequacy 233
adrenal cystic lesions 78
adrenal gland 78
air drying 19, 50, 119, 133, 144, 158, 183, 201
alcohol-fixed preparations 20, 133, 155
ancillary techniques 23, 26, 27, 105, 125, 134, 136, 142, 145, 146, 152
arm 164
aspiration techniques 15
aspirator 11, 13, 14, 15, 17, 28, 182, 219, 226, 229
axilla 118, 192

B

background 21, 22, 35, 36, 37, 38, 39, 40, 41, 42, 43, 44, 84, 109, 119, 136, 137, 139, 146, 154, 155, 159, 160, 162, 167, 172, 186, 188, 191, 194, 195, 199, 203, 205
bile ducts 12
bone 134, 155
breast 11, 21, 26, 27, 36, 37, 38, 40, 44, 46, 47, 48, 56, 81, 82, 91, 96, 99, 106, 107, 122, 123, 128, 156, 183, 184, 185, 186, 187, 188, 189, 190, 191, 192, 193, 194, 195, 196, 197, 198, 199, 200, 201, 202, 203, 204
breast 11, 107, 122, 181, 193, 204, 205, 206, 220, 225, 231, 232, 234
– apocrine changes 186, 193, 194

– fibroadenoma 182, 183, 184, 185, 186, 187, 188, 190, 191, 195, 198, 203, 204, 205, 206, 226, 233
– in situ carcinoma 198, 199
– invasive 199, 200, 201
– invasive carcinoma 186, 193, 198, 201
– lobular carcinoma 196, 233
– mucinous lesions 195
– papillary lesions 188, 189, 190, 191, 192, 193, 207, 226
– radiation changes 207
– rare lesions 202

C

carcinomas 187, 188, 190
cell arrangement 44, 45, 46, 47, 48, 49, 133, 134, 137, 195, 196, 202, 206
cell block 18, 78, 191, 227
cerebrospinal fluid 23
cervical 20
chest wall 177
clinical management (see management) 107
CNS 37, 83
complications 13, 14, 17, 80, 233
core biopsy (CB) 202, 207, 225, 226, 227
– abdominal 227
– breast 225, 226
– CB vs. FNAC 207
– gynaecology 228
– hepatic 227
– lung 227
– prostate 228
– skeletal 228
– soft-tissue 228
– thyroid 228

cost 11, 220, 226
cystic 129
– background 39
– change 62, 185, 198
– lesions 17, 59, 62, 69, 80, 122, 195, 205
– lesions of the liver 77
– lesions of the peritoneum 79
cystic 17
cystic lesions 217
– abdomen 73
– breast cysts 80
– head and neck 59, 60, 62
– lesions of the pancreas 73
– other cysts 82
– thoracic cysts 79
cysts 193, 215
cytoplasm 20, 21, 22, 69, 109, 110, 124, 133, 134, 137, 139, 140, 142, 144, 171, 172, 198, 203

D

desmoplastic small round cell tumour 143
diagnostic
– challenge 133
– principles 35
diagnostic interpretation 35
– criteria of malignancy 57
– cytology report 57, 58
– cytoplasm 53, 55, 56, 57
– nucleus 47, 49, 50, 52, 53, 54, 55
– slide background 35, 36
Diff-Quik 21, 22
dilemmas 81, 91, 99, 117, 156, 182, 188, 203
DNA amplification 27
DNA cytometry 26
duodenum 12

E

ES/PNET 134
EUS-FNAC 13, 40, 217
experience 13, 14

F

false negative diagnosis 19, 21, 66, 84, 232, 233, 234
false positive diagnosis 19, 21, 65, 77, 232, 233
fibroadenoma 191
fibrocystic change 182
fluorescence in situ hybridisation (FISH) 26, 27
FNAC 12, 126, 219
FNAC and core biopsy 108
FNAC clinic 9, 11, 28, 220
FNAC lymph node 139, 140
FNAC ovary 84, 85
FNAC skin 83
FNAC technique 7
– conventional preparations 17, 19
– cytochemistry 23
– fixation techniques 19
– inpatient FNAC 12
– location of the FNAC 8
– other stains 23
– Romanowsky staining 22
– slide preparation 7, 13, 17
– staining methods 20
– suction FNAC 15
– the capillary method 16
– transport medium 20
forearm 163

G

gene microarray analysis 26
general principles 117
gomori 24
granuloma 99, 156
granulomatous lymphadenitis 92

H

haematoxylin and eosin 23
hand 159
head and neck 24, 41, 42, 60, 61, 62, 63, 69, 73, 109, 120, 123, 124, 125, 126, 128, 129, 137, 146, 147, 166, 174
health and safety guidelines 28
histochemistry 233

HIV 24, 28, 42, 63, 71, 219
hypopharynx 12

I

image guided FNAC 12
imaging 99
immunocytochemistry 24, 104, 120, 124, 125, 136, 137, 141, 143, 144, 146, 147, 165, 172, 174, 175, 183, 194, 233
immunohistochemistry 227
informed consent 7, 8
inguinum 138

J

jugulodigastric node 154

K

kidney 23, 78, 79
kidney 217
knee 164

L

liquid-based cytology (LBC) 13, 18
liquid-based preparations 18
liver 77, 78
lung 12, 13, 19, 25, 50, 52, 53, 55, 57, 99, 124, 125, 144
lymph node 24, 25, 27, 36, 39, 41, 43, 45, 46, 53, 54, 70, 92, 93, 94, 95, 96, 98, 108, 110, 123, 143, 145
lymphoid infiltrates 80, 91, 102, 105, 109
– extranodal sites 99
– granulomatous infiltrates 91
– lymphoma 108
– solid neoplasms 109
lymphoma 27, 64
lymphoproliferative diseases 27, 103, 206

M

management 50, 117, 124, 129, 140, 172, 190, 198, 214, 217, 218, 219, 220, 232
– adrenal and kidney 217
– bone 218
– breast 214
– cost-effectiveness 219, 220
– diagnostic accuracy 217, 219
– gastrointestinal tract 217
– gynaecology 219
– head and neck conditions 216
– HIV-related lesions 219
– lymph nodes 216
– soft-tissue 218
– thyroid 215, 220
– transrectal 219
May Grünwald Giemsa (MGG) 22, 23, 206
mediastinum 12, 79, 80, 98, 110, 125, 127
medicolegal issues 231
meningioma 123
metastasis 38
metastatic 65, 136, 137, 138, 147, 152, 161, 170, 172, 192, 214, 216, 217, 218, 227
metastatic tumours 22, 23, 27, 47, 117, 134, 141, 142, 143, 204, 215, 218
– carcinoma 118, 228, 229
– metastases of non-epithelial tumours 129
methenamine silver (Grocott) 23
– staining 24
misleading 202
missed cases 232
mitoses 165
molecular markers in cytology 26
molecular studies 136, 233
mucinous 185
– carcinoma 187
multi-disciplinary team 229
myofibrosarcoma 157

N

nucleus 20, 21, 22, 23, 69, 109, 110, 134, 137, 144, 146, 155, 162, 165, 170, 172, 194, 195, 196, 198, 203

O

operation scar 119
operation site 97, 167
oral cavity 39, 41, 72
orbit 91
ovarian cysts 83
ovary 36, 43, 46, 56, 79, 83, 84, 85

Subject Index

P

pancreas   12, 41, 43, 45, 51, 52, 54, 55, 56, 73, 74, 75, 76, 77
Papanicolaou (Pap) stain   20, 21, 22, 23, 28, 156, 185
papillary carcinoma   185
paraspinal mass   136
parathyroid   71
parotid gland   21, 92, 106
PAS   23
PAS-d   23, 37
PAS distase   23
PCR   26
pelvic mass   159
periodic acid-Schiff   23
perls   23
pitfall   22, 183, 185, 188, 190, 204, 206
preparations   19, 35

R

real-time PCR   27
rectum   12
renal   217
renal cystic lesions   78
report   28, 58
retroperitoneum   140, 158
Romanowsky staining   20, 21, 22

S

safety   27, 28, 219, 227, 228, 234
salivary gland   14, 21, 36, 39, 44, 45, 62, 64, 65, 66, 67, 68, 71, 83, 91, 103, 104, 106, 119
scalp   173
scar   96, 166
shin   175
skin   16, 38, 40, 44, 47, 83
slide preparation   7
– air drying   19
– alcohol fixation   20
– ancillary techniques   23, 27
– aspiration techniques   15
– aspirator   11, 13, 14, 15, 17, 28
– capillary method   16
– cell block   18
– conventional preparations   17, 19
– cytochemistry   23
– fixation techniques   19
– FNAC clinic   9, 11, 28
– image guided FNAC   12
– immunocytochemistry   24
– informed consent   7, 8
– inpatient FNAC   12
– liquid-based preparations   18
– location of the FNAC   8
– molecular markers in cytology   26
– other stains   23
– Romanowsky staining   20, 21, 22
– safety   27, 28
– staining methods   20
– suction FNAC   15
– transport medium   20
small-cell variant of synovial sarcoma   142
small round cell tumours   133
– acute lymphoblastic leukaemia and LBL   139
– Burkitt's lymphoma   144
– desmoplastic SRCT (DS-RCT)   143
– Ewing's Sarcoma/Primitive Neuroectodermal Tumour   134
– ganglioneuroblastomas   136
– hepatoblastoma   141
– in adults   142
– lymphoglandular bodies   145
– Merkel cell carcinoma   146
– neuroblastoma   136
– of childhood   133
– of kidney   141
– olfactory neuroblastoma   147
– pleuropulmonary blastoma   142
– rhabdomyosarcoma   137
– small-cell carcinoma of the lung   144
– small-cell synovial sarcoma   142
smear background   133
soft-tissue lesions   151
– breast   157
– lung   156, 172
– myxoid and chondroid lesions   157
– pseudosarcomatous lesions   162, 165
– rare and difficult sarcomas   172
– salivary gland   156
– sarcomas mimicking other lesions   171
– soft-tissue deposits of non-sarcomatous lesions   171
– tumours of low or borderline malignancy   169
solid-organ transplant   219
spindle-cell lesions   153, 156, 157
– of the breast   82
subcutaneous mass   147
submandibular swelling   122
supraclavicular fossa   167
supraclavicular mass   98

T

techniques   35
testicular   37
testis   36, 82
thigh   136, 154, 160, 163
thyroid   9, 14, 27, 36, 38, 39, 43, 46, 47, 48, 51, 52, 53, 54, 56, 60, 68, 69, 91, 97, 98, 100, 101, 102, 123
training   36
trunk   168, 170
tuberculous lymphadenitis   92
tumour in the stomach wall   161

U

upper arm   157

Z

Ziehl Nielsen stain   23